Achieving Person-Centred Health Systems

The idea of person-centred health systems is widely advocated in political and policy declarations to better address health system challenges. A person-centred approach is advocated on political, ethical and instrumental grounds and believed to benefit service users, health professionals and the health system more broadly. However, there is continuing debate about the strategies that are available and effective to promote and implement 'person-centred' approaches. This book brings together the world's leading experts in the field to present the evidence base and analyse current challenges and issues. It examines 'person-centredness' from the different roles people take in health systems, as individual service users, care managers, taxpayers or active citizens. The evidence presented will not only provide invaluable policy advice to practitioners and policy-makers working on the design and implementation of person-centred health systems but will also be an excellent resource for academics and graduate students researching health systems in Europe.

ELLEN NOLTE is Professor of Health Services and Systems Research at the London School of Hygiene & Tropical Medicine. Her expertise is in health systems research, international health care comparisons and performance assessment. She has published widely on health systems, integrated care, European health policy and population health assessments and serves as co-editor of the *Journal of Health Services Research and Policy*. Previous books include *Caring for People with Chronic Conditions: Health System Perspective* (2008) and *Assessing Chronic Disease Management in European Health Systems: Concepts and Approaches* (2014).

SHERRY MERKUR is Research Fellow and Health Policy Analyst at the European Observatory on Health Systems and Policies, based at the LSE. She is Editor-in-Chief of *Eurohealth* and an author and editor of *HiT: Health system reviews*. Her publications include *Promoting Health, Preventing Disease: The Economic Case* (2015). With Martin McKee, Nigel Edwards and Ellen Nolte, she is co-editor of *The Changing Role of the Hospital in European Health Systems* (Cambridge, 2020).

ANDERS ANELL is Professor at Lund University School of Economics and Management, Chairman of the Board at the Swedish Agency for Health and Care Services Analysis (Vårdanalys) and a former general director of the Swedish Institute for Health Economics (IHE). He has published widely on health systems, patient choice and the role and impact of incentives in health care.

European Observatory on Health Systems and Policies

The volumes in this series focus on topical issues around the transformation of health systems in Europe, a process being driven by a changing environment, increasing pressures and evolving needs.

Drawing on available evidence, existing experience and conceptual thinking, these studies aim to provide both practical and policy-relevant information and lessons on how to implement change to make health systems more equitable, effective and efficient. They are designed to promote and support evidence-informed policy-making in the health sector and will be a valuable resource for all those involved in developing, assessing or analysing health systems and policies.

In addition to policy-makers, stakeholders and researchers in the field of health policy, key audiences outside the health sector will also find this series invaluable for understanding the complex choices and challenges that health systems face today.

LIST OF TITLES

Challenges to Tackling Antimicrobial Resistance: Economic and Policy Responses
Edited by Michael Anderson, Michele Cecchini, Elias Mossialos

The Changing Role of the Hospital in European Health Systems
Edited by Martin McKee, Sherry Merkur, Nigel Edwards, Ellen Nolte

Series Editors

JOSEP FIGUERAS Director, European Observatory on Health Systems and Policies

MARTIN MCKEE Co-Director, European Observatory on Health Systems and Policies, and Professor of European Public Health at the London School of Hygiene & Tropical Medicine

ELIAS MOSSIALOS Co-Director, European Observatory on Health Systems and Policies, and Brian Abel-Smith Professor of Health Policy, London School of Economics and Political Science

REINHARD BUSSE Co-Director, European Observatory on Health Systems and Policies, and Head of the Department of Health Care Management, Berlin University of Technology

Achieving Person-Centred Health Systems

Evidence, Strategies and Challenges

Edited by

ELLEN NOLTE
London School of Hygiene & Tropical Medicine

SHERRY MERKUR
European Observatory on Health Systems and Policies

ANDERS ANELL
Lund University, Sweden

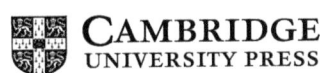 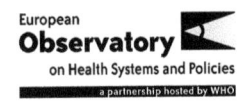 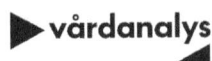

CAMBRIDGE
UNIVERSITY PRESS

University Printing House, Cambridge CB2 8BS, United Kingdom

One Liberty Plaza, 20th Floor, New York, NY 10006, USA

477 Williamstown Road, Port Melbourne, VIC 3207, Australia

314–321, 3rd Floor, Plot 3, Splendor Forum, Jasola District Centre, New Delhi – 110025, India

79 Anson Road, #06–04/06, Singapore 079906

Cambridge University Press is part of the University of Cambridge.

It furthers the University's mission by disseminating knowledge in the pursuit of education, learning and research at the highest international levels of excellence.

www.cambridge.org
Information on this title: www.cambridge.org/9781108790062
DOI: 10.1017/9781108855464

First published 2020

A catalogue record for this publication is available from the British Library.

ISBN 978-1-108-79006-2 Paperback

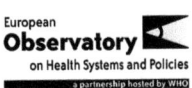

European Observatory
on Health Systems
and Policies

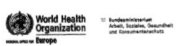 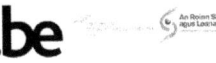

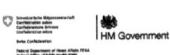 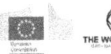

The European Observatory on Health Systems and Policies supports and promotes evidence-based health policy-making through comprehensive and rigorous analysis of health systems in Europe. It brings together a wide range of policy-makers, academics and practitioners to analyse trends in health reform, drawing on experience from across Europe to illuminate policy issues.

The European Observatory on Health Systems and Policies is a partnership hosted by the World Health Organization Regional Office for Europe which includes the Governments of Austria, Belgium, Finland, Ireland, Norway, Slovenia, Spain, Sweden, Switzerland, the United Kingdom, and the Veneto Region of Italy; the European Commission; the World Bank; UNCAM (French National Union of Health Insurance Funds); the Health Foundation; the London School of Economics and Political Science; and the London School of Hygiene & Tropical Medicine. The Observatory has a secretariat in Brussels and it has hubs in London (at LSE and LSHTM) and at the Berlin University of Technology.

Contents

Foreword I

Already in 2006, Council Conclusions by EU health ministers confirmed access to good quality health care as an overarching value for health systems across Europe. Next to effectiveness and safety, patient experience is considered a key component of health care quality. Historically, concern with patient safety has been the prime driver of EU-level rules on medical products. In the last decade, effectiveness has risen to the fore of health system analysis through EU-level processes such as the European Semester. In recent years, we have seen initiatives focusing on the patient perspective, assessing how health systems can draw on patient-reported experiences and outcomes. This book delivers a key contribution to this debate.

The book's very title, referring to 'person-centredness', raises some compelling questions on how to frame the current conceptual framework. Does a term like 'patient-centredness' cover dimensions which are more general in service delivery and not necessarily limited to experiences related to morbidity? How would this concept fit with areas such as prevention and health promotion, where the whole idea is to help people avoid becoming patients? These questions go well beyond 'petty semantics' and the discussions raised in this book are very timely.

The book presents valuable lessons from areas in health systems where persons (many of them patients) have already found ways of expressing choice, gaining a voice and more generally participating in health systems. In doing so, it convincingly makes the point that a more systematic move to person-centred care will support health systems in addressing the challenges they face. Obviously, there are barriers for health systems to overcome when pursuing a person-centred redesign, duly recognized in the book.

Current population health literacy levels across the EU will need to be raised if citizens are to take up a more active role in co-steering health systems. Also, health systems need to overcome the important information gap they face. The uptake of more holistic, person-centred health data holds great potential. The quality of care and the performance of health systems across the EU stand to gain significantly from improvements in this direction. The development of such complementary health indicators will help policy-makers and health professionals to more effectively treat patients, who are increasingly frail and suffering from multiple morbidities. The European Commission is actively supporting Member States to achieve this health system transformation.

For many years patient groups have rightfully demanded from policy-makers 'nothing about us without us'. Now it is time to push this principle to a higher level. Inspired by this book, we should strive for a person-centred redesign of health systems that will include all patient groups, as well as the wider population that health systems aim to keep healthy.

ISABEL DE LA MATA
European Commission

Foreword II

Centring health systems around people remains a major challenge for all countries. Traditionally, a fragmented landscape of health providers has determined what services to offer and how they are delivered, while patients have had limited options to choose, participate or even co-produce.

People demand now a more active role in their health care and a better response to their expectations as social values have progressed and information asymmetries have shrunk with the advent of new forms of communication and participation. Hence, it has become a health systems practitioners' mandate to walk the talk of valuing choice and the preferences of individuals, de-institutionalizing services for increased community-based care closer to home, involving individuals and their caregivers in managing long-term care needs, engaging multiple care disciplines, promoting the exercise of personal choice, and extending services beyond physical limits into virtual modalities.

This book provides a comprehensive and necessary analysis of the multi-pronged concept of people-centredness to set a common background to health reformers, practitioners and researchers. Its editors and chapter authors explore what health strategies and innovations can contribute to effectively make health systems more people-centred, empowering community participation, measuring people's perceptions and enabling choice of providers and payers. They also provide evidence-based guidance on how health services can be more person-centred by engaging patients in decision-making, empowering them as managers of their own care and, overall, fostering self-management.

It comes at a timely moment when health systems celebrate historical landmarks like the foundation of the World Health Organization in 1948. In 2018 we also commemorated the 40th anniversary of the Declaration of Alma Ata and the 10th anniversary of the Tallinn Charter that shape modern health policies aiming to achieve health for all underpinned by the vision put forward by Health 2020. They all share the vision of people-centred health systems based on the principles of equity, social justice, community participation, health promotion, the appropriate use of resources and intersectoral action.

Against this backdrop, 21st century health systems need to be rethought and strengthened to successfully face a changing world context characterized by ageing societies, globalization, climate change and technological progress. People-centred health systems based on strong primary health care and integrated health services across the life-course are vital to reach the Sustainable Development Goals and achieve universal health coverage by 2030 and this book is an accurate compass to guide the way forward.

DR HANS HENRI P. KLUGE
WHO Regional Director for Europe

Foreword III

Modern medicine has contributed to tremendous achievements in terms of expanding life expectancy, curing diseases that previously were fatal, finding new ways of alleviating pain and suffering, and improving patients' quality of life. However, when we ask patients about their experiences of the health services they use, the results are not always as positive. Patients do not always feel that they have been respected and listened to, that their needs and preferences have been taken into account and that their experiences and knowledge are valued.

Studies that compare patients' experiences in different countries show us that some countries are ahead when it comes to delivering health services that are person-centred. Person-centred care essentially entails services where patients feel that they are treated as persons, with respect and dignity, and that their needs, wants and preferences are considered. It is therefore of great value to explore how different countries, and providers in these countries, have attempted to change the way they deliver health care. The Swedish Agency for Health and Care Services Analysis has collaborated with the European Observatory on Health Systems and Policies in an attempt to shed light on possible strategies that can contribute to making our health systems more person-centred. This work rests on the assumption that it is not enough to increase person-centredness in the patients' interaction with nurses, doctors and other health professionals, but that all tiers of the health system need to consider the perspective of the user and the wider public. Managers and policy-makers at different levels need to create incentives, eliminate obstacles and show leadership in order to create services that will meet individuals' varying needs and include them in the care process. This volume has brought together some of the most experienced researchers in the field, coming from a range of disciplines, in order to outline and analyse what we know of the effectiveness of different strategies that could contribute to transforming our health systems.

Respecting patients' wants and preferences, and involving them in the care they receive, can potentially lead to better medical results. More research is, however, needed in this area to create a more comprehensive understanding of the effects of person-centred care. What is more, and perhaps more importantly, person-centredness should be seen as an important value in its own right. The process of participation, in its many different forms, has an intrinsic value as a democratic principle.

Involving patients in their own care, and in designing the health services they use, is a much overlooked resource that we, in light of the pressures our health systems face, can no longer afford to ignore. Learning from patients and their families and letting their voices be a core feature when we design, reform and evaluate our health systems sends an important message to both health professionals and policy-makers. This book can guide and inspire decision-makers, nationally, regionally and locally, in their attempts to create sustainable and inclusive health systems.

We want to thank the Observatory and the World Health Organization for this collaborative process. We are also grateful to the authors of the different chapters and to the editors for their hard work, and we lastly send our thanks to all other participants who have contributed to the book. As a next step, we intend to summarize the most important lessons from the anthology and analyse them in the context of the Swedish health system – thus hoping to increase knowledge and capacity among Swedish policy-makers.

JEAN-LUC AF GEIJERSTAM
General Director
The Swedish Agency for Health and Care Services Analysis

Acknowledgements

This volume is one of a series of books produced by the European Observatory on Health Systems and Policies. We are immensely grateful to all the authors for their hard work and enthusiasm in this study, and to Isabel de la Mata, Jean-Luc af Geijerstam and Dr Hans Henri P. Kluge for contributing the Forewords.

In addition to the authors (*see* List of contributors), we gratefully acknowledge the contributions of those who participated in a policy roundtable held in Stockholm in March 2017, to discuss contents, direction and individual draft chapters of the volume. These were: Sevim Barbasso-Helmers, Ann Catrine Eldh, Björn Hansell, Kaisa Immonen, Stefan Jutterdal, Bodil Klintberg, Fredrik Lennartsson, Johanna Lind, Tove Lindahl Greve, Veronika Lindberg, Lisbeth Löpare, Maria Montefusco, Stig Nyman, Sara Riggare, Ingrid Schmidt, and Kajsa Westling. The roundtable discussions provided an invaluable source for guiding this work further and improving its overall relevance to policy.

The information presented reflects the evidence as it stood in the spring of 2018. We would further like to thank the reviewers of individual chapters for all their comments and suggestions, which further enhanced the quality of the work. These were: Paula Blomqvist, Paul Buchanan, Sibylle Erdmann, Dominick Frosch, Tamara Hervey, Anya de Iongh, Karen Jones, Danny van Leeuwen, Cristin Lind, Maria Montefusco, Šarunas Narbutas, Catherine Needham, Jennie Popay, Sara Riggare, Sophie Staniszewska, Sarah Thomson and Sue Ziebland. We also gratefully acknowledge the time taken by the final reviewers of this volume, Dr Ann Catrine Eldh, and Professor Mike Dent. We greatly benefited from their very helpful comments and suggestions.

We are especially grateful to the Swedish Agency for Health and Care Services Analysis (Vårdanalys) for co-funding this study, and in particular to Johanna Lind (now Lumell Associates), Hanna Sjöberg, Kajsa Westling and Fredrik Lennartsson (now Director of Health and

Care, Region Skane) for their continued collaboration and support, patience and enthusiasm from the inception of this study to its final publication.

Finally, this book would not have appeared without the able and patient support throughout the project of our colleagues in the Observatory. In particular, we would like to thank Celine Démaret and Annalisa Marianecci who helped manage all administrative matters related to this work, including the organization of the author workshop in Stockholm. We are also very grateful to Jonathan North and Caroline White for managing the production process and to Sarah Cook for copy-editing the manuscript.

Contributors

Anders Anell is Professor, Department of Business Administration, Lund University, Sweden

Andrew Barnes is Associate Professor, Department of Health Behaviour and Policy, University of California (UCLA), USA

Peter Beresford OBE is Professor of Citizen Participation, School of Health and Social Care, University of Essex, UK and Co-Chair of Shaping Our Lives, the UK disabled people's and service users organization and network

Helmut Brand is Jean Monnet Professor of European Public Health and Head of the Department of International Health, School for Public Health and Primary Care (CAPHRI), Maastricht University, the Netherlands

Timo Clemens is Researcher, Department of International Health, School for Public Health and Primary Care (CAPHRI), Maastricht University, the Netherlands

Angela Coulter was chief executive of Picker Institute Europe from 2000 to 2008 and is now an independent consultant based in Oxfordshire, UK

Alizon K. Draper is Reader, School of Life Sciences, University of Westminster, UK

Marianna Fotaki is Professor of Business Ethics, Warwick Business School, University of Warwick, UK

Martin Härter is Chair of the Department of Medical Psychology, University Medical Center Hamburg-Eppendorf, University Medical Center, Hamburg, Germany

France Légaré is Tier 1 Canada Research Chair in Shared Decision Making and Knowledge Translation and Professor, Department of Family Medicine and Emergency Medicine, Faculty of Medicine, Université Laval, Québec, Canada

Andrew McCulloch was chief executive of Picker Institute Europe from 2013 to 2017 and is now an independent consultant based in London, UK

Sherry Merkur is Research Fellow and Health Policy Analyst, European Observatory on Health Systems and Policies, London School of Economics and Political Science, London, UK

Ellen Nolte is Professor of Health Services and Systems Research, London School of Hygiene & Tropical Medicine, London, UK

Herman Nys is Director, Centre for Biomedical Ethics and Law (CBMER), KU Leuven, Belgium

Willy Palm is Senior Advisor, European Observatory on Health Systems and Policies, Brussels, Belgium

Giuseppe Paparella was research officer at Picker Institute Europe and is now visiting scholar at the Hoover Institution, Stanford University, USA

Wilm Quentin is Senior Research Fellow, Department of Health Care Management, Berlin University of Technology, European Observatory on Health Systems and Policies, Germany

Thomas Rice is Professor, Fielding School of Public Health, University of California (UCLA), USA

Susan B. Rifkin is Adjunct Professor, Colorado School of Public Health, USA

Jasna Russo is Deputy Professor of Gender Studies in Rehabilitation and Education, Faculty of Rehabilitation, Technical University, Dortmund, Germany

David Shaw is Senior Researcher, Institute for Biomedical Ethics, University of Basel

Martin Smatana is General Director, Institute for Health Policies, Slovakia

Dawn Stacey is Research Chair in Knowledge Translation to Patients and Professor, School of Nursing, Faculty of Health Sciences, University of Ottawa, Canada and Senior Scientist, Ottawa Hospital Research Institute, Centre for Practice Changing Research, University of Ottawa, Ottawa, Canada

Anne M. Stiggelbout is Professor of Medical Decision Making, Department of Biomedical Data Sciences, Leiden University Medical Center, Leiden, the Netherlands

Richard Thomson is Professor of Epidemiology and Public Health, Population and Health Sciences Institute, Newcastle University, Newcastle upon Tyne, UK

David Townend is Professor of Law and Legal Philosophy in Health, Medicine and Life Sciences, School of Public Health and Primary Care (CAPHRI), Maastricht Universty, the Netherlands

Ewout van Ginneken is Hub Coordinator, European Observatory on Health Systems and Policies, Berlin University of Technology, Germany

Nick Verhaeghe is Post-doctoral Researcher, Department of Public Health and Primary Care, Ghent University, Belgium

Ruth Waitzberg is Researcher, Smokler Center for Health Policy Research, Myers-JDC-Brookdale Institute, Israel

Figures

Tables

Boxes

Appendix

1 | The person at the centre of health systems: an introduction

ELLEN NOLTE, SHERRY MERKUR, ANDERS ANELL

Introduction

[T]he people have the right and duty to participate individually and collectively in the planning and implementation of their health care.
Declaration of Alma Ata, 1978

There is now widespread acceptance, in political and policy declarations, that the individual citizen should be at the heart of the health system (OECD Health Ministerial Meeting, 2017; World Health Organization, 2016; World Health Organization Regional Office for Europe, 2015). A person-focused approach has been advocated on political, ethical and instrumental grounds and is believed to benefit service users, health professionals and the health system more broadly (Dieterich, 2007; Duggan et al., 2006; Richards, Coulter & Wicks, 2015). However, and in contrast to the political and policy emphasis placed upon 'person focus', there is continuing debate about its actual meaning in the health care context vis-à-vis concepts such as 'patient-centred', 'user-centred', 'family-centred' or 'people-centred' care, or indeed 'personalized' health care, as well as the strategies that are available and effective to promote and implement 'person focus'. There is no single definition of related concepts, and there are different views on the extent to which patient- or person-centredness:

- constitutes one of the several dimensions of delivering 'good quality care', along with effectiveness, safety, efficiency or equity, among others (Institute of Medicine, 2001; Klassen et al., 2010);
- represents a component of the broader idea of engaging patients and their carers in their health and health care (Mittler et al., 2013); or
- forms a complex strategy to innovate and implement long-lasting change in the way services in the health sectors are being delivered, involving multiple changes at multiple levels (World Health Organization, 2016).

1

The discussion around person-centredness is further complicated by more general concepts of empowerment and participation. Frequently used interchangeably (EMPATHiE Consortium, 2014; Scholl et al., 2014), the terms 'empowerment' and 'participation' have themselves defied a commonly agreed definition or framework. For example, Bravo et al. (2015), in a scoping review of patient empowerment, identified widely varying definitions. These ranged from those that viewed empowerment to be grounded in the principles of autonomy and self-determination and those that interpreted it as a transformative process that patients go through as they gain control of their health and health care, to those that simply viewed empowerment as an intervention aimed at promoting patient self-management. Similarly, participation and involvement have been described in different ways (Conklin, Morris & Nolte, 2010; Wait & Nolte, 2006). A 2014 review of reviews of consumer and community engagement described a distinct, while overlapping, set of concepts related to involvement, which included shared decision-making, self-management, community-based health promotion, participation in research, collaboration in research design and conduct, and peer support, among others (Sarrami-Foroushani et al., 2014).

Common to all these concepts is what Mittler et al. (2013) have referred to as the 'philosophical argument' (or ethical argument) and the 'performance-based argument' (or instrumental argument). The former stresses that individuals should have more say in their care as a principle: user involvement has a value in itself irrespective of its possible impact on quality of care or health. The performance-based argument expects that removing obstacles to service user involvement, such as a lack of information or motivation, will lead to an informed service user who behaves in ways which will ultimately improve the quality of their care and their health. It assumes that informed service users will select high-quality providers or help design a person-centred care plan to follow, which in turn may help enhance provider and service performance and contain care costs. If these instrumental purposes are not fulfilled, user involvement can, according to the performance-based argument, be challenged.

While intuitively, and indeed conceptually appealing, available evidence to support the premise that person-focused care and related concepts will lead to improved performance remains patchy. In brief, and as will be developed further in this book, there is good evidence at the individual user level for some aspects to be positively associated with selected measures. Examples include shared decision-making in the clinical encounter, which was shown to enhance knowledge and patients taking a more active role in decision-making (Stacey et al., 2017). Further evidence also points to the potential for interventions related to shared decision-making to contribute to reducing health inequalities (Durand et al., 2014). Similarly, self-management support can improve selected health outcomes among people with chronic disease, including health-related quality of life and healthy behaviours (Franek, 2013). Conversely, the evidence of the impact of patient and public engagement in health care decision-making more broadly remains difficult to establish (Groene et al., 2014; Mockford et al., 2012), although, in line with the philosophical argument above, it has been argued that involving the public in the health care policy process can be seen to be a value in its own right (Conklin, Morris & Nolte, 2010).

Against this background of growing policy interest and a patchy evidence base, it seems timely to revisit the idea of person-centredness, set it in a broader context and review the available evidence on strategies and interventions more coherently. Specifically, there is a need to take a systems approach to better understand and clarify the use and usefulness of strategies seeking to give individuals, their families and communities a greater role in the health system. This takes greater urgency against concerns that lack of clarity about what person-centred care and related concepts really mean can "produce efforts that are superficial and unconvincing" (Epstein & Street, 2011, p. 101), and which can, ultimately, undermine the legitimacy of a public health care system (Flood, 2015). Policy-makers seeking to improve the position of individuals, their families and communities in the health system, based on philosophical or performance-based arguments or both, are thus faced with two major policy questions to ensure person-centredness is systematically considered in decision-making:

- how to characterize and organize the range of approaches and strategies that are available; and
- what types of interventions and strategies are effective to strengthen person-centredness in different health system contexts.

This book aims to respond to these two policy concerns by exploring 'person-centred' care and its realization at the different tiers within health systems. In doing so, the study considers the various concepts that have been discussed under the headings of 'centredness' and 'involvement' and how these play out at the different levels of the system. This stretches from the broad collective population level to the individual patient level in a clinical setting, capturing strategies and policies that share the common aim of placing individuals, their families and communities at the centre and enabling them to play a more central and directing role in their own care as well as in shaping the system that serves them.

In this chapter, we first set out the challenges that a greater person-focus is expected to address. We then describe the framework that has guided this work and our methodological approach. We conclude with a brief outline of the book and who should read it.

What is the problem policy-makers want 'person-centredness' to address?

Globally, health systems are facing numerous challenges. While there have been significant advances in people's health and life expectancy in Europe and elsewhere, relative improvements have been unequal among and within countries and there remain considerable challenges across regions (GBD 2016 DALYs and HALE Collaborators, 2017). Key challenges include the rising burden of chronic health problems and of multimorbidity, along with growing consumer expectations and technological advances against a backdrop of increasing financial constraints, creating a pressing need for the efficient use of resources and a fundamental rethink in the way systems are organized and financed (Nolte, Knai & Saltman, 2014).

Thus, as populations age and advances in health care allow those with once fatal conditions to survive, the prevalence of chronic conditions is rising in many countries. In the European Union in 2014 about one-third of the adult population reported having a long-standing illness or health problem, ranging from some 20% in Romania and Bulgaria to over 40% in Estonia and Finland (Eurostat, 2016). Of particular concern is the rise in the number of people with multiple health and care needs, which tend to be more common among older people, the proportion of whom is also increasing rapidly in the population (Violan et al., 2014). An estimated two-thirds of those who have reached pensionable age have at least two chronic conditions, although the actual number of people with multimorbidity is higher at younger ages (Barnett et al., 2012; Koné Pefoyo et al., 2015; Schiøtz et al., 2017), affecting those with lower socioeconomic status in particular (Violan et al., 2014). People with multimorbidity are more likely to have poorer outcomes, along with higher use of health services and associated costs (Palladino et al., 2016; Sambamoorthi, Tan & Deb, 2015; Thavorn et al., 2017).

Chronic conditions create a spectrum of needs that require multifaceted responses over extended periods of time, from a range of professionals as well as active patient engagement (Holman & Lorig, 2000). It is clear that the traditional approach to health care, with its focus on acute, episodic illness, is not suited to meet the long-term and fluctuating needs of those with chronic illness. Instead, services should be centred on the needs of patients and grounded in partnerships between patients and providers working to optimize outcomes (Nolte & McKee, 2008). Yet, as data from an international survey among adult people with chronic conditions in 11 countries show, patient involvement in their own care remains suboptimal (Figure 1.1).

Fragmentation of services along the care continuum means that patients often receive care from many different professionals or providers, in particular when they have multiple health and care needs. As a result, they are frequently called upon to monitor, coordinate or carry out their own treatment plan. For example, in the aforementioned international survey, between 20% and 40% of respondents who had seen their provider during the past two years reported to have experienced coordination problems, such as the specialist did not have information on their medical history, or they had received conflicting information from different health professionals (Osborn et al., 2016). Failure to coordinate services along the care continuum may result in suboptimal outcomes, including potentially preventable hospitalizations, medication errors and other adverse events (Vogeli et al., 2007). In addition, there are numerous other negative patient outcomes associated with a lack of coordination that are less well documented, such as anxiety, worry and distress, along with feelings of being lost in the system, frustration and disempowerment (Sampson et al., 2015; Schiøtz, Høst & Frølich, 2016), and, ultimately, loss of trust (Pedersen et al., 2013).

Osborn et al. (2016) further found that among people who have a regular doctor or place of care, between 10% in Australia and the Netherlands and up to 36% in France reported that their doctor did not spend enough time with them and did not explain things in a way they could understand. This can be seen to be of particular concern in light of advances in medical technology, from diagnostic testing

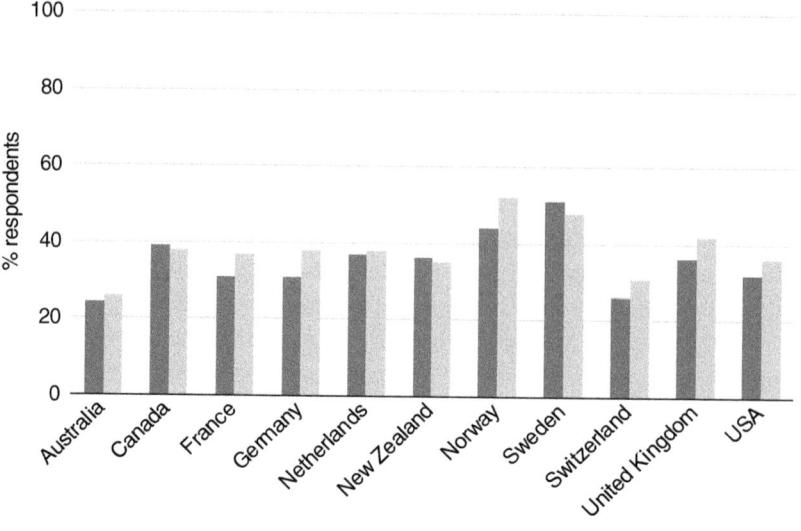

- ■ Did not discuss their main goals and priorities in caring for their condition
- ▨ Did not discuss treatment options, including side effects

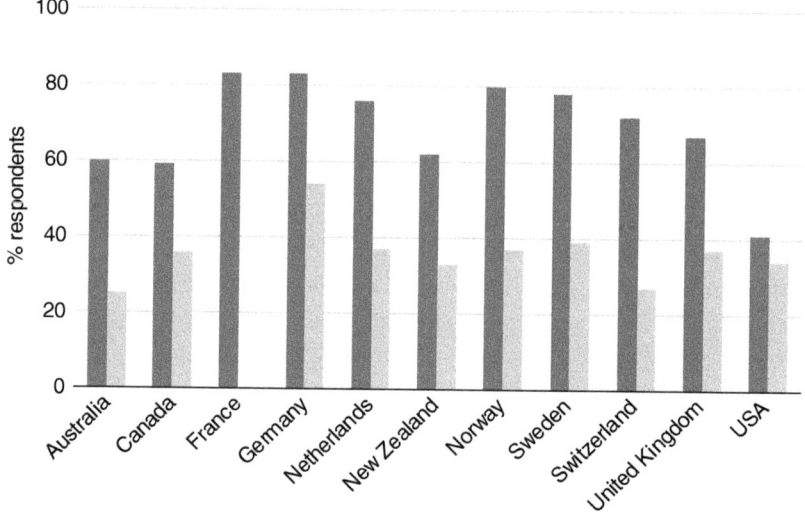

- ■ Did not talk about healthy diet, exercise and physical activity
- ▨ Did not talk about things in life that cause worry or stress

Figure 1.1 Engagement of service users with chronic conditions in their own care, 2016

Source: adapted from Osborn et al., 2016

to therapeutic treatments and procedures. These provide significant potential for new methods of delivering and organizing health care such as providing care closer to people's homes in response to changing population health and care needs. But countries have to ensure that any such technology is used effectively and appropriately and at a cost that is affordable, with associated changes carefully balancing growing consumer expectations and respecting people's needs, wants and preferences (Elshaug et al., 2017).

At the same time, a growing service user movement, facilitated by modern digital technologies, in particular social media, is challenging the traditional way in which people use health services. Examples include health-related online discussion forums and virtual patient networks for the provision of information about health and health concerns as well as for patient support; the online forum PatientsLikeMe has developed into a clinical research platform that collects and analyses data generated by patients to inform research and practice (Okun & Goodwin, 2017). Virtual user platforms were found to have both positive and negative effects on people, such as enhancing (for example through the experience of positive relations with others) but also reducing subjective well-being (for example producing negative emotions through feelings of worry and anxiety) (Smailhodzic et al., 2016). They can also affect the patient–health professional relationship, leading for example to more equal communication while also potentially undermining the interaction, such as when the professional's expertise is being challenged. Online user platforms have considerable potential to inform and promote person-centred care, and possibly person-driven care, especially for those with chronic conditions. Examples include harnessing the knowledge and lived-experiences of patients and their carers, but such approaches have yet to be integrated strategically into practice (Amann, Zanini & Rubinelli, 2016).

These challenges come against a backdrop of persistent and, in some settings, rising health inequalities and inequities in access to and utilization of health care services. Elstad (2016) analysed data on self-reported unmet need for medical care because of costs, waiting time or geographical distance from the European Union Statistics on Income and Living Conditions (EU-SILC) for the period 2008–2013. This showed that levels of unmet need for medical care increased in most countries but in particular among those populations considered most vulnerable because of their low socioeconomic status and health problems (Figure 1.2). For these populations, unmet need for medical care tended to be higher in countries with larger income inequalities. This highlights that countries with a more equal income distribution had been more able to protect their populations, and vulnerable groups in particular, against worsening access to medical care in the context of economic crises. The findings also suggest that there is a need for a shift from service delivery that simply responds to demand to a service that proactively seeks need, even when it is not voiced as demand, in the knowledge that those whose needs are greatest may be least able to access care. Such a shift will be of particular importance in light of increasing reliance on digital health technologies, which, while having considerable potential to support person-centred systems, may exacerbate social inequalities in health if not carefully designed (Latulippe, Hamel & Giroux, 2017).

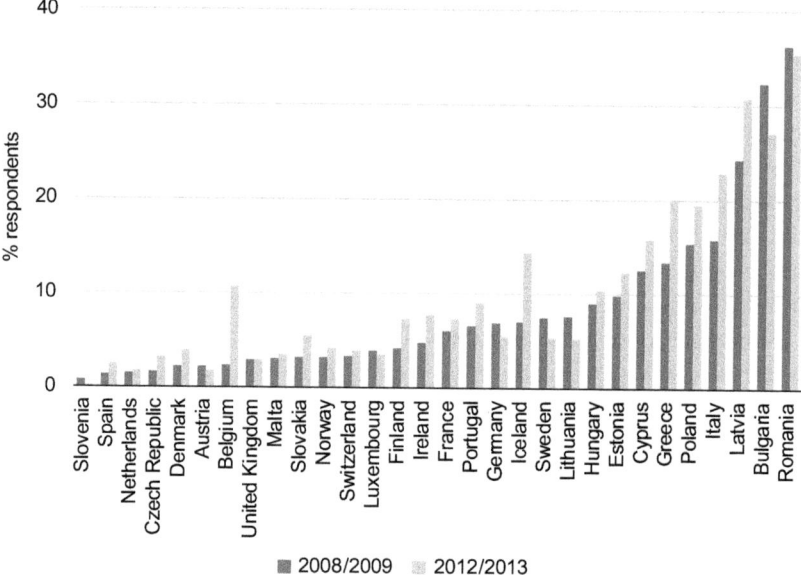

Figure 1.2 Forgone medical care (%) in 2008/2009 and 2012/2013 among disadvantaged populations in 30 countries

Note: disadvantaged defined as (i) being in the lowest income tertile (the lower third of the income distribution in the country sample, age 30–59, in the given survey), and (ii) reporting health difficulties in terms of either a long-standing (chronic) disease or self-rated overall health status as fair or bad.

Source: adapted from Elstad, 2016

A health system that is focused on the person at the centre is seen as a means to address these challenges through ensuring (World Health Organization, 2017) that:

- everyone has access to the quality health services they need, when and where they need them (*equity in access*)
- safe, effective and timely care that responds to people's needs and that is of the highest possible standard (*quality*)
- care that is coordinated around people's needs, respects their preferences and allows for their participation in health care (*responsiveness and participation*)
- ensures that services are provided in the most cost-effective setting with the right balance between health promotion, prevention, and in- and outpatient care, avoiding duplication and waste of resources (*efficiency*)
- that the capacity of health actors, institutions and populations is strengthened to prepare for, and effectively respond to, public health crises (*resilience*).

Conceptualizing person-centredness: a guiding framework

This study was initially guided by a broad framework that builds on a 'service user typology' proposed by Fotaki (2013) in the context of governing public services systems. This was developed further by Dent & Pahor (2015), who sought to conceptualize the rise of the idea of 'patient involvement' in European health care settings over past decades in an attempt to enable cross-country comparison of strategies and approaches that aim to strengthen the individual's role in the health system. The framework principally distinguishes three core roles: consumerist, deliberative and participatory, which Dent & Pahor (2015) summarized under the broad headings of 'choice', 'voice', and 'co-production' (Figure 1.3).

Choice relates to the general idea of the patient or service user as a consumer within the health system. The notion of voice represents the individual patient or service user as a citizen who is actively involved in decision-making (bodies) related to health. Co-production can be seen to be located at the interface between voice and choice and describes how patients or service users engage, individually or collectively, in the delivery of their own treatments and care in partnership with providers (Fotaki, 2013). Although the idea of co-production may be less familiar

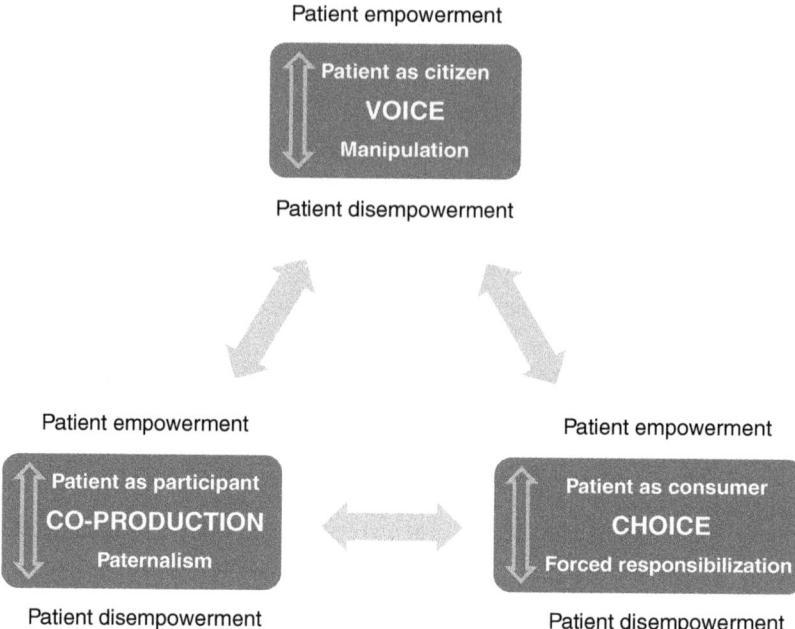

Patient empowerment

Patient as citizen
VOICE
Manipulation

Patient disempowerment

Patient empowerment

Patient as participant
CO-PRODUCTION
Paternalism

Patient disempowerment

Patient empowerment

Patient as consumer
CHOICE
Forced responsibilization

Patient disempowerment

Figure 1.3 The conceptual framework guiding the study

Source: adapted from Dent & Pahor, 2015

to readers, it is increasingly seen to be key to public services reforms (Osborne et al., 2016; Pestoff, 2014) and is gaining traction in the health services and systems literature, too (Batalden et al., 2016).

These distinctions are not clear-cut, but rather present different roles that individuals can take, at times simultaneously, as a patient, decision-maker, taxpayer and active citizen (Coulter, 2002). For example, individuals might exert their right to make decisions about the provider they wish to consult (choice), and at the same time participate in decision-making bodies about how to organize delivery (voice) and work with their own provider towards shared decision-making (co-production) to clarify acceptable medical options and choose an appropriate treatment.

The different notions of involvement or 'person focus' as conceptualized in Figure 1.3 may have positive outcomes in terms of better quality or service delivery, as well as unintended consequences. Outcomes will also depend on whether the strategy under consideration truly empowers or disempowers individuals (Dent & Pahor, 2015; Fotaki, 2013). For example, policies that use public deliberation processes to legitimize decisions rather than engage the public in a true exchange might be seen to be tokenistic or even manipulative rather than giving a 'voice'. Likewise, service users might be made responsible for their choices (forced responsibilization), or they are asked to choose from services they have little control over, which weakens the individual's role in the system.

It is important to emphasize that the framework presented in Figure 1.3 should not be interpreted as a normative model in an evaluative sense. We used it simply as a descriptive frame to categorize and guide our preliminary analyses of individual strategies and systems more broadly. In doing so, we further operationalized the three principal categories at the level of the different tiers of the health system. These include the primary process of patient care ('micro' level), the organizational ('meso') context and the financing and policy context at system ('macro') level, each with distinct rationales and perspectives concerning the delivery of health care (Plochg & Klazinga, 2002). This structure provided one way of organizing the different themes that will be reviewed in this book, while acknowledging the close links and overlaps between the different roles of service users within the system. We also recognize that alternative frameworks exist, for example focusing on themes related to the challenges of developing coordinated and integrated care from a service provider perspective. Our approach looks explicitly at roles that service users can take, which in turn will have implications for service providers in their attempts to coordinate and integrate services.

Our approach to the analysis

The study as presented in this book was led by the European Observatory on Health Systems and Policies, in collaboration with the Swedish Agency for Health and Care Services Analysis (Vårdanalys). The principal approach is an exploration of key themes of person-centredness, based on a synthesis of the theoretical and empirical evidence from a wide range of mostly high-income countries. The selection of key themes to be explored was guided by an initial expert workshop held in June 2015 and the conceptual framework described above. It is reflected in a series of themed chapters that examine 'voice' in the context of public involvement in health care decision-making and research; 'choice', of provider, of payer and of services; and 'co-production', largely revolving around the individual as a service user in the primary context of patient care.

For each of the themes covered in this book, we commissioned experts with proven expertise to contribute an overview of each selected area. Contributors were identified through a range of sources, including a track record in the relevant scientific literature and an international profile through, for example, membership in advisory groups on the topic under study, further informed by the editors' own professional networks. Contributors, or teams of contributors, were invited to produce a chapter on the given topic area in line with a set of terms of references developed by the editors. Specifically, authors were asked to set out:

(i)   the drivers behind the subject under analysis (how the topic has evolved; what the anticipated impacts in relation to health system performance are);
(ii) measurement issues (how do we know that the subject under analysis has been implemented, and what is the evidence of impact);
(iii) bottlenecks for implementation;
(iv) innovations and future developments; and
(v)   policy lessons learned.

Chapter authors were encouraged to give examples of relevant person-centred approaches that have been implemented in European countries for further illustration of the topic area being explored.

Each of the themed chapters was externally peer reviewed by an academic expert in the field and by a service user to ensure that the content of the relevant chapter is covered comprehensively, that it adequately reflects the key issues, in particular those arising from a service user perspective, and that it does not overlook important evidence. A separate review process concerned the study as a whole. It focused on the four framing chapters 1–4 in particular to ensure coherence, appropriateness, relevance and quality.

Outline of the book

While this book takes an explicit systems approach, it should be emphasized that it cannot capture the full complexity of the idea of person-centredness. We see the analyses presented as a starting point for a more critical engagement with a concept that is widely but variously used in different contexts, often without a clear understanding what it is actually meant to convey. Yet, as the brief introduction to this book has shown, a more person-centred approach is expected to address, or perhaps even solve, a wide range of challenges contemporary health systems are facing. We examine a range of perspectives on person-centred strategies to help inform whether and how available strategies are suited to meet these challenges and to guide the development of more informed policies and practices. Inevitably there are trade-offs between the breadth and depth of relevant strategies and approaches that we could have covered in this book. We opted for an in-depth analysis of selected perspectives, recognizing that other, equally relevant, perspectives will have been left out for others to address.

The book is divided into two broad parts. The first part comprises Chapters 1–4, which set out the overall conceptual framework for the work presented in this book and provide a synthesis and analysis of the key themes examined in-depth in the second part (Chapters 5–13). In brief, Chapter 2 explores the evolution of the concept of person-centredness by reviewing insights from the published academic literature and policy documents. It finds that there is wide variation in the terminology and interpretation of the idea of 'centredness', reflecting different professional disciplines, perspectives and clinical settings, as well as different regional and country contexts. At the same time, there is agreement on the fundamental ethical premise that patients and service users should be treated as persons, with respect and dignity, and that care should take into account their needs, wants and preferences. Yet beyond this, there remains considerable diversity among different stakeholders in how to translate this common understanding into practice, and it is this diversity that we will need to disentangle in order to understand and inform policy development.

Chapter 3 synthesizes the main insights and lessons that emerge from the in-depth analyses presented in Chapters 5–13, building on the principal framework of voice, choice and co-production as described above. They examine the different roles people take in health systems, from engaging in and leading on health service and system development (Chapter 5) and research (Chapter 6), evaluating the quality of health services and systems (Chapter 7), and making decisions about purchasers or providers of individual care packages and services (or choosing not to do so) (Chapters 8–10), to participating in their own care (Chapters 11 and 12), along with legal frameworks seeking to ensure that people can exercise their rights as taxpayers and citizens (Chapter 13). The synthesis of these in-depth chapters finds that there is a need to move to a more complex model of engagement that considers people's values and preferences at the level of the individual patient–professional relationship (micro level), as well as the organizational (meso) and the governance and finance, along with wider societal (macro) levels in order to systematically implement person-centred strategies. These issues are then examined further in Chapter 4, which also provides pointers to the range of options, or levers, that show promise in supporting a move to more person-centred care. It discusses some of these options, highlighting the opportunities while also considering problematic issues that need to be overcome in order to move to person-centred health systems.

Who should read this book?

The starting point for this book is the various roles people take in health systems, and it is perhaps fair to say that very few of us will go through life without being affected, directly or indirectly, by the system. This might be as service users, carers, taxpayers or voting citizens, or those working in and with the health system, whether as health professionals, managers or policy-makers, or as representatives of patients, carers or the public more widely. This book will, inevitably, be of most interest to practitioners, managers, representatives of service user organizations and policy-makers, but we hope that there will also be something useful in it for others, including the growing number of researchers in the field. The nature of health care is changing, in many cases quite rapidly. It will be ever more important for those designing, directing and governing services to implement effective approaches and strategies that place individuals, their families and communities at the centre of the health system and enable service users to play a more central and directing role in their own care as well as in shaping the system that serves them. There are no easy answers, and those working in and for different health systems must find approaches that are appropriate to their own circumstances. Yet there is also considerable scope for shared learning from successes as well as failures. This book seeks to contribute to this process.

References

Amann J, Zanini C, Rubinelli S (2016). What Online User Innovation Communities Can Teach Us about Capturing the Experiences of Patients Living with Chronic Health Conditions. A Scoping Review. *PLoS One*, 11:e0156175.

Barnett K et al. (2012). Epidemiology of multimorbidity and implications for health care, research, and medical education: a cross-sectional study. *Lancet*, 380:37–43.

Batalden M et al. (2016). Coproduction of healthcare service. *BMJ Quality & Safety*, 25:509–17.

Bravo P et al. (2015). Conceptualising patient empowerment: a mixed methods study. *BMC Health Services Research*, 15:252.

Conklin A, Morris Z, Nolte E (2010). Involving the public in healthcare policy. An update of the research evidence and proposed evaluation framework. Santa Monica: Rand Corporation.

Coulter A (2002). *The autonomous patient – ending paternalism in medical care*. London, TSO.

Dent M, Pahor M (2015). Patient involvement in Europe – a comparative framework. *Journal of Health Organization and Management Information*, 29:546–55.

Dieterich A (2007). The modern patient – threat or promise? Physicians' perspectives on patients' changing attributes. *Patient Education and Counseling*, 67:279–85.

Duggan PS et al. (2006). The moral nature of patient-centeredness: is it "just the right thing to do"? *Patient Education and Counseling*, 62:271–6.

Durand M et al. (2014). Do interventions designed to support shared decision-making reduce health inequalities? A systematic review and meta-analysis. *PLoS One*, 9:e94670.

Elshaug A et al. (2017). Levers for addressing medical underuse and overuse: achieving high-value health care. *Lancet*, 390:191–202.

Elstad J (2016). Income inequality and forgone medical care in Europe during The Great Recession: multilevel analyses of EU-SILC surveys 2008–2013. *International Journal for Equity in Health*, 15:101.

EMPATHiE Consortium (2014). Empowering patients in the management of chronic diseases. Available at: http://ec.europa.eu/health/patient_safety/docs/empathie_frep_en.pdf (accessed September 2015).

Epstein R, Street RJ (2011). The values and value of patient-centred care. *Annals of Family Medicine*, 9:100–3.

Eurostat (2016). Self-perceived health statistics. Available at: http://ec.europa.eu/eurostat/statistics-explained/index.php/Self-perceived_health_statistics#Further_Eurostat_information (accessed 18 November 2017).

Flood C (2015). Scoping the shape of an iceberg: the future of public involvement in health policy: reflecting on 'Public involvement policies in health: exploring their conceptual basis'. *Health Economics, Policy and Law*, 10:381–5.

Fotaki M (2013). Towards developing new partnerships in public services: users as consumers, citizens and/or co-producers in health and social care in England and Sweden. *Public Administration*, 89:933–55.

Franek J (2013). Self-management support interventions for persons with chronic disease: an evidence-based analysis. *Ontario Health Technology Assessment Series*, 13:1–60.

GBD 2016 DALYs and HALE Collaborators (2017). Global, regional, and national disability-adjusted life-years (DALYs) for 333 diseases and injuries and healthy life expectancy (HALE) for 195 countries and territories, 1990–2016: a systematic analysis for the Global Burden of Disease Study 2016. *Lancet*, 390:1260–1344.

Groene O et al. (2014). Involvement of patients or their representatives in quality management functions in EU hospitals: implementation and impact on patient-centred care strategies. *International Journal for Quality in Health Care*, 26:81–91.

Holman H, Lorig K (2000). Patients as partners in managing chronic disease. Partnership is a prerequisite for effective and efficient health care. *BMJ*, 320:526–7.

Institute of Medicine (2001). *Crossing the quality chasm: a new health system for the 21st century*. Washington, DC: National Academies Press.

Klassen A et al. (2010). Performance measurement and improvement frameworks in health, education and social service systems: a systematic review. *International Journal for Quality in Health Care*, 22:44–69.

Koné Pefoyo A et al. (2015). The increasing burden and complexity of multimorbidity. *BMC Public Health*, 15:415.

Latulippe K, Hamel C, Giroux D (2017). Social health inequalities and eHealth: a literature review with qualitative synthesis of theoretical and empirical studies. *Journal of Medical Internet Research*, 19:e136.

Mittler J et al. (2013). Making sense of 'consumer engagement' initiatives to improve health and health care: a conceptual framework to guide policy and practice. *Milbank Quarterly*, 91:37–77.

Mockford C et al. (2012). The impact of patient and public involvement on UK NHS health care: a systematic review. *International Journal for Quality in Health Care*, 24:28–38.

Nolte E, McKee M (eds.) (2008). *Caring for people with chronic conditions: a health system perspective*. Maidenhead: Open University Press.

Nolte E, Knai C, Saltman R (eds.) (2014). *Assessing chronic disease management in European health systems. Concepts and approaches*. Copenhagen: WHO Regional Office for Europe on behalf of the European Observatory on Health Systems and Policies.

OECD Health Ministerial Meeting (2017). The next generation of health reforms. Available at: http://www.oecd.org/health/ministerial/ministerial-statement-2017.pdf (accessed 20 August 2017).

Okun S, Goodwin K (2017). Building a learning health community: By the people, for the people. *Learning Health Systems*, 1:e10028.

Osborn R et al. (2016). In New Survey Of Eleven Countries, US Adults Still Struggle With Access To And Affordability Of Health Care. *Health Affairs (Millwood)*, 35:2327–36.

Palladino R et al. (2016). Associations between multimorbidity, healthcare utilisation and health status: evidence from 16 European countries. *Age Ageing*, 45:431–5.

Pedersen J et al. (2013). *The puzzle of changing relationships*. London: The Health Foundation.

Pestoff V (2014). Collective action and the sustainability of co-production. *Public Management Review*, 16:383–401.

Plochg T, Klazinga N (2002). Community-based integrated care: myth or must? *International Journal for Quality in Health Care*, 14:91–101.

Richards T, Coulter A, Wicks P (2015). Time to deliver patient centred care. *BMJ*, 350:h530.

Sambamoorthi U, Tan X, Deb A (2015). Multiple chronic conditions and healthcare costs among adults. *Expert Review of Pharmacoeconomics & Outcomes Research*, 15:823–32.

Sampson R et al. (2015). Patients' perspectives on the medical primary-secondary care interface: systematic review and synthesis of qualitative research. *BMJ Open*, 5:e008708.

Sarrami-Foroushani P et al. (2014). Key concepts in consumer and community engagement: a scoping meta-review. *BMC Health Services Research*, 14:250.

Schiøtz M, Høst D, Frølich A (2016). Involving patients with multimorbidity in service planning: perspectives on continuity and care coordination. *Journal of Comorbidity*, 6:95–102.

Schiøtz M et al. (2017). Social disparities in the prevalence of multimorbidity – a register-based population study. *BMC Public Health*, 17:422.

Scholl I et al. (2014). An integrative model of patient-centeredness – a systematic review and concept analysis. *PLoS One*, 9:e107828.

Smailhodzic E et al. (2016). Social media use in healthcare: a systematic review of effects on patients and on their relationship with healthcare professionals. *BMC Health Services Research*, 16:442.

Stacey D et al. (2017). Decision aids for people facing health treatment or screening decisions. *Cochrane Database of Systematic Reviews*, 4:CD001431.

Thavorn K et al. (2017). Effect of socio-demographic factors on the association between multimorbidity and healthcare costs: a population-based, retrospective cohort study. *BMJ Open*, 7:e017264.

Violan C et al. (2014). Prevalence, determinants and patterns of multimorbidity in primary care: a systematic review of observational studies. *PLoS One*, 21:e102149.

Vogeli C et al. (2007). Multiple chronic conditions: prevalence, health consequences, and implications for quality, care management, and costs. *Journal of General Internal Medicine*, 22:391–5.

Wait S, Nolte E (2006). Public involvement policies in health: exploring their conceptual basis. *Health Economics, Policy and Law*, 1:149–62.

World Health Organization (2016). Framework on integrated, people-centred health services. Report by the Secretariat. Available at: http://apps.who.int/gb/ebwha/pdf_files/WHA69/A69_39-en.pdf?ua=1 (accessed 17 December 2017).

World Health Organization (2017). Framework on integrated people-centred health services. Available at: http://www.who.int/servicedeliverysafety/areas/people-centred-care/framework/en/ (accessed 17 December 2017).

World Health Organization Regional Office for Europe (2015). Priorities for health systems strengthening in the WHO European Region 2015–2020: walking the talk on people centredness. Available at: http://www.euro.who.int/__data/assets/pdf_file/0003/282963/65wd13e_HealthSystemsStrengthening_150494.pdf (accessed 15 June 2017).

2 Person-centredness: exploring its evolution and meaning in the health system context

ELLEN NOLTE, SHERRY MERKUR, ANDERS ANELL

Introduction

The right of citizens and patients to participate in the decision-making process affecting health care, if they wish to do so, must be viewed as a fundamental and integral part of any democratic society.
Council of Europe, 2000

As we have seen in the introduction to this book, there remains a lack of consensus about the actual meaning of patient or person 'centredness' in the context of health systems. There is considerable overlap with concepts such as 'empowerment' and 'participation'. Some view empowerment as a core principle or dimension of patient-centred care (Docteur & Coulter, 2012; International Alliance for Patients' Organizations, 2006), while others define centredness as a foundation or prerequisite for achieving empowerment (Castro et al., 2016; Lhussier et al., 2015).

A wide range of reviews have been carried out over the past two decades to better understand patient- and person-centred care and related concepts. Yet uncertainty remains, mainly because reviews tend to differ on a number of characteristics, such as:

- *the methodological approach*: including scoping review (Constand et al., 2014), systematic review (Kogan, Wilber & Mosqueda, 2016), meta-narrative review (Kitson et al., 2013), and integrative review (Sidani & Fox, 2014), as well as dimensional (Hobbs, 2009) or concept analysis (Castro et al., 2016; Lusk & Fater, 2013; Morgan & Yoder, 2012; Holmstrom & Roing, 2010), discourse analysis (Pluut, 2016), or a combination of these (Hughes, Bamford & May, 2008; Mead & Bower, 2000; McCormack & McCance, 2006; Scholl et al., 2014);
- *the disciplinary perspective*: mainly medicine (Lhussier et al., 2015; Mead & Bower, 2000; Scholl et al., 2014) and nursing (McCormack & McCance, 2006), although several studies looked across disciplines

(Castro et al., 2016; Constand et al., 2014; Hughes, Bamford & May, 2008; Kitson et al., 2013; Morgan & Yoder, 2012; Sidani & Fox, 2014);

- *the setting*: considering for example general practice or family medicine (Hudon et al., 2012; Mead & Bower, 2000), acute or post-acute inpatient care (Castro et al., 2016; Morgan & Yoder, 2012; McCormack & McCance, 2006; Hobbs, 2009), rehabilitation (Leplege et al., 2007), dentistry (Mills et al., 2014), or across settings (Constand et al., 2014; Hughes, Bamford & May, 2008; Scholl et al., 2014; Sidani & Fox, 2014); or
- *the patient population or service area*: such as chronic care (Hudon et al., 2012), older people (Kogan, Wilber & Mosqueda, 2016) or maternity services (de Labrusse et al., 2016).

As a consequence, it remains challenging to arrive at an overarching common conceptual framework relevant to policy-making. At the same time, seminal work in the field has informed key policy documents at national and international levels, embracing the notion of patient- or person-centredness as fundamental to the delivery of health care that is accessible, effective and of high quality (Australian Commission on Safety and Quality in Health Care, 2011; Department of Health, 2010; Institute of Medicine, 2001; International Alliance for Patients' Organizations, 2006; International College of Person-centered Medicine, 2011).

In this chapter, we explore the evolution of patient- or person-centredness and seek to synthesize the insights emerging from existing reviews in the academic literature and policy documents. We begin by briefly tracing the emergence of the different notions and their objectives in the health and care sectors. We then critically examine the range of definitions and conceptualizations and consider the role of the perspective of different stakeholders and disciplines in shaping the understanding of these concepts. We close this chapter with some overarching observations and conclusions.

Informed by the review of the different concepts in this chapter, we use the term 'person-centred' throughout the entire volume. This decision was driven, mainly, by a recognition that the term 'patient-centred' may too narrowly focus on the patient–provider interaction within the individual (clinical) consultation and insufficiently take account of the social context within which people live and that influences disease trajectories and care choices (Hobbs, 2009; Starfield, 2011). More importantly perhaps, the notion of 'patient' may unduly reduce the individual to one affected by a given health problem (or disability) within the medical care system while within the context of this book we consider the broader context of health systems with the individual person at the centre in terms of exercising voice and choice and actively involved in shaping health services at the different tiers in the system (*see* Chapter 1). However, when reviewing the academic literature and policy documents we have considered both patient- and person-centredness because of their frequent and, at times, interchangeable use in the health care context.

Tracing the evolution of patient- and person-centredness as a concept in the health care context

The roots of some of the core principles underlying the idea of patient- and person-centredness date back to ancient civilizations that conceptualized health holistically and viewed respect for individuals as a key value (Mezzich et al., 2009). It is only more recently that either notion has emerged as a distinct term, although descriptions and interpretations of the evolution of these concepts vary among authors. This largely reflects the underlying differences in disciplines and perspectives (Hobbs, 2009; Kitson et al., 2013; Leplege et al., 2007; Mead & Bower, 2000; Laine & Davidoff, 1996; Stewart et al., 2003). For example, in the UK and Canada the terms patient-centredness and patient-centred medicine have been most closely linked to family medicine and general practice (Levenstein et al., 1986; Mead & Bower, 2000). Here, the concept can be traced to the writings of Balint in the 1960s, who described patient-centredness in medicine in the context of the physician–patient encounter, arguing for the physician to understand the patient as a whole person and "unique human-being" (Balint, 1969, p. 269). Similar developments have occurred elsewhere in Europe from around the mid-20th century, including in France, Switzerland and Sweden. Here, the approach to the medical encounter that emphasizes the whole person has been more commonly referred to as person-centred medicine (Leplege et al., 2007; Pfeifer, 2010; Mezzich et al., 2009).

In the USA the emergence of patient-centredness in medicine can be traced to the patient rights movement since the 1960s, and the concept is seen to have evolved at different paces in different aspects of medical care, from the process of patient care, to medical law, medical education and quality assurance (Laine & Davidoff, 1996). Some of the most influential work in the field that eventually led to the establishment of the Picker Institute and the formulation of the Picker principles of patient-centred care (*see* below) originated from empirical research undertaken in the hospital setting in the USA during the 1980s (Gerteis et al., 1993; Picker Institute, 2013). That work also informed the formulation of patient-centred care as one of the core components of high quality care as advanced by the US Institute of Medicine's influential 2001 report, 'Crossing the Quality Chasm' (Institute of Medicine, 2001).

The nursing literature has linked the idea of 'centredness' more closely to the notion of caring, tracing its origins to Florence Nightingale and the emergence of modern nursing, with its focus on the patient, in contrast to medicine with its focus on the disease (Morgan & Yoder, 2012). This understanding is most often, although not always, expressed through the use of the term person-centred care (McCormack, 2003; McCormack & McCance, 2006; Morgan & Yoder, 2012). In this context, a number of scholars both in the medical and the nursing literature have referred to the writings of Carl Rogers in the 1940s on client-centred psychotherapy, which are seen to have influenced the understanding of the relationship between the professional (doctor, nurse, therapist) and the patient in building a therapeutic alliance as a key component of person-centred care (Hughes, Bamford & May, 2008; Morgan & Yoder, 2012; Leplege et al., 2007; Mead & Bower, 2000).

The concept has evolved and expanded over time, with a broad range of terminologies, definitions and multiple dimensions discussed in the literature. Thus, Scholl et al. (2014) identified, in a systematic review of patient-centredness in health care, 417 articles that contained a definition of the concept. Their review also noted that over 80% of reviewed papers had been published after 1999, pointing to the exponential increase in recognition of the notion of this and associated concepts in both research and the policy context. Box 2.1 presents a selection of definitions of patient- and person-centred care that have been proposed since the late 1960s.

The range of definitions presented in Box 2.1 is not meant to be exhaustive but rather serves to illustrate the variety of understandings of the concept and the different emphasis placed on particular aspects. However, notwithstanding the differences between definitions and characterizations, a number of common themes can be identified. These relate to the fundamental ethical premise that patients should be treated as persons, with respect and dignity, and that care should take

---

Box 2.1 Selected definitions of patient- and person-centred care

Balint (1969)	Patient-centred medicine understands the patient "as a unique human-being" (p. 269)
Gerteis et al. (1993)	Patient-centred care is "an approach that consciously adopts the patient's perspective" (p. 5)
Laine & Davidoff (1996)	"Patient-centered care is health care that is closely congruent with and responsive to patients' wants, needs and preferences" (p. 152)
Institute of Medicine (2001)	"Patient-centered – providing care that is respectful of and responsive to individual patient preferences, needs, and values, and ensuring that patient values guide all clinical decisions" (p. 6)
International Alliance for Patients' Organizations (2006)	"[T]he essence of patient-centred healthcare is that the healthcare system is designed and delivered to address the healthcare needs and preferences of patients so that healthcare is appropriate and cost-effective." (p. 1)
Berwick (2009)	Patient-centred care is "the experience (to the extent the informed, individual patient desires it) of transparency, individualization, recognition, respect, dignity and choice in all matters, without exception, related to one's person, circumstances, and relationships in health care." (p. w560)
Canadian Medical Association (2010)	"The essential principle is that health care services are provided in a manner that works best for patients. Health care providers partner with patients and their families to identify and satisfy the range of needs and preferences. Health providers, governments and patients each have their own specific roles in creating and moving toward a patient-centred system" (p. 8)
International College of Person-Centered Medicine (2011)	"Person-centered medicine is dedicated to the promotion of health as a state of physical, mental, social and spiritual wellbeing as well as to the reduction of disease, and founded on mutual respect for the dignity and responsibility of each individual person" (p. 1)

Box 2.1 (cont.)	
The Health Foundation (2014)	"Person-centred care supports people to develop the knowledge, skills and confidence they need to more effectively manage and make informed decisions about their own health and health care. It is coordinated and tailored to the needs of the individual. And, crucially, it ensures that people are always treated with dignity, compassion and respect" (p. 3)
Haut Autorité de Santé (2015)	"The patient-centred approach is based on a partnership of the patient, their relatives and the health care professional or a multi-professional team to achieve the development of a care plan, the monitoring of its implementation and its adjustment over time" (p. 1)

into account their needs, wants and preferences (Duggan et al., 2006; Entwistle & Watt, 2013), which reflect the key concerns that the idea of patient- or person-centredness is expected to address.

Indeed, the emergence of patient-centredness in medicine has been linked to the perceived shortcomings of the conventional way of providing medical care, in particular the physician–patient interaction (Duggan et al., 2006; Laine & Davidoff, 1996; Mead & Bower, 2000). This interaction was seen to be too disease- or illness-oriented, where the patient is "reduced to a set of signs and symptoms" (Mead & Bower, 2000, p. 1008) and the health care professional to a technician who delivers a given intervention and performs procedures (Duggan et al., 2006). The traditional model was also viewed as too paternalistic and system- or staff-centred, that is, inappropriately focused on the needs and interests of those providing the services, thus giving insufficient attention to the needs, preferences and values, and autonomy of the individual patient (Entwistle & Watt, 2013). A patient- or person-centred approach, then, is seen to provide a strategy to overcome or correct for these limitations as reflected in the range of characterizations shown in Box 2.1.

It is against this background that different authors have proposed conceptualizations of patient-centred care that distinguish a set of dimensions or domains from specific perspectives and Table 2.1 presents a selection of influential frameworks. The most commonly known is

Table 2.1 *Dimensions of patient-centred care as identified by selected seminal frameworks*

Gerteis et al. (1993)	Stewart et al. (1995)	Mead & Bower (2000)
Conceptual framework that explicitly adopts the patient's perspective; developed from empirical research with recently discharged patients, their families and hospital staff	Model of the patient-centred clinical method, building on both theoretical and empirical research	Conceptual framework focused on the physician–patient relationship, based on a review of the published literature
• *Respect for patients' values, preferences and expressed needs*: paying attention to patient's quality of life, dignity, needs and autonomy; involvement in decision-making • *Coordination and integration of care*: clinical care, ancillary and support services, front-line patient care • *Information, communication and education*: on clinical status, progress and prognosis; on processes of care; information and education to facilitate autonomy, self-care and health promotion	• *Exploring both the disease and the illness experience* (history, physical, lab; dimensions of illness [feelings, ideas, effects on function and expectations]) • *Understanding the whole person*: the person, the proximal (e.g. family, employment, social support) and the distal context (e.g. culture, community, ecosystem) • *Finding common ground*: problems and priorities; goals of treatment and/or management; roles of patient and doctor	• *Bio-psychosocial perspective*: perspective on illness that includes consideration of social and psychological (as well as biomedical) factors • *Patient-as-person*: an understanding of the personal experience of the illness for each individual patient within their unique context • *Sharing power and responsibility*: recognition of patients' needs and preferences and respect for patient autonomy, encouraging active patient involvement

Table 2.1 (*cont.*)

Gerteis et al. (1993)	Stewart et al. (1995)	Mead & Bower (2000)
• *Physical comfort*: pain management; help with activities of daily living; surroundings and hospital environment • *Emotional support and alleviation of fear and anxiety* • *Involvement of friends and family*: accommodation; involvement in decision-making; involvement as caregivers; recognizing needs of the family • *Transition and continuity*: provision of information; coordination and planning of ongoing treatment and services; ongoing support	• *Incorporating prevention and health promotion* • *Enhancing the patient–doctor relationship*: compassion, power, healing; self-awareness; transference and counter-transference • *Being realistic*: time and timing; teambuilding and teamwork; wise stewardship of resources	• *Therapeutic alliance*: developing common therapeutic goals and enhancing the personal bond between the doctor and the patient • *Doctor-as-person*: awareness of the influence of the personal qualities and subjectivity of the doctor on the practice of medicine

perhaps the conceptualization which was developed within the Picker-Commonwealth Program for Patient-Centered Care. This programme began in the 1980s in the USA to promote the movement of patient-centredness into a comprehensive health care system as a way to deliver better health care services (Gerteis et al., 1993). Adopting an explicit patient perspective, the framework put forward by Gerteis et al. (1993) identified seven dimensions of patient-centred care (Table 2.1). As noted earlier, these dimensions became the Picker principles of patient-centred care, with an eighth dimension (access to care) added subsequently to emphasize the need for care to be available and accessible in a timely manner (Picker Institute, 2013). This programme was the first to identify that patient-centred care should not only occur at the interpersonal level, between care provider and patient, but also at the organizational level (Kitson et al., 2013). As noted earlier, it informed the US Institute of Medicine's programme on health care quality, as well as health policy internationally.

In Canada, at around the same time, Stewart et al. (1995) developed a model of the patient-centred clinical method in the context of primary care, building on both theoretical and empirical research. This work identified six dimensions of the patient-centred process and it has been seen to be influential in stimulating patient-centred research in primary care, in particular around effective doctor–patient communication (Kitson et al., 2013). The model developed by Stewart et al. (1995) also informed work by Mead & Bower (2000), who proposed a conceptualization of patient-centred medicine that focused on the physician–patient relationship. This framework identified five key dimensions with each representing a particular aspect of the physician–patient relationship (Table 2.1).

The nursing literature has evolved in parallel but is less frequently referred to in the writings about patient-centred care. Indeed, the nursing perspective has tended to use the term 'person-centred' rather than patient-centred care, reflecting its focus on caring rather than diagnosis and treatment options, as highlighted above. Work by McCormack and colleagues (McCormack, 2003; McCormack & McCance, 2006) is seen to have been particularly influential in informing the development of person-centred nursing (Kitson et al., 2013). Arguing from the perspective of nursing theory and influenced by Donabedian's work on quality of care, McCormack & McCance (2006) proposed a person-centred nursing framework that comprises these constructs:

the characteristics and attributes of the nurse; the context in which care is delivered; person-centred process: how care is delivered; and expected outcomes.

Similar to the aforementioned work of the Picker-Commonwealth Program for Patient-Centered Care, McCormack & McCance (2006) highlighted the importance of the care environment in enabling the delivery of person-centred care. Indeed, the care environment is seen to have a "major impact on the operationalization of person-centred nursing, and has the greatest potential to limit or enhance the facilitation of person-centred processes" (p. 476). We will return to this issue below.

Patient-centredness and person-centredness: the same but different?

So far, we have considered the terms patient-centredness and person-centredness in parallel, as if they were interchangeable. However, as indicated above, this is not necessarily the case and here we explore the similarities and differences between these two notions in order to encourage a more nuanced debate of their actual meaning.

As noted earlier, based on our assessment of the available literature, we have observed that differences in the usage of these terms appear to reflect, to a great extent, different disciplinary traditions, perspectives and settings. For example, considering the perspective of the medical encounter, we have seen that the Anglo-American literature has, at least traditionally, tended to emphasize the notion of patient-centredness and patient-centred medicine (and more recently, patient-centred care) (Australian Commission on Safety and Quality in Health Care, 2011; Berwick, 2009; Gerteis et al., 1993; Laine & Davidoff, 1996; Mead & Bower, 2000; Picker Institute, 2013), whereas some of the continental European literature has tended to use the notion of person-centred medicine (Leplege et al., 2007; Mezzich et al., 2009; Pfeifer, 2010) and person-centred care (Ekman et al., 2011).

This is, in part, reflected by the frequency with which either term is used in the predominantly medical literature as compiled in PubMed, the archive of biomedical and life sciences journal literature at the US National Institutes of Health's National Library of Medicine, and illustrated further in Figure 2.1.

Clearly, the number of mentions of a particular term in the biomedical and life sciences literature can only be seen as an approximation of

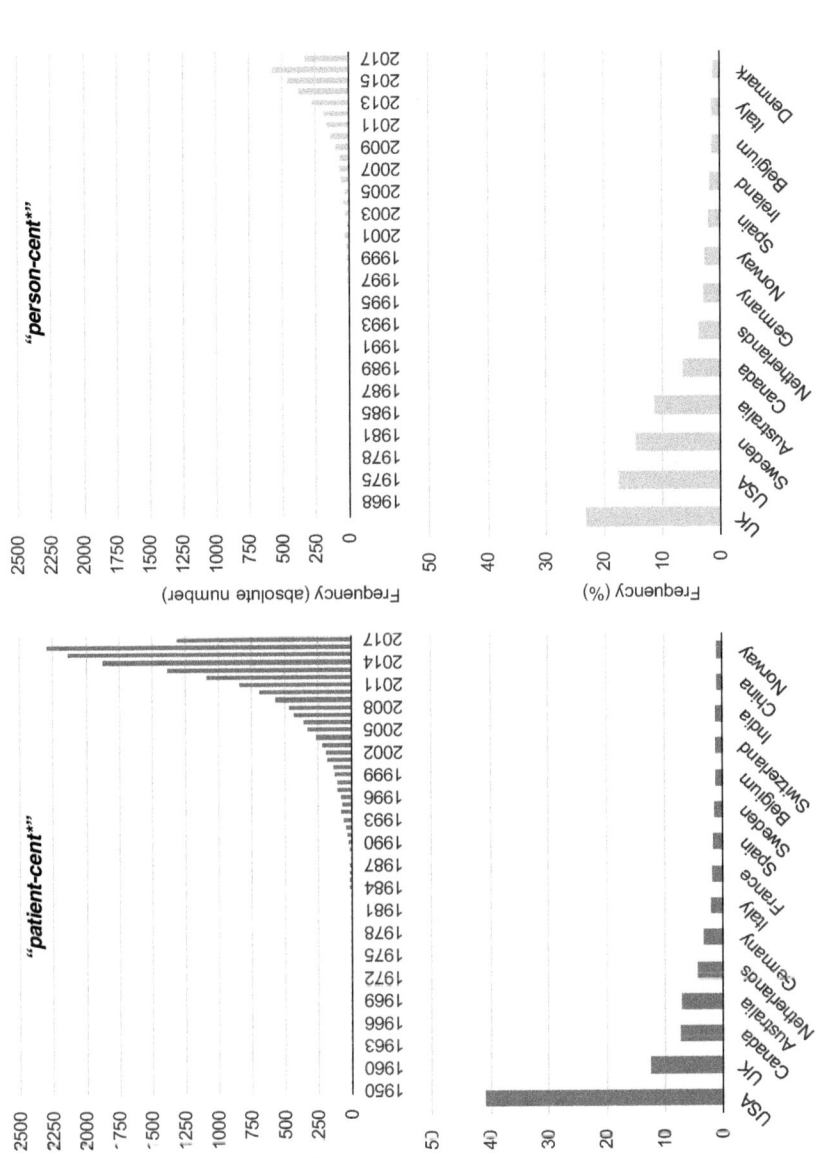

Figure 2.1 Frequency of articles mentioning versions of 'patient-centred' or 'person-centred' in the biomedical and life science database PubMed by July 2017

Source: authors' compilation based on PubReMiner, 2017

the use of a given term in practice; however, Figure 2.1 indicates that 'patient-centred' is by far the most commonly used term in the literature overall, and in particular in studies originating from the USA, reflecting, at least in part, the predominance of US-based papers in PubMed (Xu, Boggio & Ballabeni, 2014).

The nursing literature has tended to more explicitly use the term person-centred care (Kitson et al., 2013). This view is confirmed by, for example, the Royal College of Nursing in the UK, which uses the notion of 'person-centredness' deliberately to bring the different roles of service users (as patients in health care; clients in mental health care; residents in residential care homes) together using one term (Royal College of Nursing, 2015). Yet this is not consistent, with some nursing work also using 'patient-centred' care, although that work tends to focus on the acute, inpatient setting (Hobbs, 2009; Lusk & Fater, 2013).

It may be worth noting in this context that the Royal College of General Practitioners, also in the UK, highlighted in a 2014 report the importance of using the term patient-centred (Royal College of General Practitioners, 2014). It argued that the term patient was easily under-stood by professionals and the public and, notably, it would "challenge any negative associations that the word patient may suggest in today's NHS" (p. 10). However, at the same time the report emphasized the desirability of using 'person-centred' to describe the vision of an indi-vidualized, whole person approach to care.

The Health Foundation, an independent charity based in the UK, promoted a widely cited conceptualization that explicitly promotes the use of the term person-centred care as an approach that takes into account the whole person and "their preferences, wellbeing and wider social and cultural background" (Health Foundation, 2014, p. 9) – the very same characteristics that were identified to be among the core dimensions of patient-centredness as proposed in the seminal work by Mead & Bower (2000) (*see* below).

Are patient- and person-centredness the same, then? Hughes, Bamford & May (2008) carried out a review of the term 'centredness' across health care more broadly, to help clarify the use of the different concepts that have been emerging over recent decades, including client-, family-, patient-, person- and relationship-centred care (Table 2.2).

They found that the different types of 'centredness' contained, at a conceptual level, similar themes, and these, they argued, "could be used to characterize any particular type of centredness in health and

Table 2.2 *Types of 'centredness' identified by Hughes, Bamford & May (2008)*

Type of centredness	Description
Client-centredness	Initially focus on empathic understanding, unconditional positive regard and therapeutic genuineness as (necessary and sufficient) conditions for therapeutic relationships; subsequently broadened to also include wider aspects of communication, in particular the provision of information to help inform decisions
Family-centredness	Emphasizes partnerships among providers, patients and families that are mutually beneficial; primarily used within paediatrics although considered to be applicable to all patient groups; linked to the practice of family therapy
Patient-centredness	Originated in large part from general practice with a focus on fostering joint understanding of illness and its management
Person-centredness	Originated in client-centred psychotherapy and subsequently adopted in other fields, such as dementia care, emphasizing communication and the relationship
Relationship-centredness	Intended to support the central role of relationships in modern health care; suggestion that the patient-centred model may not be sufficiently inclusive

Source: adapted from Hughes, Bamford & May, 2008

social care settings" (p. 461). This view might indicate the need to further specify the definition of the different concepts, a call that has been made by a number of authors in order to enable operationalization and measurement of patient-centredness in particular (Kogan, Wilber & Mosqueda, 2016; Mead & Bower, 2000; Scholl et al., 2014). However, given the multidimensionality of each of the concepts, Hughes, Bamford & May (2008) argued that it may not be possible to identify one single aspect that defines, say, patient-centredness as a whole. Also, existing measurement tools of, for example, patient-centredness address only some of the dimensions that are seen to be relevant to this concept, such as patient trust and satisfaction. As a consequence, most empirical studies of impacts of patient-centredness have only been able to identify evidence for some aspects of patient-centredness (McMillan et al., 2013; Rathert, Wyrwich & Boren, 2013; de Silva, 2014). Indeed, as argued by Hughes, Bamford & May (2008), given the complexity of the concept it may be unrealistic to measure it in its entirety within a single study.

Similarly, Sidani & Fox (2014) considered a wide range of disciplines and settings in their review of patient-centred care. They noted that while there were slight variations in, for example, the terminology used, they found more similarities than differences with regard to the components distinctive of patient-centred care. Hobbs (2009), in her review of patient-centred care, also noted that the (nursing) literature did not appear to fundamentally differ in terms of defining underlying constructs. At the same time, she asserted that the term person-centred care may more adequately reflect the shift of focus away from illness and disease towards the person experiencing illness. Hobbs further suggested that the core element of recognizing the patient as a person with the ability to make autonomous decisions was common to literature that used either term but that this element was more developed in the literature using the label 'person'. Based on this observation, she proposed that moving away from the use of 'patient' to that of 'person' "may enable broader conceptualizations of the individual experiencing illness" (Hobbs, 2009, p. 58). This latter view was reinforced in a commentary by Lines, Lepore & Wiener (2015), who highlighted the importance of terminology in recognizing that the social context within which people live can affect disease trajectories and care choices and ought to be taken account of in order to improve outcomes.

A similar view was offered by Starfield (2011), who, based on a review of the evidence, noted that definitions of patient-centred care tended to be organized around patient–provider interactions within individual consultations, which may be episode-oriented. Conversely, conceptualizations of care focused on the person would typically stress the longitudinal nature of the patient–provider relationship, which would see diseases and body systems as "interrelated phenomena" (p. 63) and which would be concerned with understanding people's experienced problems. This was seen to be of particular relevance in the context of chronic and multiple care needs, which also highlights the role of collaboration and coordination as a key feature of person-focused care.

Finally, the late 1990s also saw the emergence of a new concept of 'people-centredness'. This was first discussed in the context of health reforms in the UK at that time, which envisaged enhancing efficiency and maximizing health gain, alongside offering patients greater choice and calls for local communities to be more engaged in setting health care priorities (Williams & Grant, 1998). The notion of people-centred health systems was subsequently taken up by the World Health Organization in the context of efforts to address the continued pressures facing health systems, in particular equitable access to care that is both of high quality and responsive to the needs of people (World Health Organization, 2016; World Health Organization Regional Office for Europe, 2012; World Health Organization Western Pacific Region, 2007). These documents explicitly identify patient-centred care as focusing on the individual seeking care, while people-centred care would also consider the health of people in their communities and their crucial role in helping to shape health policy and services (World Health Organization Regional Office for Europe, 2012). More specifically, people-centred care is interpreted as an approach to care that "consciously adopts individuals', carers', families' and communities' perspectives as participants in, and beneficiaries of, trusted health systems that are organized around the comprehensive needs of people rather than individual diseases, and respects social preferences" (World Health Organization, 2016, p. 2). This approach would require that people have the education and support to enable them to make decisions and participate in their own health and care, while also supporting carers.

Implications and conclusions

This chapter set out to synthesize some of the key insights emerging from the evidence around the concepts of patient- and person-centredness in the health care context. In line with other authors, we have shown that there remains considerable debate about the specific meanings of the different concepts, reflecting the different professional disciplines, perspectives and clinical settings, as well as different regional and country contexts, within which either notion has been approached and discussed. However, we have also seen that despite variations in terminology, when considering seminal texts from different disciplinary backgrounds (e.g. health policy, medicine and nursing), these tend to be fairly consistent regarding broad themes (Hughes, Bamford & May, 2008; Kitson et al., 2013; Sidani & Fox, 2014). These themes relate to the fundamental ethical premise that patients and service users should be treated as persons, with respect and dignity, and that care should take into account their needs, wants and preferences (Duggan et al., 2006; Entwistle & Watt, 2013).

Much of the literature on patient- and person-centredness has tended to focus on the interpersonal level between the care provider and the individual patient. Indeed, according to Kitson et al. (2013), it is only the health policy and nursing literature that has tended to focus explicitly on wider system and contextual issues, whereas the medical discourse tended to be "constructed around a very clearly delineated relationship between the individual medical professional and the patient" (p. 12). Hobbs (2009) highlighted the importance of the organizational and institutional context for providing person-centred care, with the distribution of authority and interaction of systems found to be of particular relevance. For example, organizations that relied primarily on a command-and-control style of leadership were less likely to provide person-centred care compared to those with shared governance. Few analyses and conceptualizations go beyond this meso-level awareness, however, with a subsequent systematic review noting that of the various dimensions characterizing patient-centred care, none addressed the macro-level of health systems (Scholl et al., 2014).

In this context, it is notable that there is considerable variation across the reviews and documents considered in this chapter as to whether patient- or person-centredness is to be seen as a concept or a framework that helps inform the delivery of care (e.g. McCormack & McCance, 2006; Mead & Bower, 2000; Stewart et al., 2003), a complex intervention (Sidani & Fox, 2014), a means to enhance the quality of care more broadly (e.g. Institute of Medicine, 2001) or an end, that is, a principle guiding the design of health systems more widely (e.g. World Health Organization, 2016; World Health Organization Regional Office for Europe, 2012; World Health Organization Western Pacific Region, 2007). Each of these perspectives, also linked to the philosophical and performance-based arguments as discussed previously (*see* Chapter 1), is of course legitimate but they will have different implications for the further development of health services and systems.

Finally, although work reviewed in this chapter has covered different disciplines, perspectives and settings in interpreting the conceptual foundations of patient- and person-centredness, few studies have explicitly considered the views of different stakeholders (Kitson et al., 2013). For example, Gillespie, Florin & Gillam (2004) found, in an interview study of clinical, managerial and lay stakeholders in the

UK, that each group tended to place different emphasis on different aspects of patient-centred care. Notably, health professionals were more likely to interpret this notion as communication skills in terms of explaining and eliciting information (but not necessarily in terms of shared decision-making) within the individual consultation, while managerial stakeholders tended to view patient-centred care to be grounded in quality assurance measures. Conversely, lay groups viewed patient-centredness in the context of a social or whole person model of health, and this was frequently expressed to occur at the level of patient involvement in planning and delivery of services rather than within the individual clinical encounter. This reflects only one study in a specific health system context but similar findings have been reported in a study set in Switzerland (Gachoud et al., 2012).

These observations illustrate that while different stakeholders all agree that patient- or person-centredness is important, the concept very much remains subject to debate, with different perspectives attaching different meanings and with different implications. To help inform policy development it will be important to better understand this diversity of interpretations of centredness at the different tiers within the health system and backgrounds in order to achieve the goal for health systems to take a more person-focused approach.

References

Australian Commission on Safety and Quality in Health Care (2011). *Patient centred care: Improving quality and safety through partnerships with patients and consumers*. Sydney: ACSQHC.

Balint E (1969). The possibilities of patient-centred medicine. *Journal of the Royal College of General Practitioners*, 17:269–76.

Berwick D (2009). What 'patient-centered' should mean: confessions of an extremist. *Health Affairs*, 28:w555–65.

Canadian Medical Association (2010). Health care transformation in Canada. Available at: http://policybase.cma.ca/dbtw-wpd/PolicyPDF/PD10-05.PDF (accessed 12 September 2016).

Castro EM et al. (2016). Patient empowerment, patient participation and patient-centeredness in hospital care: a concept analysis based on a literature review. *Patient Education and Counseling*, 99:1923–39.

Constand MK et al. (2014). Scoping review of patient-centered care approaches in healthcare. *BMC Health Services Research*, 14:271.

De Labrusse C et al. (2016). Patient-centered Care in Maternity Services: a Critical Appraisal and Synthesis of the Literature. *Womens Health Issues*, 26:100–9.

De Silva D (2014). *Helping measure person-centred care. A review of evidence about commonly used approaches and tools used to help measure person-centred care*. London: The Health Foundation.

Department of Health (2010). *Equity and Excellence: liberating the NHS*. London: Department of Health.

Docteur E, Coulter A (2012). *Patient-centeredness in Sweden's health system: an assessment and six steps for progress*. Stockholm: Vårdanalys.

Duggan PS et al. (2006). The moral nature of patient-centeredness: is it "just the right thing to do"? *Patient Education and Counseling*, 62:271–6.

Ekman I et al. (2011). Person-centered care – ready for prime time. *European Journal of Cardiovascular Nursing*, 10:248–51.

Entwistle V, Watt I (2013). Treating patients as persons: a capabilities approach to support delivery of person-centered care. *American Journal of Bioethics*, 13:29–39.

Gachoud D et al. (2012). Meanings and perceptions of patient-centeredness in social work, nursing and medicine: a comparative study. *Journal of Interprofessional Care*, 26:484–90.

Gerteis M et al. (eds.) (1993). *Through the patient's eyes. Understanding and promoting patient-centred care*. New York: John Wiley & Sons, Inc.

Gillespie R, Florin D, Gillam S (2004). How is patient-centred care understood by the clinical, managerial and lay stakeholders responsible for promoting this agenda? *Health Expectations*, 7:142–8.

Haut Autorite de Sante (2015). Démarche centrée sur le patient: information, conseil, éducation thérapeutique, suivi. Available at: http://www.has-sante.fr/upload/docs/application/pdf/2015-06/demarche_centree_patient_web.pdf (accessed 12 September 2016).

Health Foundation (2014). *Person-centred care made simple. What everyone should know about person-centred care*. London: The Health Foundation.

Hobbs JL (2009). A dimensional analysis of patient-centered care. *Nursing Research*, 58:52–62.

Holmstrom I, Roing M (2010). The relation between patient-centeredness and patient empowerment: a discussion on concepts. *Patient Education and Counseling*, 79:167–72.

Hudon C et al. (2012). Patient-centered care in chronic disease management: a thematic analysis of the literature in family medicine. *Patient Education and Counseling*, 88:170–6.

Hughes J, Bamford C, May C (2008). Types of centredness in health care: themes and concepts. *Medicine, Health Care and Philosophy*, 11:455–63.

Institute of Medicine (2001). *Crossing the quality chasm: a new health system for the 21st century*. Washington, DC: National Academies Press.

International Alliance for Patients' Organizations (2006). Declaration on: Patient-centred healthcare. Available at: https://www.iapo.org.uk/sites/default/files/files/IAPO_declaration_ENG_2016.pdf (accessed 12 September 2016).

International College of Person-Centered Medicine (2011). By-Laws of the International College of Person-centered Medicine. Available at: http://www.personcenteredmedicine.org/doc/ICPCM_ByLaws_Oct_11-2011.pdf (accessed 12 September 2016).

Kitson A et al. (2013). What are the core elements of patient-centred care? A narrative review and synthesis of the literature from health policy, medicine and nursing. *Journal of Advanced Nursing*, 69:4–15.

Kogan AC, Wilber K, Mosqueda L (2016). Person-Centered Care for Older Adults with Chronic Conditions and Functional Impairment: A Systematic Literature Review. *Journal of the American Geriatrics Society*, 64:e1–7.

Laine C, Davidoff F (1996). Patient-centred medicine. A professional evolution. *JAMA*, 275:152–6.

Leplege A et al. (2007). Person-centredness: conceptual and historical perspectives. *Disability and Rehabilitation*, 29:1555–65.

Levenstein J et al. (1986). The patient-centred clinical method. 1. A model for the doctor–patient interaction in family medicine. *Journal of Family Practice*, 3:24–30.

Lhussier M et al. (2015). Care planning for long-term conditions – a concept mapping. *Health Expectations*, 18:605–24.

Lines L, Lepore M, Wiener J (2015). Patient-centered, person-centered, and person-directed care: They are not the same. *Medical Care*, 53:561–3.

Lusk J, Fater K (2013). A concept analysis of patient-centered care. *Nursing Forum*, 48:89–98.

McCormack B (2003). A conceptual framework for person-centred practice with older people. *International Journal of Nursing Practice*, 9:202–9.

McCormack B, McCance T (2006). Development of a framework for person-centred nursing. *Journal of Advanced Nursing*, 56:472–9.

McMillan SS et al. (2013). Patient-centered approaches to health care: a systematic review of randomized controlled trials. *Medical Care Research and Review*, 70:567–96.

Mead N, Bower P (2000). Patient-centredness: a conceptual framework and review of the empirical literature. *Social Science & Medicine*, 51:1087–110.

Mezzich J et al. (2009). The international network for person-centered medicine: Background and first steps. *World Medical Journal*, 55:104–7.

Mills I et al. (2014). Patient-centred care in general dental practice – a systematic review of the literature. *BMC Oral Health*, 14:64.

Morgan S, Yoder L (2012). A concept analysis of person-centered care. *Journal of Holistic Nursing*, 30:6–15.

Pfeifer H (2010). Paul Tournier and 'Médecine de la Personne' – The man and his vision. *International Journal of Integrated Care*, 10:e022.

Picker Institute (2013). Principles of person-centered care. Available at: http://www.picker.org/about-us/picker-principles-of-person-centred-care/.

Pluut B (2016). Differences that matter: developing critical insights into discourses of patient-centeredness. *Medicine, Health Care and Philosophy* [Epub ahead of print].

PubReMiner (2017). PubMed PubReMiner. Available at: http://hgserver2.amc.nl/cgi-bin/miner/miner2.cgi (accessed 19 July 2017).

Rathert C, Wyrwich MD, Boren SA (2013). Patient-centered care and outcomes: a systematic review of the literature. *Medical Care Research and Review*, 70:351–79.

Royal College of General Practitioners (2014). *An inquiry into patient centred care in the 21st century. Implications for general practice and primary care*. London: Royal College of General Practitioners.

Royal College of Nursing (2015). What person-centred care means. Available at: http://rcnhca.org.uk/sample-page/what-person-centred-care-means/ (accessed 12 September 2016).

Scholl I et al. (2014). An integrative model of patient-centeredness – a systematic review and concept analysis. *PLoS One*, 9:e107828.

Sidani S, Fox M (2014). Patient-centered care: clarification of its specific elements to facilitate interprofessional care. *Journal of Interprofessional Care*, 28:134–41.

Starfield B (2011). Is patient-centred care the same as person-focused care? *Permanente Journal*, 15:63–9.

Stewart M et al. (1995). *Patient-centred medicine. Transforming the clinical method*. Thousand Oaks, CA: SAGE Publications, Inc.

Williams B, Grant G (1998). Defining 'people-centredness': making the implicit explicit. *Health and Social Care in the Community*, 6:84–94.

World Health Organization (2016). Framework on integrated, people-centred health services. Report by the Secretariat. Available at: http://apps.who.int/gb/ebwha/pdf_files/WHA69/A69_39-en.pdf?ua=1 (accessed 12 September 2016).

World Health Organization Regional Office for Europe (2012). *Towards people-centred health systems: an innovative approach for better health outcomes*. Copenhagen: WHO.

World Health Organization Western Pacific Region (2007). *People centred health care: a policy framework*. Geneva: World Health Organization.

Xu Q, Boggio A, Ballabeni A (2014). Countries' Biomedical Publications and Attraction Scores. A PubMed-based assessment. Version 2. *F1000Res*, 3:292.

3 | Person-centred health systems: strategies, drivers and impacts

ELLEN NOLTE, ANDERS ANELL

Introduction

Patient/citizen participation should be an integral part of health care systems and, as such, an indispensable component in current health care reforms.

Council of Europe, 2000

As the notion of person-centredness of health services and systems is becoming more established in national and international policy declarations and commitments, there is a need to better understand and clarify the use and usefulness of relevant strategies and approaches that seek to improve the position of individuals, their families and communities in the health system.

This book takes as a starting point the various roles people take in health systems, while recognizing that these roles overlap and may be performed simultaneously (*see* Chapter 1). Indeed, as Coulter (2002) suggested, the 21st-century health service user is at once "a decision-maker, a care manager, a co-producer of health, an evaluator, a potential change agent, a taxpayer and an active citizen whose voice must be heard by decision-makers" (p. 6). Viewed through this lens, a greater person focus can contribute to advancing equity, efficiency and the responsiveness of health systems. For example, service user choice of provider may increase satisfaction because individuals choose the provider they prefer; it may increase efficiency because people are using their voice (and, where possible, exit) to express dissatisfaction, which then may lead to enhanced service quality to better meet individuals' needs; and it may decrease inequity because more knowledgeable service users may be better equipped to exercise choice. Likewise, involving people in health care planning and decision-making may positively impact service user satisfaction as it might increase the likelihood that their views are taken seriously; it may also impact on equity if lay involvement is representative of the views of the local population in provider governance and service delivery.

However, the degree to which any of these aspirations will be met will depend, to a great extent, on how relevant strategies and policies are designed and implemented, and by whom. Inevitably there will be trade-offs and there may be unintended consequences. Thus, it is conceivable that policies that seek to involve people in health care decision-making but where the decision making space is driven by policy and clinical priorities, rather than by patients or the public, may be perceived as tokenistic or not making a difference, and so lead to disengagement (Peckham et al., 2014). This is likely to weaken rather than strengthen the individual's role in the system. Likewise, where lay involvement is not representative of the wider population, those participating might constrain their contributions and so inadvertently reduce, rather than enhance, public influence on health service decisions (Martin, Carter & Dent, 2017).

Building on the principal framework of voice, choice and co-production as described in Chapter 1, Chapters 5–13 explore these issues further. They examine the different roles people take in health systems, from engaging in and leading on health service and system development (Chapter 5) and research (Chapter 6), evaluating the quality of health services and systems (Chapter 7), and making decisions about purchasers or providers of individual care packages and specific services (or choosing not to do so) (Chapters 8–10), to participating in their own care (Chapters 11 and 12), along with legal frameworks seeking to ensure that people can exercise their rights as taxpayers and citizens (Chapter 13). Each chapter contributes a different perspective on person-centred strategies and describes the outcomes, both positive as well as unintended.

This chapter synthesizes the main insights and lessons that emerge from the in-depth analyses presented in Chapters 5–13. Inevitably there will be overlap between the individual chapters that are being presented here. This is intended: this chapter is aimed at extracting the main messages for readers who wish to gain an instant overview of the key issues that are being discussed in the detailed syntheses in the second part of the book. In examining the different perspectives we identify a number of common themes which we then summarize and analyse in further detail in Chapter 4.

The person at the centre of the health system: insights from different roles individuals can take

Engaging in health service and system development and research

In Chapter 5 Draper & Rifkin explore the contribution of community participation to health systems and to people's health, and highlight the core role that has been ascribed to participation both as a means to improve service provision and utilization and to achieve greater equity in health care, a main driver behind the Alma Ata Declaration of 1978 (World Health Organization, 1978). Yet the authors caution that while the evidence to support policies addressing equity has successively strengthened, policies to promote community participation have struggled to find strong supporting evidence and direction. One major reason for the relative lack of robust evidence around the contribution of community participation to health improvements is that relevant strategies often fail to account for a number of factors. These include defining realistic outcomes of what could be achieved, considering the complex reasons why people do or do not wish to participate, and understanding the degree to which a given strategy empowers people to actively engage and to engage in ways that lead to the desired outcomes (Rifkin, 2012). Policies advocating community participation tend to combine different rationales. They often simultaneously seek to achieve more effective (and potentially more efficient) health services by incorporating public or community views while also recognizing that people have the right to be involved in those decisions that affect them. However, this can lead to tensions inherent in the underlying political and societal values, representing utilitarian or consumerist views on one hand, and a democratic or rights-based perspective on the other. Furthermore, the extent to which power should be devolved to community members remains contested.

Draper & Rifkin highlight the renewed interest in community participation internationally, and by exploring a range of experiences in European settings they find that community participation in the context of health service design and delivery is very variable in terms of who is engaged, for what, how and why. They highlight that the reasons for people to get involved, and the subjective benefits gained, are complex, ranging from personal benefits (e.g. achieving a sense of purposeful action) to considerations of contributing to the 'public good'. Yet there is also evidence of unintended negative consequences, such as stress and fatigue caused by demands placed upon people. This underlines the need for community participation programmes to be realistic and take account of the ability of marginalized people in particular to participate. Importantly, the authors show that community participation can make a difference, but not always. Factors that have been associated with positive outcomes include appropriate financing of the initiative, logistics and systems of communication, and partnerships with relevant organizations (Tempfer & Nowak, 2011). Overall, the evidence of impact of involving people in health service planning and development, and health care decision-making more broadly, remains difficult to establish. At the same time, the authors emphasize that while there is a lack of clear empirical evidence on the outcomes, the process of participation in itself can have its own benefits and intrinsic value.

Moving forward, it will be important for all stakeholders involved in the development of community participation in health services and systems to agree what it is they seek to achieve and how. Central to any such effort will be ownership by the community, with power-sharing identified as key to enable transformation of community action that is sustainable (Marston et al., 2016). Participation should be conceptualized as a *process* that facilitates a given intervention or strategy, rather than as an intervention in itself that can then be studied in terms of its effects on health outcomes. This would enable reflection on how intended beneficiaries view their role in the process. There is a need to take account of the wider context within which communities operate and function and this should be core to any evaluation to strengthen the evidence base for community participation in health systems development, with successes as well as failures to be shared widely to inform learning.

The rationales identified as key drivers for community participation can also be seen to have shaped much of the emergence of patient and public involvement (PPI) in research, although, as Beresford & Russo note in Chapter 6, this evolution needs to be interpreted in the context of broader social and political developments. Focusing on the UK initially, the authors contrast the influence of the emancipatory disability research emerging in the 1970s, which sought, among other things, to equalize the relationships of research production between researcher and the researched, with more recent researcher and service system-led initiatives. It is, however, the latter that has tended to dominate contemporary approaches to user involvement in research nationally and internationally, and the authors illustrate this with a small number of examples of PPI initiatives in research, such as INVOLVE within the UK National Institute for Health Research (National Institute for Health Research, 2017).

PPI in health and social care research takes place at different levels and intensities, from no involvement to consultation, contribution, and collaboration, through to user control. PPI also takes place at different stages within the research process (from identifying the research topic and designing the research to writing-up findings and dissemination), as well as the wider research infrastructure (from identifying and setting research agendas and research priorities to editorial roles in research journals and speaking on research platforms). However, as Beresford & Russo clarify, while there are isolated examples for each of these, PPI in research still has some way to go towards becoming an accepted feature in the research landscape. Importantly, the authors highlight that the research process and infrastructure remain dominated by professional expertise. This is confirmed in an analysis by Nasser et al. (2017) of efforts by 11 research funding organizations in seven countries to reduce waste in research. It found that grant-awarding committees continued to be dominated by academics and clinicians.

Evidence of the impact of PPI in research suggests that involving patients and the wider public can have beneficial effects on service users, researchers and communities (Brett et al., 2014b), as well as on the quality and appropriateness of the research itself (Brett et al., 2014a). However, it will be important to understand whose perspective is being measured, as this will determine the criteria used for assessment and what will eventually be referred to as 'evidence'. The quality of research is traditionally assessed on grounds of scientific criteria (from applications for funding to academic dissemination of findings). This approach may risk undermining and devaluing participation and the systematic incorporation of experiential knowledge generated from lived experiences of users in the research process. This, the authors highlight, is increasingly seen as problematic, especially with regard to the engagement (or lack thereof) of vulnerable populations such as older people, people from minority backgrounds, refugees and asylum seekers, and others.

Thus, as Beresford & Russo conclude, if PPI in research is to develop effectively as part of the mainstream, there is a need for a series of strategies that systematically address identified tensions. Similar to what we have learned from the review of community participation in health service and system development (Chapter 5), there is a need for strengthening the theoretical underpinnings of research with patient and public involvement, and of the evidence base more broadly. This process requires the comprehensive evaluation of user involvement in research, taking due account of the context within which any such approach is being implemented and improving the sharing of learning from PPI in research. Ensuring greater PPI in research structures will be of particular importance, as will be adequate resourcing if PPI in research is seen as a means to improve the appropriateness and relevance of health research. This includes building capacity to support the development of PPI and user-controlled research, improving access to PPI in research especially for vulnerable or marginalized populations, and supporting user-controlled organizations.

Evaluating the quality of health services and systems

Coulter, Paparella & McCulloch in Chapter 7 focus on the role of the individual (as a patient, a service user, member of the public or citizen more broadly) in the evaluation of the degree to which a given health system is person-centred. People's views on the quality of care and their experiences of care constitute key indicators of person-centred care (*see also* Chapter 2). The authors highlight that measuring people's views and experiences is important for both intrinsic reasons (person-centred care is a dimension of quality in its own right, i.e. the philosophical argument) and extrinsic motivations (person-centred care is a means to improve the quality of care, i.e. the performance-based argument) (Berwick, 2009).

Person-centred care includes both functional aspects, such as access to care, waiting times, physical environment and amenities, and interpersonal or relational aspects, especially communication between service users and professional staff. The authors note that while both are important, relational aspects are likely to have the greatest influence on the way people evaluate the care they receive (Entwistle et al., 2012). It is these aspects that are more closely linked to positive outcomes, such as self-rated health, adherence to recommended treatments, and lower health care resource use such as hospitalizations and primary care visits, among others (Doyle, Lennox & Bell, 2013). Yet despite their key role, interpersonal characteristics such as the quality of care relationships do not tend to be covered by existing health care quality frameworks (Entwistle et al., 2012).

Coulter, Paparella & McCulloch further highlight that capturing public and patients' perspectives on health care is becoming increasingly important as systems strive to be more responsive to the needs of those using their services. Many European countries now have implemented related measurement programmes and policies on the public release of quality data at national or regional levels. They illustrate these approaches with a number of country examples, finding that the publication of data on patient satisfaction, patient-reported experience and patient-reported outcomes (PROMs) (Box 3.1) is widely seen as an important way to hold providers to account for the quality of care they deliver ('voice') and for providing patients with information to act as 'discerning consumers' ('choice'). The evidence of whether or not these aspirations are being met remains scant, however (Roland & Dudley, 2015; Schlesinger et al., 2014) (*see also* Chapters 8 and 9).

Box 3.1 Approaches to collect data on people's views and experiences of care

Approaches to collect data on people's views and experiences are often focused on measuring satisfaction, that is the extent to which health care fulfils people's expectations (e.g. by answering the question, 'how satisfied were you with your care in hospital x?'). Yet, as Coulter, Paparella & McCulloch caution, such assessments are unlikely to reliably capture the complexities of modern health care and the diversity of patients' expectations and experiences. There is increasing interest in gathering factual reports on what actually happened to people during, for example, a particular service or an episode of care, such as through surveys of patient-reported experience measures (PREMs). Alongside these, patient-reported outcome measures (PROMs) are receiving attention as a potential means to improve process and outcomes of care, and to reduce

Box 3.1 (cont.)

inappropriate care (High Level Reflection Group on the Future of Health Statistics, 2017). PROMs measure patients' perceptions of their health status, clinical outcomes, mobility and quality of life, using standardized questionnaires. They are currently mostly used for clinical research and to facilitate shared decision-making between clinicians and patients to improve clinical practice; their wider use for performance measurement or to inform decision-making is not yet common.

A key challenge that remains concerns the timeliness of survey data to inform improvement activity, given the time that is required to collect experience data that are representative and reliable. This has led to a search for briefer, easy to implement measures, such as the collection of real-time feedback during routine clinical activities. These ask patients (or their carers) about their experiences while they are still in a given service setting (hospital, clinic, GP practice, etc.) or shortly thereafter. However, such methods remain problematic because of their unsystematic approach to data collection, which reduces their reliability as a performance indicator (Coulter, 2016; Sizmur, Graham & Walsh, 2015).

An increasingly important source of data on people's experiences of health care is social media. As Coulter, Paparella & McCulloch highlight, there is an increasing number of websites that collect unstructured feedback from patients about their experiences, such as PatientsLikeMe (patientslikeme, 2017), while health care providers have been setting up social network pages such as through Facebook inviting their patients to review the care they have been receiving. There is some evidence of a positive association between objective quality measures and Facebook reviews of hospitals, with Lagu & Greaves (2015) proposing that hospitals that are active on social media and that "encourage patients to provide ratings and feedback are the hospitals that are most concerned with patient-centeredness" (p. 1397). However, they also caution that patient-generated ratings on social media face the same limitations as real-time feedback data in terms of unsystematic elicitation which reduces generalizability and reliability of data, at least if these are to be used to compare performance across providers.

It is against this background that the authors argue that it is unethical to not act upon information derived from asking people to report their health care experiences. Promising examples of local initiatives that have made systematic use of large-scale surveys of user experiences to improve quality do exist (Haugum et al., 2014), as does the understanding of the key enablers for rolling-out this learning across whole health systems. These, as Coulter, Paparella & McCulloch highlight, include, among other factors, the active engagement of patients and families and workforce policies that embed quality improvement skills in training and staff development, along with adequate resourcing and effective institutional support.

Reflecting on their insights, the authors outline a set of key lessons to be taken forward if the collection of data on people's views on and experiences of care is to effectively inform service and system improvement. They emphasize a number of key principles for establishing national systems of patient experience measurement, if measurement is expected to lead to actual, measurable improvements in the quality of health care. These include, among other things, that measurement should be patient-based, with relevant instruments developed with patient input. Further, the goals of measurement should be clear. For example, is the goal to provide information for consumer choice, for public accountability or pay-for-performance, or for internal use by providers as part of quality improvement schemes or even research? The actual measurement and analyses of patient experiences should be standardized and reproducible, and reporting methods of experience data should be carefully designed and tested. Coulter, Paparella & McCulloch emphasize that national systems for the measurement of patient experiences should be supported by appropriate infrastructure and they call for countries to work together to develop and test methods for ensuring that survey findings are taken seriously and incorporated into quality improvement initiatives.

Making decisions about purchasers or providers of individual care packages and services

Chapters 8–10 look at person-centredness from the perspective of service users as 'customers' who make decisions about purchasers or providers of care packages and individual services (or choose not to do so). Fotaki in Chapter 8 begins by setting the wider context for the 'choice' debate, drawing on the theoretical underpinnings and empirical evidence to understand the rationale for and objectives of choice policies more broadly, along with their impacts. Focusing on choice of health care provider, the author then identifies the likely tensions between choice and the other values that societies (wish to) pursue and some of the practical challenges of implementing any such strategy.

Similar to public involvement policies discussed above, and the more general discussion about arguments to support person-centredness presented in Chapter 1, the introduction of choice policies in the health context can be seen to have both intrinsic value, that is, choice is a 'good thing' that speaks to philosophical principles of individual autonomy and user empowerment, while the utilitarian or performance-based motive views choice as a means to achieving desirable goals such as improving efficiency and quality of care. The former recognizes the need for health systems to respond to the demands of user groups for greater control of health care resources that are available to them, while the utilitarian argument is based on the assumption that service users rationally select high-quality providers based on their needs and preferences. Fotaki traces the evolution of choice of provider policies in a small number of single-payer health systems in northern Europe, highlighting that both arguments permeated relevant approaches. Yet it is perhaps fair to say that the strive for greater quality and efficiency of health services was the key driver in most settings. Thus, in Denmark, England and Sweden choice policies were driven, at least initially, by policy concerns about waiting times in accessing specialist care, with improving access to primary care becoming a greater focus from the 2000s onwards, dominating the choice agenda in Norway and Sweden in particular.

Fotaki then examines the evidence base on the degree to which choice policies have achieved desired impacts. This analysis finds that the majority of people value having the possibility of choice. However, perceptions of choice are influenced by individuals' characteristics and circumstances such as age, gender and health status, and these factors also determine whether they exercise choice at all. For example, evidence from Sweden suggests that highly educated young people, especially women, both exercise and favour choice more when compared to other population groups (Rosén, Anell & Hjortsberg, 2001). Access to information is equally important, and this tends to be worse for people with low educational attainment. This latter point will be particularly pertinent for policies that introduce or strengthen choice of provider as a means to improve equity in access. Fotaki cites evidence from England, Norway and Sweden that choice can lead to improved access to certain services for some populations and in some settings, but warns about potentially negative impacts for those who are less able to exercise choice, a finding confirmed in a systematic review by Aggarwal et al. (2017). Thus, choice policies may exacerbate existing inequalities if they are not designed carefully with the appropriate structures in place to support vulnerable population groups in particular.

Robust evidence of whether choice of provider improves the quality or efficiency of care remains scant. Overall, it remains difficult to attribute observed outcomes to choice policies as such, given that these tend to be introduced as part of a larger set of reforms. For example, limited work from Sweden and Norway points to increases in patient satisfaction and trust in primary care services, although it is unclear whether this reflects increased choice, or greater capacity and access, or both. The evidence that patient choice of provider leads to greater efficiency is also weak, and it will be important to interpret observed findings in the context in which they were generated (Goddard, 2015).

Based on these observations, Fotaki emphasizes that policy-makers should consider the suitability of provider choice for promoting the goals of health systems and for supporting person-centred care. There is so far no evidence to support that choice policies have increased efficiency or welfare at population level. There is also a need to better understand the information needs of people to help inform choices, and their preferences for choice, including the option of choosing not to choose.

Similar conclusions are drawn by van Ginneken et al. in Chapter 9, which focuses on choice of payer, and more specifically, choice of health insurance. Again noting that choice is generally valued by people, the authors find that the evidence of whether insurance choice leads to higher quality care remains weak. However, it is this latter feature that has largely driven the introduction of choice and competition between insurers in a number of health systems. Reviewing the experiences in Germany, Israel, the Netherlands, Slovakia, Switzerland and the USA, the authors describe considerable variation in the types of choice offered to individuals, highlighting the difficulty people face in making informed insurance choices.

As with provider choice, a core question is whether people exercise choice and their motivations for doing so, or choosing not to. Here the authors cite empirical evidence from Germany, the Netherlands, Switzerland and the USA that finds that people who change between insurers tend to be young, male, healthy and well-educated. However, as van Ginneken et al. highlight, reasons for moving ('switching') between insurers vary and, importantly, switching does not appear to be motivated by the quality of contracted care providers, or by costs, two of the key assumptions underpinning insurer choice and competition policies. This may be because of the complexity of the information that people have to comprehend in order to make choices, in particular where there are multiple options of what is covered. For example, the authors cite data from Switzerland showing that in 2013 there were 58 insurers offering some 287 000 different policies. Countries have put in place strategies and tools to support people through providing comparative information. Yet the provision of meaningful data that would allow people to make inferences about the quality of care of providers contracted by insurers remains a challenge, as does their presentation in a transparent and easy-to-understand manner.

Concerning the impact of insurance choice and competition, it may thus not seem surprising to find that evidence of improvements in the quality of care is largely absent. This is in part because of the lack of robust empirical research. More importantly perhaps, and similar to what we have seen for choice policies more broadly, it remains challenging to attribute a specific outcome to a specific policy, with the latter typically forming part of a wider reform package. However, the authors point to some evidence suggesting that insurance choice may have led to increased satisfaction with insurance services and, possibly, insurance policies that are better tailored to the needs of individuals in terms of benefits and services. It remains equally uncertain to determine the degree to which insurance choice may have led to more person-centred care. Here the authors point to conflicting impacts, with evidence from the Netherlands and Slovakia suggesting that some insurers have pursued strategies to attract more 'profitable' individuals such as young professionals; contracting for more person-centred care approaches may not be financially attractive to insurers. Many countries are experimenting with new ways of organizing and delivering care to better meet the needs in particular of those with (multiple) chronic conditions. But these strategies are typically driven by motivations other than insurance choice. Risk-adjustment schemes may provide an opportunity to incentivize insurers to focus their attention on those population groups that would benefit the most from more integrated, person-centred care arrangements, such as those with chronic conditions and vulnerable groups more broadly.

Like Fotaki in Chapter 8, van Ginneken et al. conclude that if insurer choice and competition are to lead to the expected outcomes of improved care quality and person-centred care, there is a need for more strategic consideration of the needs of those who are meant to choose through involving them in the governance, design, operations, learning and purchasing decisions of insurers. In addition, their review suggests that there is also a need to better understand the nature of the information and its presentation that most appropriately meet individuals' needs, by involving people in the design and operation of relevant tools such as comparison websites. The authors further highlight the need for regularly improving and updating the risk-adjustment system to minimize gaming and optimize incentives for contracting for person-centred services. Overall, however, it will be important for decision-makers to be considerate of the wider implications of insurer choice for health systems, including the administrative burden, incentives that may undervalue public health, and possible further system fragmentation, which is likely to undermine rather than promote more person-centred systems.

Finally, Verhaeghe in Chapter 10 explores the evidence around personal budgets and similar schemes that are viewed as an alternative way of purchasing elements of health and social care services. Somewhat in contrast to wider choice policies, and similar to what we have learned about the evolution of public and patient involvement in research (Chapter 6), the origins of personal budgets are closely linked to the independent living and disability rights movement in western countries during the 1970s. This movement argued for greater self-determination and the right of people with disabilities to make decisions about the services that affect their lives. It was only more recently that personal budget schemes gained greater attention as part of a move towards personalization of care to promote choice, with an expectation that greater choice will lead to greater independence and autonomy, which, it is assumed, will then result in improved outcomes that are achieved at lower costs (Gadsby et al., 2013).

Reviewing experiences in Australia, Belgium, England, the Netherlands, Scotland, Sweden and the USA, Verhaeghe finds wide variation regarding the nature and scope of related schemes (Box 3.2), as well as in the drivers behind these. While all seek to place the individual 'at the centre' of the process of identifying needs and making choices about the services they expect to best meet their health and/or social care needs, there is also a range of other policy goals. These include cost savings (Australia), reducing care home admissions (Belgium), or strengthening the private sector and diversification in the care market, so increasing service options (the Netherlands).

Box 3.2 Personal budgets and related schemes: an overview

The terminology used under the broad heading of personal budgets varies widely. It includes 'direct payments' (England), 'cash and counseling' (United States), 'personal assistance budgets' (Belgium), 'assistance allowances' (Sweden), and 'consumer directed care' (Australia), among others. Based on the commonalities between schemes, Verhaeghe uses 'personal budgets' as an overarching concept, defining it as 'an amount of money to be spent by individuals to purchase services to tailor care to meet specific needs'.

Verhaeghe identifies four principal approaches to the way personal budgets are managed. These are:

- direct payment models, in which the individual as the budget holder receives a cash payment or vouchers to purchase services or support;
- third-party payment models in which a third party holds the budget (e.g. a professional, care worker, 'broker') who will then assist the individual to access funding; service provision is monitored according to an approved care plan;
- notional budget models in which commissioners are responsible for purchasing services, but the individual is aware of the treatment or service options and the corresponding costs; and
- a combination of one or more features of the above models.

Among the countries reviewed, Verhaeghe finds that most operate direct payments and third-party payment models (England, the Netherlands, Scotland, Sweden, USA), while Belgium uses direct payments and notional budgets. In Australia the self-directed care scheme operates on a model in which the provider holds the budget.

Box 3.2 (cont.)

Schemes in place in different countries also vary in terms of the populations targeted. These differ by age range ('older people' in Australia, USA; 'youth' in the Netherlands) or the nature of needs (e.g. 'long-term care needs' in Belgium, England, the Netherlands, USA; 'physical or mental disabilities' in Sweden; 'psychiatric problems' in the Netherlands). Most schemes are located in the social care or long-term care sectors, with more recent moves also introducing health-related support in the form of personal health budgets. For example, in England people who are eligible for NHS Continuing Healthcare had the right to have a personal health budget from October 2014 onwards (NHS England, 2017b).

Personal budgets and related schemes permit individuals to determine how to spend an allocated budget on care and support services that best meet their needs, such as therapies, personal care and equipment, and so offer individuals more choice and control. Whether this is realized in practice will, however, depend on a number of factors. As Verhaeghe points out, while personal budgets can enhance an individual's sense of control and allow for flexibility in terms of selecting services thought to best meet their needs, there is a risk that people choose services that are not in their own best interest. Also, greater choice brings with it greater personal responsibility, which may disadvantage those who are less able to act upon this without appropriate support, for example older people with complex health and care needs. Family members or third parties can provide this support for those lacking the capacity to manage budgets themselves, but there are concerns about potential financial exploitation by family members or aggressive marketing tactics by third party organizations. Importantly, personal budgets may challenge established ways of working, in particular in the health sector. An inquiry into personal budgets in the UK noted that health care staff can find it difficult to support service users in experimenting with novel ways to meet their health needs, in particular where these counter their own experiences (House of Commons Committee of Public Accounts, 2016) or where these require additional capacity that is not available.

Similar to what we have seen for choice of provider and insurance, access to comprehensive information will be crucial to help inform choices but countries vary in terms of the data that are made available (Gadsby et al., 2013). Overall, as Verhaeghe notes, there is a lack of evidence about 'best practices' regarding the nature and scope of information that should be provided, or the training or support needs of service users. Likewise, while there is some evidence that personal budgets can improve choice, control, well-being and quality of life, evidence of their impact on health outcomes, costs and value for money remains scarce. There is thus a need for better understanding of what strategies work best for whom and under what circumstances, and of what people want. Available evidence suggests that while people wish to be informed about available options they do not necessarily want to make decisions themselves without adequate (professional) support (Davidson et al., 2013). Verhaeghe asserts that the provision of financial support through the use of personal budgets is only one way towards more personalization in health and social care and that any such scheme must be embedded in wider policies towards people with health and social care needs.

Partnering in the care process

Chapters 11 and 12 explore the role of individuals as participants in their own care. Légaré et al. focus on the role of shared decision-making (SDM) in the clinical encounter, which they define as an "interpersonal, interdependent process in which health professionals, patients and their caregivers relate to and influence each other as they collaborate in making decisions about a patient's health care" (p. 284). They trace the origins of SDM to the early 1970s in the USA as a potential solution to address observed practice variation as well as over-, under- and misuse of services through enabling people to choose alternative treatments in line with their preferences. The concept has subsequently been taken up widely in national and international policy, and it is generally seen to form a core component of person-centred care (Coulter, 2017), along with self-management (*see* below) and personalized care planning (Coulter et al., 2015). Yet, as Légaré et al. caution, while we know much about the impacts of SDM tools (such as decision aids), our understanding of the full complexity of SDM and its implementation in clinical practice remains inadequate, and this might explain why its adoption by physicians has been slow.

Reviewing the experience in Europe and elsewhere, the authors find widespread acceptance of the 'ethical imperative' for health care professionals to share important decisions (Salzburg Global Seminar, 2011). Many countries have formally recognized SDM in policy and regulatory frameworks as part of a move towards more person-centred care, typically in the context of legislation on patients' rights to informed consent and information (Chapter 13). Moreover, countries are also stepping up their efforts to develop broader strategic policy frameworks for SDM, such as through formally incorporating SDM in medical education and training, the promotion of coordinated, nationwide implementation bringing together professional associations and patient organizations, or national initiatives to make available patient decision aids (Härter et al., 2017). Yet despite this progress, the routine implementation of SDM into daily practice or at the system level has yet to be achieved (*see also* Box 3.3). They cite evidence of barriers at the level of the individual patient and health care provider as well as the organizational and system levels. These barriers, they argue, result from a combination of individual attitudes, beliefs and trust, but more importantly perhaps, the inconsistent evidence base about the risks and benefits of SDM and a continued lack of agreement on 'best practices' that would enable systemic support for the routine implementation of SDM at the different tiers of the system.

A particular challenge identified by Légaré et al. relates to the issue of power, which we have seen to be of concern also for the implementation of patient and public involvement in service development and research discussed earlier (Chapters 5 and 6). Thus, the authors argue, SDM requires an explicit sharing of power and knowledge in a relationship that has traditionally been dominated by the clinician, and this might be difficult to achieve in more deferential cultural contexts. This highlights the need for the development of approaches that take account of context and that involve stakeholders from diverse backgrounds, in particular those groups that may find it challenging to understand risk–benefit information. The authors further note that much of the work on SDM has focused on the doctor–patient relationship and there is lack of understanding about perceptions at organizational and system-level decision-making.

It is against this background that Légaré et al. support the need to move to a more complex model of engagement that considers people's values and preferences at the level of the individual patient–professional

Box 3.3 Assessment of the 2015 Patient Act, Sweden

The Swedish Patient Act came into force in 2015. Its overarching aim was to strengthen and clarify the position of the patient and further promote their autonomy, self-determination and participation (Vardanalys, 2017). Seeking to protect patients' rights and interests, it stipulates that individuals are to be informed about their health problem and the treatment options that are available. Patients have the right to participate in all decisions about their care and they must also be informed about where they can obtain the care they need (1177 Vardguiden, 2016).

An assessment of the implementation of the Patient Act over the period 2014–2017 found, however, that the patient's position had not perceptively strengthened since its introduction (Vardanalys, 2017). Drawing on a survey of patients, legal guardians of children and the population more widely pre- and post-implementation of the law, the analysis found that respondents' perceptions of some aspects had actually worsened between 2014 and 2016. Examples include the perceived accessibility of health services, the provision of adequate information, or their participation in their own care. In seeking to explain this observed lack of impact, the authors suggested that the Act had failed to strengthen the legal position of patients overall. This was in part attributed to a lack of clarity in terms of legal provisions, but more importantly perhaps, to a lack of enforcement, that is the implementation of some form of supervision, control or other type of monitoring of adherence to the legislation, both at the national level and at the level of the health service itself. Furthermore, the stipulations as set out by the Patient Act did not take the form of granting individuals legal rights that they could then use for enforcement themselves. The authors also noted that there had been little concerted effort at the different administrative tiers of the system to raise awareness and institute support tools to facilitate access to information and active participation. Based on these insights, the assessment called for a collective strategy to consolidate and strengthen the patient's position further, through both strengthening their legal position and accelerating health services' efforts to help implement and enforce these rights.

relationship (micro level), as well as the organizational (meso) and the governance and finance, along with wider societal (macro) levels in order to systematically implement SDM. Such an approach, they argue, would require the development of social and cultural norms that systematically consider public views and participation at the various tiers of the system. While SDM is mostly applicable to the individual clinical encounter, its effective implementation into routine practice will require concurrent efforts at meso and macro levels, including investment in supporting the public, as patients, clinicians or decision-makers, in acquiring the skills and competencies to critically engage, ask questions, express values and preferences, and understand risks.

The need to consider the individual, organizational and societal levels in the design and implementation of effective person-centred strategies is also emphasized in Chapter 12 by Nolte and Anell, who review the evidence base for self-management and support. As indicated above, self-management is widely regarded to be a core component of person-centred care, along with SDM. Support for self-management is important in enabling service users to move from passive recipients to active partners in care, and essential to providing high-quality care for those with chronic disease (Wagner, 1998).

Somewhat similar to the evolution of public and patient involvement in research (Chapter 6) and of personal budgets (Chapter 10), the emergence of self-management in the health field can be linked to the self-care and self-help movements of the 1970s in particular. The focus was on achieving equality between the provider and service user in terms of making decisions and the capacity to determine the direction of their own care. However, more recently, as self-management and support have entered national, regional or local strategies, there is an expectation that supporting service users increases their confidence, strengthens preventive activities and ensures appropriate use of services, and will thus reduce costs and make service delivery more sustainable. There is also an expectation that it will improve service users' experiences of health care, give people more control over their lives, empower them as partners, and improve health outcomes and well-being.

Whether and how these varied ambitions can be achieved remains uncertain, however, as the authors argue. Similar to what we have seen for SDM, one main reason is an inconsistent evidence base, with only some forms of support for self-management found to impact positively on some of these anticipated outcomes and only for some service user groups. Importantly, robust evidence that self-management efforts will reduce service utilization has so far been established for selected (hospital) services and specific conditions only (Taylor et al., 2014). There are several reasons for this. For example, existing outcome measures are frequently developed without appropriate service user input; also, interventions may not be suited to achieve desired outcomes such as reduced service use. A strong focus has so far been on psychological mechanisms, which tend to neglect the social context within which people live (Ong et al., 2014). As a result, relevant approaches might benefit only those who are capable of taking up these roles and this is likely to further disadvantage more vulnerable groups, who are already at a higher risk of multiple health problems (Barnett et al., 2012) and such approaches might thus inadvertently increase health inequities.

Nolte and Anell highlight that among the key challenges remains a disjoint of interpretations of self-management among lay people, health care professionals, managers and decision-makers, although the views of the latter two groups are inadequately understood. For example, while individual patients tend to emphasize the quality of the relationship between themselves and the professional, seeing self-management as a collaborative partnership, health professionals frequently view it as a tool to promote compliance with expert advice and treatment. Contemporary approaches to self-management and support tend to focus on managing people's condition/s in terms of biomedical outcomes or disease-control ('narrow approach'), rather than emphasizing supporting people to manage well (or live well) with their condition/s ('broad approach') (Morgan et al., 2016). This divergence may cause tensions, in particular, where it involves differing understandings of the responsibility for self-management, along with what is understood to be 'good' self-management. For example, the patient's wishes and preferences might not align with what the professional considers as the 'right' course of action, or user choices might lead to increased costs to the system (Harvey et al., 2015).

Nolte and Anell caution that there may be a risk that contemporary strategies and approaches to self-management and support continue to emphasize the 'narrow' focus, which stresses individual responsibility for management and behavioural change 'in order to function optimally'. This conclusion could also be drawn from a review of support efforts in Europe as described in Box 3.4. It finds that contemporary approaches to self-management support tend to emphasize medical and behavioural management with less or little attention on the wider social context within which people live.

Box 3.4 Self-management support strategies in European countries

Decision-makers across Europe have recognized the need for implementing policies and strategies to support self-management mainly in the context of chronic diseases (Nolte & Knai, 2015). But approaches vary widely between and within countries in terms of content, format, provider and availability. A review of diabetes self-management arrangements in Bulgaria, Greece, the Netherlands, Norway, Spain and the UK found that the majority of approaches comprises educational or training programmes, typically, although not always, emphasizing behavioural change as an important goal (Kousoulis et al., 2014). Similar variation in levels of support provided was demonstrated by Nolte, Knai & Saltman (2014) in a review of some 50 approaches across 13 countries in Europe. Here, the focus tended to be on education for self-management, which was frequently delivered in a group-based context or on a one-to-one basis and most often in the context of disease management programmes. The education offered tended to focus on disease control through the provision of information about the disease, healthy behaviours and practical instructions concerning, for instance, blood glucose monitoring, foot examination, or insulin injection. Most approaches used support materials in the form of information brochures to complement patient education programmes, with a smaller number using interactive websites or telephone-based support services to provide patients with personalized information on how to manage their disease. In the majority of cases, self-management support was provided by health professionals including physicians, or, more frequently, by trained nurses within primary care settings, highlighting that, with a few exceptions, approaches in place tended to be professional- or service-driven. Most aimed at disease control rather than offering more general support strategies that target the wider social context within which people live and that draw on a wider potential support network including other patients, peers or volunteers, among others.

Overall, there is a need for self-management support strategies to be based on social models that specifically address differences in expectations and abilities to take responsibility in terms of learning self-management skills, and to tailor professional support accordingly. Better understanding of managers' and policy-makers' views and priorities will be important, given their role in developing and funding services that support self-management. Strategies have to go beyond the immediate health care context in order to take full account of the broader influences that impact self-management activities.

Exercising rights as taxpayers and citizens

Finally, in Chapter 13 Palm et al. examine the role of legal frameworks in seeking to ensure that people can exercise their rights as taxpayers and citizens. Drawing on a mapping of provisions for patients' rights in 30 countries in 2015, the authors explore the role of patients' rights for person-centred care, and what is needed to realize their potential to contribute to achieving person-centred health systems. Locating their origins within the human rights movement, the authors explain the specifics of patients' rights within this broader context, distinguishing the right to health and the right to health care, along with individual rights (protecting the individual from harm) and social rights (safeguarding people's entitlement to, and ability to access, care). Most commonly, patients' rights are defined within the context of health care and the relationship with the individual health care provider while also noting wider responsibilities at the organizational and system levels.

Based on an analysis of four influential European frameworks, the authors identify six categories of patients' rights, which are reproduced in Table 3.1. These, they argue, require specific action or measures for implementation, as opposed to other aspects also seen to be core to person-centred care, such as treating people with respect, which, the authors argue, cannot be reinforced by legal means. Similarly, the authors do not consider the right to collective participation here as, they argue, it should be considered a 'basic citizen right' that goes beyond the individual as a patient.

The review finds that countries in Europe vary considerably in the implementation of legal frameworks to ensure patients' rights, with most having instituted specific legislation dedicated to this purpose. Using the rights' categories described in Table 3.1, Palm et al. report that patients'

Table 3.1 *Principal categories of patients' rights based on a review of four European frameworks**

Principal category	Individual patients' rights
Self-determination	The right to (informed) consent
	The right to participate in (clinical) decision-making/ to choose treatment options
Confidentiality	The right to data confidentiality
	The right to access one's medical record
Access to health care	The right to benefit from medical treatment according to needs
	The right to safe and high-quality treatment received in a timely manner
Choice	The right to choose health care provider
	The right to a second opinion
Information	The right to information about one's health
	The right to information about health care providers
	The right to information about rights and entitlements
Redress	The right to complain
	The right to compensation

Source: Chapter 13

Note: * The four European frameworks are the Amsterdam Declaration on the promotion of the rights of the patient in Europe (1994); the Convention on Human Rights and Biomedicine (1997); the European Charter on Patients' Rights (2002); and the EU Directive on the application of patients' rights in cross-border health care.

rights frameworks in European countries generally seek to ensure the right to self-determination, including shared decision-making (Chapter 11) and confidentiality. However, the right to access care and provider choice is intrinsically related to the provisions of the statutory health system more broadly (Chapter 8) and as such is typically addressed outside specific patients' rights legislation. Differences remain regarding the status of rights afforded, for example, whether the rights are directly legally enforceable, are enforceable via wider public sector regulation (quasi-legal), or take the form of a charter or code of conduct (moral rights). This may impact the way patients' rights are implemented in practice. For example, we have seen from the assessment of the 2015 Swedish Patient Act as described in Box 3.3 that the observed lack of impact of this law has, at least in part, been attributed to the failure to define patients' rights as a legal right (Vardanalys, 2017). However, as Palm et al. note, enforcement can also be ensured through other means, such as through formal dispute settlement mechanisms.

 A key aspect is the right to information to enable individuals to make informed decisions about their health and care, an issue we have seen to be core to any strategy that seeks to ensure person-centred services. Palm et al. distinguish the right to information about the individual's health status as a prerequisite to inform the right to consent and shared decision-making; the right to information about health care providers as a requirement to help inform provider choice; and the right to information about rights and entitlements as a condition to enable people to exercise their rights in the first place. It remains unclear to what degree national frameworks make the provision of this information a legal requirement, although the 2011 EU Directive on the application of patients' rights in cross-border health care requires EU Member States to make available relevant information as far as cross-border health care is concerned.

 Crucially, while most countries have implemented patients' rights frameworks, evidence of their impact remains largely absent, with a few notable exceptions (*see* Box 3.3). At the same time, recognition of the importance of this issue as evidenced by the widespread introduction of dedicated patients' rights frameworks could be seen as a significant step towards establishing the prerequisites for health systems that are more person-centred and that see the individual as an active partner rather than a passive recipient of care. However, as Palm et al. caution, the main challenge remains in reinforcing provisions for patients' rights, which may render this strategy possibly less effectual than it could be and it would be important to monitor progress and identify examples of good practice.

Summary and conclusions

In this chapter we have synthesized the evidence of different strategies seen to promote more person-centred care at the different tiers of the health system through examining the different roles people take as service users, active members of the community and citizens, evaluators, decision-makers and care managers. Building on the principal framework of voice, choice and co-production, we find that each perspective can contribute to the advancement of more person-centred health systems while highlighting challenges and possible unintended consequences for related policies and strategies. It is important to reiterate that the notions of voice, choice and co-production are not mutually exclusive, but they co-exist and are frequently performed simultaneously.

In synthesizing this evidence, we identify a series of common themes, and these relate to:

- the drivers behind relevant strategies and policies, and how they have evolved over time;
- the evidence of their impact and the role of context in interpreting this evidence; and
- the implications of lessons learned for the further advancement of person-centred health systems.

We discuss these themes briefly in turn and examine some of the pertinent issues in further detail in Chapter 4.

There are several drivers behind person-centred strategies which are conflicting and potentially undermine the goal of achieving a person-centred health system

At the risk of simplifying what is inherently complex, we can observe that person-centred strategies as conceptualized in this book have evolved, largely, from broader social movements that emerged in the western world in the 1960s and 1970s. Most notably, although not exclusively, the independent living and disability rights movement and self-care and self-help movements more widely have been important. These have argued for greater self-determination and emphasized equality between the provider and service user in terms of making decisions about the services that affect their lives. The Alma Ata Declaration of 1978 explicitly linked this debate to inequalities and called for health care to be made "universally accessible to individuals and families in the community through their full participation" (World Health Organization, 1978).

At the same time, there has also been recognition of a 'democratic deficit' more generally in public services and this has initiated the notion of deliberative democracy and interest representation in the political process. For example, the Council of Europe interpreted the rights of patients and citizens to participate fully and to determine the goals and targets in health care as an integral part of any democratic society and proposed that governments should promote policies that foster citizen participation (Council of Europe, 2000). The democratic perspective tends to assume that involvement is a good thing either in itself (an intrinsic value), or else impacts positively on public decisions or protects citizens from others making decisions against their interest (Conklin, Morris & Nolte, 2010). It relates to people or 'the public' in their capacity as citizens and taxpayers with rights to use public services and duties to contribute to and participate in society (Lupton, Peckham & Taylor, 1997).

The arguments based on the 'intrinsic' value of participation, along-side the rights-based approach, are in contrast to an emphasis on what has variously been described as the utilitarian or performance-based approach. In the neo-liberal agenda from the early 1990s, this became the consumerist approach, which introduced a greater focus on mar-ketization of health care and consumer choice, along with increased 'responsibilization' in many systems (Bevan, Helderman & Wilsford, 2010; Jacobs, 1998). The underlying assumption was that involving people will correct for the inherent failures in health care markets, including information asymmetry, and ultimately lead to reduced cost, greater efficiency and performance of public services (Wait & Nolte, 2006). Consumer preferences are viewed as the lever to enhance com-petitiveness between providers and, in doing so, reaffirm the rights of users to information, access, choice and redress in relation to a specific service or product (Lupton, Peckham & Taylor, 1997). It presumes that the removal of obstacles to participation, such as lack of information or lack of motivation, will lead to an informed service user who behaves in ways that will ultimately improve the quality of their care and their health (Mittler et al., 2013).

Considering the overall evidence as presented in this book, it is the utilitarian or performance-based perspective that appears to have domi-nated the different person-centred strategies. While some strategies may have initially had a focus on the intrinsic value of person-centredness, this has often been replaced by the performance-based perspective in the implementation phase. This transformation is particularly visi-ble in the area of choice reforms and can be linked to how different stakeholders view person-centredness and what they have to gain or lose. This process involving competing views across stakeholders may also explain some of the continued challenges that systems face in systematically translating promising strategies into routine practice. The dominance of stakeholders representing professional, organizational and policy-maker views is also linked to the available evidence base, which we examine next.

The evidence of impact of person-centred strategies remains inconclusive

A key insight emerging from the reviews of person-centred strategies in this book is that the evidence of impact remains largely inconsistent. In most instances we only find that *some strategies* impact positively on *some anticipated outcomes* for *some populations* in *some settings*. More broadly, the evidence tends to be stronger for individual-level approaches such as shared decision-making and self-management support and in the context of a 'narrow' perspective on person-centredness. This is in sharp contrast to the call for 'broader' approaches developed in Chapter 2.

Clearly, evidence of impact needs to be interpreted in the context within which individual studies have been carried out, as well as the design of both the relevant strategy and its evaluation. A core challenge is that many strategies lack a clear formulation of the theoretical basis that would explain how activities will lead to anticipated outcomes. There is a need for rigorous evaluation that takes account of context, and systematically considers equality and diversity. This need is echoed in the wider literature that has examined public and patient involvement in health services and systems and in public services more widely (Madden & Speed, 2017; Martin, 2009). Examples include patient safety (Ocloo et al., 2017), commissioning of health services (Peckham et al., 2014), health service reconfiguration (Dalton et al., 2016; Martin, Carter & Dent, 2017), and health care decision-making more broadly (Conklin, Morris & Nolte, 2015), including health technology assessment (Weeks et al., 2017).

The lack of consistency in the evidence base can be seen to undermine the wider roll-out or 'routinization' of potentially promising initiatives, as has been argued for shared decision-making in particular (Chapter 11). However, various authors have also highlighted that available policy instruments and strategies may not be suitable to achieve the (often implicit) aims of cost reduction and greater efficiency, at least in the short term. They thus could inadvertently undermine meeting the broader goals of enhancing person-centredness in the system overall. For example, there is so far no evidence to support that choice policies have increased efficiency or welfare at a population level (Chapters 8 and 9). Likewise, evaluations of personal budgets have thus far failed to produce robust evidence of their impact on costs and value for money (Chapter 10). However, there is some evidence that personal budgets can improve control, well-being and quality of life, and such improvements do offer value, even if they do not reduce costs.

Overall, we find that there is a need to better understand what strategies work best for whom, under what circumstances and in what settings. Crucially, there remains an urgent need to systematically consider the voice of individuals as service users, carers and members of the community in research and that seeks to inform health services and systems design more broadly. We observe that much of the evidence presented in this book remains dominated by professional, organizational and policy-makers' perspectives. Alongside this, there is a need to better understand what people want, whether and how they wish to be involved, the nature and scope of information they desire in order to support them in making decisions, including the option of choosing not to choose, and their support needs more broadly.

What are the implications for the further advancement of person-centred health systems?

Based on the evidence reviewed in this book we observe that existing models and strategies continue to fall short of systematically including the 'public voice' in health services and systems. There is a need to move to a more complex model of engagement that considers people's values and preferences at the level of the individual patient–professional relationship as well as at the organizational and the governance and finance, along with wider societal levels in order to systematically implement person-centred strategies.

Achieving truly person-centred services and systems will require a shift of the power balance away from a sole focus on professional knowledge and authority towards "negotiated participatory spaces" between lay and professional actors (Dean, 2017, p. 4). Here, careful attention needs to be given to the degree to which the range of strategies to enhance person-centredness leaves the dominant culture and practices of provider-centric and expert-based health services and systems essentially unchanged and structurally unchallenged (Dunston et al., 2009). This is most likely to be the case for choice policies and public involvement approaches that perhaps seek public input, for example through consultation, such as through patient surveys, but where the process of service production remains profession-led. A shift of power will require moving to a system where the individual as a service user or a citizen becomes *part* of this process.

There is a wealth of experience already as shown in several contributions to this volume, but initiatives that are being undertaken tend to be disjointed and lack an overarching strategic approach. Madden & Speed (2017) pointed to the rich experience of social movements, charities and non-governmental organizations in different types of participatory mechanisms that have helped to bring together citizens and experts in new forms of cooperative inquiry. These used a range of participatory techniques that seek to strengthen civil society while also critically reflecting on how participation works. There is potential to learn from these activities in order to strengthen engagement initiatives within the health system.

Services and systems will need to systematically invest in supporting the public, as patients, clinicians or decision-makers, in acquiring the skills and competencies to critically engage, ask questions, express values and preferences, and understand risks. Such investment also requires careful attention to the interlinkages between the different tiers of the health system and how these can be optimized in order to ensure systematic and systemic implementation of effective person-centred strategies and minimize unintended consequences.

Decision-makers need to consider the wider implications of individual policy options and how they may require potential compromises between different options. These are perhaps most obvious for choice policies where it has been argued that they involve trade-offs between the degree of choice and the principle of equity of access and service. Further, choice of provider and/or payer might increase system fragmentation and undervalue wider public health interventions, so undermining person-centred systems. At the same time, while provider or payer choice might not increase efficiency or reduce costs, it might still be seen as a value in itself. In either case, any such option needs to be firmly embedded within the wider policy context.

References

1177 Vardguiden (2016). Patient Act. Available at: https://www.1177.se/
Other-languages/Engelska/Regler-och-rattigheter/Patientlagen/ (accessed
21 December 2017).

Aggarwal A et al. (2017). Patient mobility for elective secondary health care
services in response to patient choice policies: a systematic review. *Medical
Care Research and Review*, 74:379–403.

Barnett K et al. (2012). Epidemiology of multimorbidity and implications
for health care, research, and medical education: a cross-sectional study.
Lancet, 380:7–43.

Berwick D (2009). What 'patient-centered' should mean: confessions of an
extremist. *Health Affairs*, 28:w555–65.

Bevan G, Helderman J, Wilsford D (2010). Changing choices in health care:
implications for equity, efficiency and cost. *Health Economics, Policy and
Law*, 5:251–67.

Brett J et al. (2014a). Mapping the impact of patient and public involvement
on health and social care research: a systematic review. *Health Expectations*,
17:637–50.

Brett J et al. (2014b). A systematic review of the impact of patient and
public involvement on service users, researchers and communities. *Patient*,
7:387–95.

Conklin A, Morris Z, Nolte E (2010). *Involving the public in healthcare policy.
An update of the research evidence and proposed evaluation framework.*
Santa Monica: Rand Corporation.

Conklin A, Morris Z, Nolte E (2015). What is the evidence base for public
involvement in health-care policy? Results of a systematic scoping review.
Health Expectations, 18:153–65.

Coulter A (2002). *The autonomous patient – ending paternalism in medical
care*. London, TSO.

Coulter A (2016). Patient feedback for quality improvement in general
practice. *BMJ*, 352:i913.

Coulter A (2017). Shared decision making: everyone wants it, so why isn't it
happening? *World Psychiatry*, 16:117–18.

Coulter A et al. (2015). Personalised care planning for adults with chronic or
long-term health conditions. *Cochrane Database of Systematic Reviews*,
3:CD010523.

Council of Europe (2000). The development of structures for citizen and
patient participation in the decision-making process affecting health care.
Recommendation Rec(2000)5 adopted by the Committee of Ministers

of the Council of Europe on 24 February 2000. Strasbourg: Council of Europe.

Dalton J et al. (2016). Service user engagement in health service reconfiguration: a rapid evidence synthesis. *Journal of Health Services Research & Policy*, 21:195–205.

Davidson J et al. (2013). Choosing health: qualitative evidence from the experiences of personal health budget holders. *Journal of Health Services Research & Policy*, 18:50–8.

Dean R (2017). Beyond radicalism and resignation: the competing logics for public participation in policy decisions. *Policy & Politics*, 45:213–30.

Doyle C, Lennox L, Bell D (2013). A systematic review of evidence on the links between patient experience and clinical safety and effectiveness. *BMJ Open*, 3:e001570.

Dunston R et al. (2009). Co-production and health system reform – from re-imagining to re-making. *Australian Journal of Public Administration*, 68:39–52.

Entwistle V et al. (2012). Which experiences of health care delivery matter to service users and why? A critical interpretive synthesis and conceptual map. *Journal of Health Services Research & Policy*, 17:70–8.

Gadsby E et al. (2013). Personal budgets, choice and health: a review of international evidence from 11 OECD countries. *International Journal of Public and Private Healthcare Management and Economics*, 3:15–28.

Goddard M (2015). Competition in healthcare: good, bad or ugly? *International Journal of Health Policy and Management*, 4:567–9.

Härter M et al. (2017). Shared decision making in 2017: international accomplishments in policy, research and implementation. *Zeitschrift für Evidenz, Fortbildung und Qualität im Gesundheitswesen*, 123–124:1–5.

Harvey J et al. (2015). Factors influencing the adoption of self-management solutions: an interpretive synthesis of the literature on stakeholder experiences. *Implementation Science*, 10:159.

Haugum M et al. (2014). The use of data from national and other large-scale user experience surveys in local quality work: a systematic review. *International Journal for Quality in Health Care*, 26:592–605.

High Level Reflection Group on the Future of Health Statistics (2017). Recommendations to OECD ministers of health from the High Level Reflection Group on the Future of Health Statistics. Strengthening the international comparison of health system performance through patient-reported indicators. Available at: https://www.oecd.org/els/health-systems/

Recommendations-from-high-level-reflection-group-on-the-future-of-health-statistics.pdf (accessed 28 November 2017).

House of Commons Committee of Public Accounts (2016). Personal budgets in social care. Second report of session 2016–2017. Available at: https://publications.parliament.uk/pa/cm201617/cmselect/cmpubacc/74/74.pdf (accessed 21 December 2017).

Jacobs A (1998). Seeing difference: market health reform in Europe. *Journal of Health Politics, Policy and Law*, 23:1–33.

Kousoulis A et al. (2014). Diabetes self-management arrangements in Europe: a realist review to facilitate a project implemented in six countries. *BMC Health Services Research*, 14:453.

Lagu T, Greaves F (2015). From public to social reporting of hospital quality. *Journal of General Internal Medicine*, 30:1397–9.

Lupton C, Peckham S, Taylor P (1997). *Managing public involvement in healthcare purchasing*. Buckingham, Open University Press.

Madden M, Speed E (2017). Beware zombies and unicorns: toward critical patient and public involvement in health research in a neoliberal context. *Frontiers in Sociology*, 2:7.

Marston C et al. (2016). Community participation for transformative action on women's, children's and adolescents' health. *Bulletin of the World Health Organization*, 94:376–82.

Martin G (2009). Public and user participation in public service delivery: tensions in policy and practice. *Sociology Compass*, 3:310–26.

Martin G, Carter P, Dent M (2017). Major health service transformation and the public voice: conflict, challenge or complicity? *Journal of Health Services Research & Policy* [Epub ahead of print].

Mittler J et al. (2013). Making sense of "consumer engagement" initiatives to improve health and health care: a conceptual framework to guide policy and practice. *Milbank Quarterly*, 91:37–77.

Morgan H et al. (2016). We need to talk about purpose: a critical interpretive synthesis of health and social care professionals' approaches to self-management support for people with long-term conditions. *Health Expectations* [Epub ahead of print].

Nasser M et al. (2017). What are funders doing to minimise waste in research? *Lancet*, 389:1006–7.

National Institute for Health Research (2017). About INVOLVE. Available at: http://www.invo.org.uk/about-involve/ (accessed 20 November 2017).

NHS England (2017). What are personal health budgets (PHBs)? Available at: https://www.england.nhs.uk/personal-health-budgets/what-are-personal-health-budgets-phbs/ (accessed 20 December 2017).

Nolte E, Knai C (eds.) (2015). *Assessing chronic disease management in European health systems. Country reports.* Copenhagen: WHO Regional Office for Europe on behalf of the European Observatory on Health Systems and Policies.

Nolte E, Knai C, Saltman R (eds.) (2014). *Assessing chronic disease management in European health systems. Concepts and approaches.* Copenhagen: WHO Regional Office for Europe on behalf of the European Observatory on Health Systems and Policies.

Ocloo J et al. (2017). Exploring the theory, barriers and enablers for patient and public involvement across health, social care and patient safety: a protocol for a systematic review of reviews. *BMJ Open*, 7:e018426.

Ong B et al. (2014). Behaviour change and social blinkers? The role of sociology in trials of self-management behaviour in chronic conditions. *Sociology of Health & Illness*, 36:226–38.

patientslikeme (2017). Home. Available at: https://www.patientslikeme.com/ (accessed 28 November 2017).

Peckham S et al. (2014). Commissioning for long-term conditions: hearing the voice of and engaging users – a qualitative multiple case study. *Health Services and Delivery Research*, 2.

Rifkin S (2012). Translating rhetoric to reality: a review of community participation in health policy over the last 60 years. Available at: http://www .wzb.eu/sites/default/files/u35/rifkin_2012_rhetoric_to_reality_a_review_ of_cp_and_health_policy.pdf (accessed 19 November 2017).

Roland M, Dudley R (2015). How financial and reputational incentives can be used to improve medical care. *Health Services Research*, 50:2090–115.

Rosén P, Anell A, Hjortsberg C (2001). Patients' views on choice and participation in primary health care. *Health Policy*, 55:121–8.

Salzburg Global Seminar (2011). Salzburg statement on shared decision making. *BMJ*, 342:d1745.

Schlesinger M et al. (2014). Complexity, public reporting, and choice of doctors: a look inside the blackest box of consumer behavior. *Medical Care Research and Review*, 71:38S–64S.

Sizmur S, Graham C, Walsh J (2015). Influence of patients' age and sex and the mode of administration on results from the NHS Friends and Family Test of patient experience. *Journal of Health Services Research & Policy*, 20:5–10.

Taylor S et al. (2014). A rapid synthesis of the evidence on interventions supporting self-management for people with long-term conditions: PRISMS – Practical systematic Review of Self-Management Support for long-term conditions. *Health Services and Delivery Research*, 2.

Tempfer C, Nowak P (2011). Consumer participation and organizational development in health care: a systematic review. *Wiener klinische Wochenschrift*, 123:408–14.

Vardanalys (2017). *Act without impact. Assessment of the Swedish Patient Act 2014–2017. Summary*. Stockholm: Vardanalys.

Wagner E (1998). Chronic disease management: What will it take to improve care for chronic illness. *Effective Clinical Practice*, 1:2–4.

Wait S, Nolte E (2006). Public involvement policies in health: exploring their conceptual basis. *Health Economics, Policy and Law*, 1:149–62.

Weeks L et al. (2017). Evaluation of patient and public involvement initiatives in health technology assessment: a survey of international agencies. *International Journal of Technology Assessment in Health Care*, 10:1–9.

World Health Organization (1978). Declaration of Alma-Ata. International Conference on Primary Health Care, Alma-Ata, USSR, 6–12 September 1978. Available at: http://www.who.int/publications/almaata_declaration_en.pdf (accessed 20 December 2017).

4 Achieving person-centred health systems: levers and strategies

ELLEN NOLTE, ANDERS ANELL

Introduction

Traveller, there is no path. The path is made by walking.

Antonio Machado

As we have seen in Chapter 2 of this book, the terminology and interpretations of person-centredness vary across disciplines, professionals and stakeholders. A common theme underlying the diverse understandings is the ethical premise that people as patients and service users, and, by extension, family members, members of the community and citizens more broadly, should be treated as persons, with respect and dignity, and that care should take into account their needs, wants and preferences. However, expectations regarding the outcomes of enhanced person-centred care vary among stakeholders. Thus, managers and decision-makers might anticipate increased efficiency and wider system level effects, while others emphasize more effective engagement at the interpersonal level. Different understandings and perspectives will significantly impact on the translation of principles into practice, and on the perceived or demonstrated effectiveness of relevant initiatives and strategies. This is especially relevant since person-centred policies and strategies involve trade-offs and the implementation of policies will be heavily influenced by how stakeholders balance goals and trade-offs, and, ultimately, existing power relations.

Based on our exploratory review of the evolution of person-centredness (Chapter 2) we can distinguish three perspectives; the interpersonal level of care (micro level), quality of care more broadly (meso level) and health systems (macro level). The micro-level perspective sees person-centredness as a concept or a framework that helps inform the (interpersonal) delivery of care, a view that is most likely held by health professionals. The meso-level perspective interprets person-centred care as a means to enhance the quality of care more broadly, as reflected in the seminal 2001 report *Crossing the Quality Chasm* by the Institute of Medicine (Institute of Medicine, 2001). This is a view most likely held by managers and decision-makers. Conversely, as Gillespie, Florin & Gillam (2004) showed, lay groups tend to view person-centredness in the context of a social or whole person model of health that occurs at the level of people involvement in the planning and delivery of services rather than within the individual clinical encounter, although this perspective may vary among people (*see also* Box 4.1). This broader view is more closely linked to those perspectives that see person-centredness as a principle that guides the design of what some have referred to as people-centred health systems (World Health Organization, 2016; World Health Organization Regional Office for Europe, 2015).

This chapter summarizes the key insights from individual chapters in this book. We conclude that contemporary approaches to organizing and governing health services and systems have largely failed to deliver person-centred care, although some progress has been made. We note that there is a need for policies to strengthen the capabilities for engagement across all stakeholders concerned, and we discuss some of these options, including the challenges that need to be overcome in order to move to more person-centred health systems.

Why different understandings and interpretations of person-centredness matter

Depending on the perspective, person-centredness will be understood and interpreted in different ways, and the implications for the further development of health services and systems will differ. Importantly, those that view person-centredness as a means to inform service delivery and to enhance care quality more broadly tend to be narrower in their approach as they rest on the assumption, or indeed postulate, that service providers play an important role in people's lives. Yet this is not necessarily the case from an individual service user (or carer) perspective, even among those who use services more frequently because of chronic health problems. For example, Foss et al. (2016) highlighted that, among people with type 2 diabetes, encounters with health care are often experienced as "yet another demand in their lives" (p. 681). Indeed, the need to navigate services and clinical appointments, interact with different health and care professionals and engage in self-management and other treatment activities creates a 'treatment burden', as the work of managing ill health ('patient work' – Shippee et al., 2012) has shifted as part of a wider agenda of increased patient responsibility for their own health and care (May et al., 2014). Treatment burden has been associated with poor adherence and unfavourable outcomes. Demain et al. (2015) also highlighted that among people with a range of conditions, treatments may lead to physical symptoms and side-effects (such as pain and nausea), yet it is often not the severity of symptoms that people struggle with but the impacts arising from those symptoms and side-effects, such as on identity, independence and interaction with others. While the interaction and the nature of the relationship with health professionals can help address and reduce these impacts (May, Montori & Mair, 2009), much of the adaptive work people undertake to "psychologically normalise treatments to their lives and their lives to the treatment" (p. 11) takes place without formal care providers' involvement (Vassilev et al., 2016). It could thus be argued that interpreting person-centredness in the context of the current mode of service delivery only reinforces existing structures. A move to 'truly' person-centred systems requires the redesign of services and systems more broadly.

This conclusion is corroborated throughout the individual contributions to this book (*see also* Chapter 3). For example, Draper and Rifkin (Chapter 5) and Beresford and Russo (Chapter 6), looking respectively at user engagement in health service and system development and in research, find that relevant strategies have been and appear to remain dominated by professional and service-led motives, which might explain the lack of measurable impact on outcomes. Similar observations are noted by Nolte and Anell (Chapter 12), citing evidence that contemporary approaches to self-management support tend to focus on managing people's conditions in terms of biomedical outcomes or disease control. This focus is driven largely by professional perceptions of self-management when instead there is a need to support people to manage well (or live well) with their conditions within the wider context within which they live. The reviews by Fotaki, Van Ginneken et al. and Verhaeghe in Chapters 8–10, which explore the role of the individual as a consumer in making decisions about purchasers or providers of individual care packages and services, all find that enabling people to exercise choice requires appropriate support structures at the different tiers of the system. Yet what is available has tended to be designed without user input. Indeed, as Verhaeghe argues, the nature and scope of what people actually would want in terms of information and support remains poorly understood. Overall, there is a more general lack of understanding of whether and how people want to be involved in decision-making at the different tiers of the system (Box 4.1).

Box 4.1 What do we know about whether people want to engage in health care decision-making at individual and collective levels?

Fredriksson, Eriksson & Tritter (2017) examined preferences for involvement in health care decisions at individual and collective levels among adults in Sweden and the UK. Using a general population survey (people aged 15 years and older) in 2014, they explored (i) the extent to which individuals wanted to make the final decision about their treatment, and (ii) whether they wished to be involved in decision-making about local health services. They also asked whether people believed that they can influence decisions about the health service more broadly. The survey found that, overall, two-thirds of respondents preferred that a health professional makes the decision about their treatment (Sweden: 70%; UK: 66%), and only a minority wanted to make this decision themselves (10% vs. 13%). The finding that people in both countries preferred their health professional to make the treatment decision may perhaps seem surprising, although it is important to note that the question was about the *final* treatment decision. The authors acknowledged that their finding did not imply that people do not wish to be involved in the process overall. Indeed, Coulter & Jenkinson (2005), in a 2002 survey of people aged 16 and over in eight European countries (including Sweden and the UK) about treatment decisions found that about one-quarter of respondents wanted to make the decision themselves (albeit after consultation with their doctor). However, the majority favoured a shared decision-making model, in which the doctor and patient are jointly responsible for making treatment decisions. Predictors for desiring a shared role include familiarity with a clinical condition, while level of trust in the physician, age and education also influence whether individuals prefer an active over

---

Box 4.1 (cont.)

a more passive role in the decision-making process (Kraetschmer et al., 2004; Deber et al., 2007).

Concerning decisions about local health care organization and delivery, Fredriksson, Eriksson & Tritter (2017) found that 44% of respondents wanted to be involved, and this was more common among people in Sweden compared to the UK (55% vs. 33%). Respondents from Sweden were also somewhat more likely to believe that their involvement in decision-making could improve services (39% vs. 36%), although a considerable minority did not believe this to be the case (30% vs. 24%). Those who wanted to be involved in decisions about their own care were more likely to also want to be involved in health care decision-making in either country. The higher propensity among Swedish respondents for wanting to be involved was explained by relative levels of dissatisfaction with the health system overall, which was found to be higher in Sweden, and this might prompt people to want to influence decision-making to improve services. However, there are various reasons for people's willingness to actively engage (Martin, 2008), reflecting a combination of individual beliefs, interests and knowledge, as well as wider contextual factors and norms, and effective involvement will need to take account of this complexity.

There has been more progress in the understanding of how people view the quality of services, with recent moves to the collection of patient-reported experiences and outcomes measures (PREMs and PROMs). Yet as Coulter, Paparella & McCullough note in Chapter 7, lay involvement in the development of such measures remains inadequate, and this observation is confirmed by a scoping review of patient involvement in the development of PROMs (Wiering, De Boer & Delnoij, 2017). More importantly, there is very limited use of such data and understanding of how people view the quality of services to support redesign of services. Overall, as Légaré et al. summarize in Chapter 11, there is a need to move to a more complex model of engagement that systematically considers people's values and preferences at all tiers of the system, from the individual patient–professional relationship to the organizational, the governance and finance, and wider societal levels in order to systematically implement person-centred strategies.

The question, then, is about how to get there. It is conceivable that progress has to be thought of as incremental, considering the various strategies that have been reviewed in this volume. Each chapter has provided useful pointers of what is needed to move towards a more person-centred approach in a given area. However, given the nature and pace of challenges facing health systems today, as discussed in the introduction to this book, and the impact this will have on people's lives, more fundamental and, by implication, more difficult change may be needed. As noted, a health system that is focused on the person at the centre is expected to address the varied challenges by ensuring accessible health care that is of high quality, responsive, affordable and financially sustainable. Yet the review of the evidence of a diverse range of strategies in this book raises a number of critical questions about the readiness of decision-makers at the various tiers of the system to truly wish to move towards more person-centred strategies. Doing so will require confronting established relationships and a rethink of some of the more fundamental processes that have traditionally governed the provider-centric and expert-based organization and financing of health services and systems. This chapter explores some of these critical questions. While not providing answers to how to solve these questions, it aims to help the various stakeholders to reflect on what person-centredness will mean in their individual system context and consider the options that may be available to them.

Are decision-makers ready to support people to actively engage at the different tiers of the system?

We have suggested that a continued focus on conceptualizing person-centredness from a professional or service delivery perspective only is likely to reinforce existing structures, thus undermining the central idea of person-centredness as a design principle. Indeed, it could even be argued that contemporary narrow strategies or approaches cater to 'dysfunctional' systems. This is exemplified by a continued focus on the traditional approach to health care organization and financing that emphasizes a biomedical model of service delivery that centres on managing and measuring biomedical indicators, such as blood sugar levels in people with diabetes, or intermediate indicators such as behaviour change that will lead to changes in the biomedical indicator. This focus is perhaps not surprising given that much of the available literature on person-centredness addresses the interpersonal level between the care provider and the patient or service user more broadly, while the organizational and system contexts are rarely discussed (Chapter 2). Yet, this 'narrow' or biomedical focus tends to be unnecessarily reinforced at the meso and macro levels, too. Examples include contemporary pay-for-performance schemes in primary care such as those implemented in the UK or France, or disease-management programmes in various European countries that incentivize control of mainly biomedical indicators (Nolte, Knai & Saltman, 2014). While such vertical, disease-oriented indicators are of course perfectly valid as a means to monitor the progress of a given disease, complementary horizontal measures that focus on outcomes that matter to people may be more important at the organizational and systems level.

This discussion raises a number of more fundamental questions. One relates to power relationships between different actors and stakeholders, most prominently perhaps at the individual level between the service user and the health professional (Box 4.2).

Box 4.2 The role of 'power' in the physician–patient interaction

Much of the work around the doctor–patient relationship has focused on the role of power, knowledge and status, dating to the work of Parsons (1951) and the notion of the 'sick role', where the patient is a passive recipient of care who responds to medical authority. Freidson (1970) pointed to the principal 'conflict' in the relationship, with doctors and patients having different agendas and formal medical knowledge competing with the patient's lay or 'folk' knowledge. Improvements in medical technology further reinforce the power imbalance between physicians and patients. Parsons' work has been challenged, inter alia, on the grounds of its medico-centric approach and the limited applicability of the 'sick role' to chronic illness. However, contemporary debate has reinterpreted Parsons' work as remaining fundamental to the understanding of the interaction between the patient and the health professional (Shilling, 2002).

Box 4.2 (cont.)

Related work has explored the role of the physician with the emergence of a 'new professionalism' against a rapidly changing context within which health care is being provided and a changing society more widely (Irvine, 1999). This has involved the redefinition of what it means to be a medical professional, such as within the US/European Charter on Medical Professionalism. This builds on three principles: those of the primacy of patient welfare, of patient autonomy and of social justice (Medical Professionalism Project, 2002). The Charter sets out professional responsibilities. These include, inter alia, a commitment to honesty whereby patients "must be empowered to decide on the course of therapy"; patient confidentiality; maintaining appropriate relations with patients; improving quality of and access to care; a just distribution of finite resources; and maintaining trust by managing conflicts of interest. This change is reflected by evidence that doctors generally seem to support shifts away from paternalism towards a new type of relationship with the patient that emphasizes partnership (Hilton, 2008). However, as the various contributions in this volume have shown, it remains challenging to translate this notion into daily practice (*see also* Chapters 11 and 12).

The move to more person-centred strategies is seen as a way to overcome these challenges, with a desire to shift from a paternalistic approach to a (more) equal partnership, but this remains difficult to realize in practice. For example, as highlighted by Légaré et al. in their review of shared decision-making (Chapter 11), and Nolte and Anell in relation to self-management (Chapter 12), numerous tensions arise, for example, where the service user wishes to pursue a course of action that costs more or may even be harmful for patients or others. The evidence about the extent to which this is happening in practice is, however, largely absent. Similar challenges related to individuals' capabilities of making good decisions have been highlighted by van Ginneken et al. (Chapter 9) in relation to insurance choice, pointing to instances where individuals have made choices of insurer that may not be in their own best interest, a challenge also highlighted by Verhaeghe in the context of personal budgets (Chapter 10).

Whose expertise 'counts'?

This then raises the question about professional authority, 'expertise' and whose experience and knowledge counts in judging whether a given decision is 'good' or appropriate. This question is not limited to the individual service user and professional interaction (Hamilton et al., 2017), but also extends to the organizational and macro or system levels. While a 'poor' decision at the individual service user level may impact the individual and their immediate carers, a 'poor' decision at the organizational or systems level may have negative consequences for populations more widely. In the context of individual service users, Renedo, Komporozos & Marston (2017) and others have highlighted the role of evidence-based medicine as a central principle of clinical practice, which can create tensions for health professionals who are asked to tailor their practice to individual service user's needs and preferences. Yet individual tailoring of services may run counter to standardized approaches, which are underpinned by ideas about hierarchies of evidence and where scientific and technical evidence is ranked above clinicians' practical or experiential evidence (Pope, 2003) and above patient or carer experience (Greenhalgh et al., 2015).

Fundamental here is the role and status of lay experience and expertise within the clinical encounter specifically and in the health service and system more broadly. This issue comprises different layers of complexity. These include the degree to which service user experiences might be ignored or excluded, because individuals are unable to articulate these, or health professionals are unable or unwilling to accept the patients' expertise as a legitimate input, as they might override the clinician's perspective on a given issue and requires them to reflect on their role as 'experts' (Carr et al., 2014). It also concerns the systematic collection of patient experience data to evaluate the quality of services (Chapter 7), information which, as Coulter, Paparella & McCulloch observed, is often not acted upon to improve services. This is despite evidence showing that among the key enablers for successful learning from service user experience to improve care quality is their active engagement. Renedo, Komporozos & Marston (2017) warned about a possible 'commodification' of patient experiences for other commercial purposes, which in turn raises ethical questions about how patient experiences are used and re-articulated by others. Importantly, it concerns questions about the nature and conceptualizations of evidence as such, what is considered to be a legitimate source of evidence and who decides on this in the context of participatory initiatives (*see* Box 4.3 for an illustrative example).

The question about what evidence counts, and whether it counts at all, has been shown to be of particular relevance in the context of patient and public involvement in research (Chapter 6). The research process, infrastructure and evaluation of public involvement remain dominated by professional expertise, and this is also reflected in research priorities (Crowe et al., 2015). This imbalance may risk undermining and devaluing participation and the systematic incorporation of experiential knowledge generated from lived experiences of users in the research process and it will be particularly problematic where vulnerable populations are concerned.

Box 4.3 Whose experience counts? Patient involvement in health technology assessment decisions in Australia

Lopes, Carter & Street (2015) examined patient involvement in health technology assessment decisions in Australia, based on 12 semi-structured interviews with patient organization representatives and members of Advisory Committees that provide advice to the Australian Department of Health. This found that participants viewed the involvement processes to be inadequate, but for different reasons that were linked to how different stakeholders conceptualized evidence. Thus, Advisory Committee members viewed evidence as encompassing clinical outcomes and patient preferences, while patient organizations focused on aspects not directly related to a given health condition but instead on "the social and emotional aspects of patients' experiences in living with illness" (p. 84). The study further highlighted that patient representatives reported having interacted with other stakeholders (in particular industry) to advocate for their conception of evidence on decision-making, illustrating existing power differentials within the decision-making process, an issue that would need to be addressed if the public is to be involved meaningfully.

The role of wider developments outside the immediate grasp of the health system

A further challenge for contemporary health systems lies in the role of new and innovative practices that are beyond the immediate control of care providers, and that role is only beginning to be understood. This applies in particular to the rapidly changing digital world, ranging from innovative devices, e- and m-health tools and technologies (mobile communication and network technologies) (Iribarren et al., 2017) to social networking sites (Rozenblum, Greaves & Bates, 2017), including online health fora and peer-to-peer support networks. These are already reshaping the way individuals and citizens are engaging with health care and systems more widely, with online resources now established as a primary route to health information. For example, a 2014 Eurobarometer study found that about 60% of adult Europeans go online when looking for health information (TNS Political & Social, 2014). Seeking health information online can improve the relationship between service users and providers, although the degree to which this is happening in practice will depend to a great degree on the willingness of the health professional to engage with the patient and the nature of their prior relationship (McMullan, 2006; O'Connor et al., 2016; Tan & Goonawardene, 2017). Online communities have become an increasingly important source and platform for finding and exchanging information and experiences around health and for providing a space for building relationships and support (Ziebland & Wyke, 2012). Social ties established online were shown to provide people living with chronic health problems with ready access to support to help self-manage their conditions and address aspects of self-management that are particularly difficult to meet offline (Allen et al., 2016). We will return to the potential of digital technology in supporting and enabling person-centred services and systems below.

Where to go from here?

The preceding sections have highlighted how contemporary approaches to organizing and governing health care and health systems largely fail to deliver person-centred care at the different tiers of the system. This is not to say that no progress has been made since the 1978 Alma Ata declaration, which advocated for the "right and duty to participate individually and collectively in the planning and implementation of their health care". Indeed, as this book has illustrated, countries have engaged and are engaging in a range of activities that aim to strengthen person-centredness at the different tiers of the system, but approaches tend to be disjointed, often focusing on the micro-level of the individual service user–professional relationship while neglecting the need to embed such approaches within the organizational and system context more broadly. More importantly perhaps, person-centred strategies, where implemented, often tend to take a professional, or service provider perspective, which may take service user views into consideration, but more often than not without involving people in the actual design of involvement processes, support and measurement tools that are meant to benefit the service user. Overall, such narrow approaches heavily constrain any true development towards person-centredness. Services are provided more or less as before, while support at organizational or system levels tends to remain haphazard. Inconsistent or poorly aligned policy frameworks at meso and macro levels are likely to further undermine the successful redesign of services that take user experiences and preferences into account.

We have highlighted that there is a need to move to a more complex model of engagement that considers people's values and preferences at each level of the system; from the individual patient–professional relationship (micro level) to the organizational (meso) and the governance, finance and wider societal (macro) levels in order to systematically implement person-centred strategies (Chapter 3). This means that we have to challenge the traditional approach to organizing and governing health care and systems by moving away from the profession- and expert-led approach towards enabling and participatory strategies which emphasize respectful and enabling partnership working. Thus, if we accept this challenge and are committed to taking a broader perspective that recognizes people's social context within which they live and make decisions, we need to reconsider the 'boundaries' between service providers and service users and people more broadly. This includes giving due consideration to the experiences of (or, more specifically, experiential evidence generated by) individuals as patients, carers, taxpayers and citizens, and ensure that these are being used strategically to inform the redesign of services at the different tiers of the system.

To achieve this, there will be a need for more general policies that seek to strengthen the capabilities for engagement across all stakeholders concerned, along with a need to make better use of existing levers, such as digital technologies. This needs to be accompanied by more supply-side oriented strategies that include investment in education and training along with measurement and monitoring to understand what matters to people and how this can be used strategically in the (re)design of service organization and delivery at the different tiers of the system. As noted earlier, we here discuss some of these options, highlighting the opportunities while also considering the barriers that need to be overcome in order to move to more person-centred health systems.

Strengthening and enabling capabilities of people at the different tiers of the system

Making sure that people are able to access information about health and health care that they can understand is seen to be key in supporting them to be involved in decisions and to make choices that benefit their health and well-being and the system more broadly (Kickbusch et al., 2013; Nutbeam, 2000). The inability to do so has been linked to poorer health outcomes among older people, increased service use such as hospitalizations and emergency care, and lower use of disease prevention services (Berkman et al., 2011), and it is viewed as an important determinant of health inequalities (Kickbusch et al., 2013).

The concept of 'health literacy' has been gaining increasing traction among policy-makers, practitioners and researchers alike. Better understanding of the potential that enhancing related skills and competencies can have on improving the health and well-being of individuals and populations and on reducing inequities in health has contributed to its inclusion as an important dimension in national and international health strategies, such as the Health 2020 health policy framework for the World Health Organization European Region (World Health Organization Regional Office for Europe, 2013). At the same time, among countries in the European Union, health literacy is only beginning to be addressed through relevant policies and initiatives, and the available evidence does not yet allow drawing firm conclusions about their impacts (Heijmans et al., 2015).

Health literacy has been, and continues to be, variously defined. A widely used understanding refers to the knowledge, motivation and competencies of accessing, understanding, appraising and applying health-related information within health care, disease prevention and health promotion settings (Sørensen et al., 2012), with Dodson, Good & Osborne (2015) emphasizing the social resources needed to enable people realizing this vision in practice. These interpretations place health literacy in a broader public health model that highlights the complex interdependencies between health understanding, health attitudes and behaviours. They also consider the social determinants of health, such as income, education, the material environment and gender, as well as the design and delivery of health services, in turn highlighting the requirement for a system-wide response to meet individual needs (Greenhalgh, 2015) (*see also* Box 4.4). The importance of the broader context has been conceptualized as health literacy responsiveness, which describes "the way in which services, environments and products make health information and support available and accessible to people with different health literacy strengths and limitations" (Dodson, Good & Osborne, 2015, p. 12). This wider interpretation implies that interventions that rely solely on educational programmes to advance health literacy are likely to fail (Greenhalgh, 2015); instead a strategic response will be needed that not only takes account of individuals' and communities'

Box 4.4 Health literacy levels in European countries

The first European comparative survey on health literacy was conducted in 2011 in eight European countries (Austria, Bulgaria, Germany, Greece, Ireland, the Netherlands, Poland and Spain) (Sørensen et al., 2015). It found that across all eight countries, almost half of all respondents showed very low ('inadequate') or low ('problematic') levels of health literacy, ranging from just under 29% in the Netherlands to around 60% in Spain and Bulgaria. The strongest predictor for low levels of health literacy across all countries was financial deprivation, followed by low social status, low educational attainment and older age. Similar findings were reported for the adult working-age population in England, highlighting that people most in need for health information appear to have least access to it (Rowlands et al., 2015).

strengths and the constraints that influence how effectively they engage with health information and services, but also introduces change in ways that reduce health inequalities.

There is a persuasive argument that addressing health literacy at the community level holds great potential for improving health knowledge, skills and behaviours, which in turn is expected to lead to better health outcomes (Beauchamp et al., 2017). Yet it remains unclear, for now, what a health literate population should look like and the approaches that would be suitable for its measurement (Guzys et al., 2015). More importantly perhaps, it remains unclear how 'the public' thinks about the idea of health literacy and there appears to be a suspicious absence of the public voice in contemporary conceptualizations of health literacy. By the same token, it is important to recognize that in order to be effective, strategies to strengthen and further advance health literacy should go beyond the individual as a (potential) service user and communities. Effective strategies also need to incorporate professionals and providers, as well as managers and decision-makers at organizational and national levels. This is an emergent field although work is ongoing that can provide useful guidance.

Rowlands et al. (2017) noted that among the health workforce, health literacy appropriate skills, knowledge and attitudes tend to be low, often reflecting the lack of inclusion of health literacy in education and training (Groene et al., 2017). Initiatives to build such skills and competencies among professionals are emerging, but more work needs to be done to better understand the impacts of a more skilled workforce in health literacy on quality of care and service efficiency more broadly (Rowlands et al., 2017).

To help operationalize the shift to a systems perspective, members of the US National Academies of Sciences, Engineering, Medicine Roundtable on Health Literacy defined 10 attributes of a health literate health care organization (Brach et al., 2012). These recognize that health literacy improvement is increasingly being viewed as a systems issue and that action is required on multiple levels. While developed in the context of the USA, the attributes have been adapted in other system contexts, including Australia and New Zealand. Trezona, Dodson & Osborne (2017) advanced the idea of health literate organizations further by developing the Organisational Health Literacy Responsiveness (Org-HLR) framework. Involving professionals from across the health and social services sectors in Australia using a series of workshops, the authors identified seven domains of health literacy responsiveness:

(i)   *External policy and funding environment*: relates to the role of governments and other relevant bodies in providing adequate funding for programmes, flexible services agreements, incentives and health literacy-specific policy frameworks and standards.

(ii) *Leadership and culture*: describes "the necessary ethos, philosophy and values of a health literacy responsive organisation, which includes being inclusive, person-centred and equity driven" (p. 7) and which recognizes health literacy as an organizational priority.

(iii) *Systems, processes and policies*: refers to intraorganizational measures such as data collection and needs assessment, performance monitoring and evaluation, service planning and quality improvement, communication systems and processes, and internal policies and procedures that are required to provide responsive services.

(iv) *Access to services and programmes*: reflects the need for organizations to ensure that services are accessible to all people, with access defined in terms of geography, physical access, financial access and cultural access. It incorporates the need for providing support for people to navigate the system and outreach.

(v)   *Community engagement and partnerships*: describes the need for organizations to "undertake meaningful consultation" and involve individuals and communities in all aspects of service planning, delivery and evaluation. It further stresses the need for organizations to engage in and develop partnerships with other organizations across the health and social care sectors to promote the design and delivery of coordinated services.

(vi) *Communication practices and standards*: refers to the range of strategies and approaches that organizations would need to develop and implement to ensure effective communication across all levels of the organization. These include communication principles, the provision of health information, use of media and technology, and health education programmes.

(vii) *Workforce*: describes the responsibility of organizations to ensure a skilled, competent and motivated workforce through appropriate recruitment and retention policies and the provision of a supportive working environment, practice resources and professional development opportunities.

The Org-HLR framework includes a range of domains that have been identified elsewhere as characteristics of organizations with a reputation of improving patient experience (e.g. Luxford, Safran & Delbanco, 2011). The key defining feature is that all domains consider health literacy as a priority and that the framework recognizes the role of the macro-level – that is, the external and funding environment – as a core element that can enable or constrain organizations in their efforts to become more responsive to local population needs. Indeed, as we have illustrated in the context of self-management support specifically (Chapter 12) and care coordination efforts more broadly (Nolte, Knai & Saltman, 2014), available evidence points to the challenges organizations can face when implementing local improvement strategies that are not appropriately resourced or that run counter to the demands placed upon them by the wider system context.

The Org-HLR framework may provide useful guidance for policy-makers, managers and practitioners seeking to strategically embed advancing the engagement of people at all levels within the system. Examples of system-wide approaches to embedding health literacy are provided by Austria (Box 4.5) and Scotland (NHS Scotland, 2017), which may usefully inform policy development elsewhere.

Box 4.5 A national strategy to strengthen health literacy at all levels in Austria

Austria included strengthening health literacy among its 2012 ten national health targets (Bundesministerium für Gesundheit und Frauen, 2017) and introduced, in 2013, the 'Österreichische Plattform Gesundheitskompetenz (ÖPG)' (Austrian Platform Health Literacy), which is tasked with the coordination, further development and support of implementation of this target by means of three strategic goals (Österreichische Plattform Gesundheitskompetenz, 2017):

1. *To strengthen the health literacy of the health system*
   This goal focuses mostly on (i) improving the quality of communication and information on health care, prevention and health promotion and (ii) embedding health literacy in the form of health-in-all-policies across all organizations and institutions that impact health.

Box 4.5 (cont.)

2. *To strengthen individual health literacy with particular consideration of vulnerable groups*
   This goal includes a range of measures seeking to impact the health literacy of individuals both directly and indirectly through measures that aim to strengthen a health literate environment through health-in-all-policies and equal opportunities in health.
3. *To embed health literacy in service provision*
   Measures are yet to be defined.
   An evaluation of the ÖPG in 2016 found that it had established itself as a 'learning platform' that successfully embedded the notion of health literacy across stakeholders, with active engagement of its members (a wide range of national and state governmental institutions and non-governmental organizations across sectors) (Gutknecht-Gmeiner & Capellaro, 2016). The platform was credited with great potential to systematically develop and embed health literacy in Austria and to lead to lasting changes.

Digital technologies to support person-centred care: potential and challenges

Digital health technologies have become increasingly important and they are at times claimed to be the main route into person-centred health services and systems through strengthening empowerment (European Commission, 2012). The available evidence on the benefits of many innovative technologies remains somewhat patchy, however (Castle-Clarke & Imison, 2016). We have seen earlier that the majority of people in Europe uses the internet for health-related information, but only about one-fifth have as yet used health and care services that are provided online, such as getting a prescription or an online consultation (TNS Opinion & Social, 2017). In 2017 the share of those using online health services varied substantially across EU Member States, with people in Estonia, Finland and Denmark most likely to have done so (between 40% and 50%), compared to fewer than 10% in Malta, Germany and Hungary. This variation is likely to reflect, at least in part, the actual availability of online health and care services, along with knowledge about their existence in a given setting, although there are few robust data on this issue. The same study also showed that just over half of

---

Box 4.6 Access to and use of e-health portals in Australia, Denmark and Estonia

Nøhr et al. (2017) examined access to e-health portals for residents in Denmark, Estonia and Australia, three countries that have implemented nationwide access to people's health records online. Looking at data for 2015 they found the proportion of those actually logging into the system to be rather low, ranging from less than 1% in Australia and 1–2% in Estonia to about 3–5% in Denmark. Younger people were more likely to access the portal in all countries, as were women in Denmark and Australia, but the proportions varied. For example, in Estonia the highest usage was among men and women aged 20–49, at around 5–7%, with the share steadily declining as people are older. In Denmark the highest levels of usage were seen among women aged 20–69, at around 5%, while among men the share was around 3%, and in both cases the share fell rapidly among those aged 70 and older. Overall usage levels tended to be low, raising questions about the degree to which investment in e-portals that provide residents access to personal health data alone contributes to patient empowerment.

---

respondents would like to have online access to their medical and health records, with those in Estonia, Denmark and Finland most likely to say so (72–82%), compared to respondents in Hungary, Germany and Austria (32–38%) (*but see* Box 4.6).

A crucial challenge remains the continued digital divide, ranging from principal access to the internet (primary divide) and its use (secondary divide) to comprehension of information on health (tertiary divide) (Latulippe, Hamel & Giroux, 2017). Principal access to the internet has increased across the EU, with, in 2014, about 70% of homes in Member States having a fixed broadband subscription (62% in rural areas) (European Parliament, 2015). The share was highest in the Netherlands and Luxembourg, at over 90%, and lowest in Bulgaria and Romania, at under 60%. About three-quarters of the population reported using the internet on a regular basis (43% almost daily) but some 58 million people did not use it; these were mostly older people and those with disabilities (*see also* Figure 4.1). Some 70% of those who lack basic digital skills were over the age of 55 and the proportion of 55–74-year-olds who reported to have never used the internet was highest in Bulgaria, Cyprus, Greece and Romania, at around 70%, and lowest in Denmark, Luxembourg, the Netherlands and Sweden, at around 10%. The latter set of countries are also those which, in 2017, scored highest on the Digital Economy and Society Index in the EU, while Bulgaria, Greece and Romania, along with Italy, scored lowest (European Commission, 2017).

This matters because those who are least likely to use the internet tend to be most vulnerable in terms of health risks and chronic illness, and vice versa. This means that e-health strategies could exacerbate social inequalities in health if not carefully designed (Latulippe, Hamel

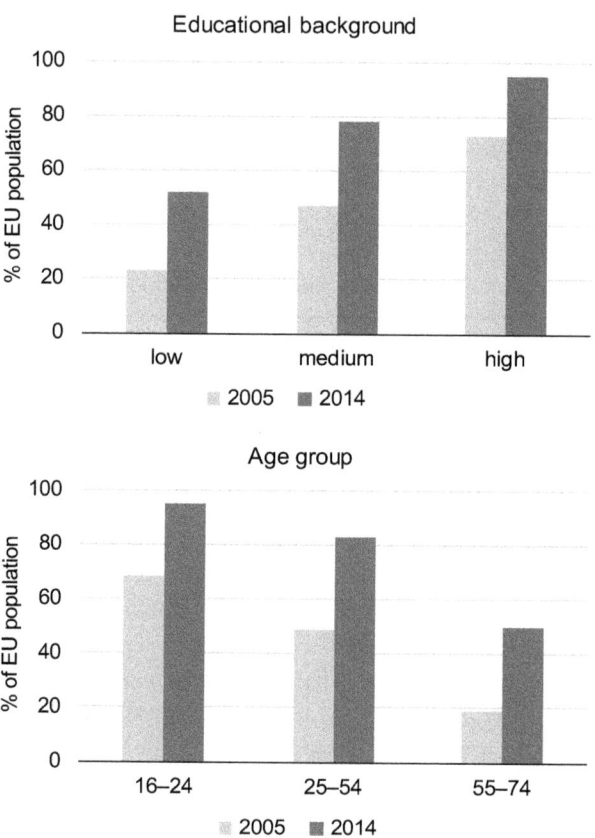

Figure 4.1 Regular internet use among EU citizens, 2005 and 2014

Source: adapted from European Parliament, 2015

& Giroux, 2017), especially where policies envisage online communities as one way for people to engage in self-management for example. Older people increasingly engage in social media and networks (Anderson & Perrin, 2017), and data from Europe suggest that this is particularly common in the Nordic countries and the Netherlands. Some evidence points to a positive association between use of social networking sites and well-being among older people (Nef et al., 2013; Sims, Reed & Carr, 2017), although others have noted that as their health declines, older people tend to engage less with technology, especially those with new-onset dementia, low physical performance or who have relocated to a nursing home (Levine, Lipsitz & Linder, 2017). Better understanding of the patterns of use may help target digital technology-based solutions, although context remains important (Peek et al., 2017). Thus, as Levine, Lipsitz & Linder (2017) cautioned, "complex everyday and digital health technology reaches few seniors in general" (p. 4).

The implementation and scaling-up of e-health technologies remains challenging

A 2012 review of reviews of the evidence of the implementation of e-health systems found that the 37 included studies that had been published between 1995 and 2009 had largely focused on organizational factors that would enable or hinder implementation (Mair et al., 2012). Studies neglected the wider social framework that should be considered when introducing new technologies. These include the purpose and benefits of e-health systems, along with their anticipated value to users; factors promoting or inhibiting engagement and participation; the impacts of e-health technologies on roles and responsibilities; risk management; and "ways in which implementation processes might be reconfigured by user-produced knowledge" (Mair et al., 2012, p. 357).

Lack of attention to the wider context within which digital health technologies are being introduced was also found to be a major impediment to the implementation of a national digital health innovation programme in the United Kingdom (Lennon et al., 2017). The programme aimed to stimulate a consumer market for person-centred digital technologies, which involved a wide range of products and services (apps, personal health records, telecare, telehealth, wearable activity trackers, etc.) to enable preventive care, self-care and independent living at scale.

Capturing the experiences of a wide range of stakeholders and over time, an evaluation of the programme found that while there was a general receptiveness to digital health, there remained numerous barriers to routinization of technologies into daily practice at all tiers of the system. Identified barriers included lack of IT infrastructure, uncertainty around information governance, lack of incentives to prioritize interoperability, lack of precedence on accountability within the commercial sector, and a market perceived as difficult to navigate by consumers. These findings highlight a need for greater investment in national and local infrastructure, the implementation of guidelines for the safe and transparent use and assessment of digital health, incentivization of interoperability, and investment in training of professionals and the public.

These observations were broadly confirmed in a subsequent update of the above-mentioned 2012 review (Ross et al., 2016). It highlighted that successful implementation of e-health systems requires multiple factors to be present, including the need for supportive legislation, and recognized standards, as well as the 'fit' of e-health systems with current organizational workflow. The review further noted that although e-health is a rapidly moving field, many factors that are relevant for effective implementation remain fairly consistent over time. These include the need for adequate resources, in particular financial and policy support, as well as standards and interoperability. Based on these findings, Ross et al. (2016) formulated a set of recommendations for the implementation of e-health systems, which are summarized in Box 4.7.

Box 4.7 Recommendations for implementation of e-health systems based on a systematic review of systematic reviews

Updating and re-analysing the systematic review of the e-health implementation literature by Mair et al. (2012), Ross et al. (2016) identified a set of recommendations to help guide more successful implementation of e-health systems. The recommendations are:

- Select an appropriate e-health system, taking into account:
    - Complexity
    - Adaptability
    - Compatibility with existing systems and work practices
    - Cost

Box 4.7 (cont.)

- Include key stakeholders and implementation champions as early as possible in the implementation process.
- Make available sufficient financial and legislative support to support implementation.
- Establish standards for technology which address interoperability, security and privacy to improve acceptability and implementation.
- Plan implementation, ensuring that organizations are in a state of readiness.
- Provide training and education to all those involved with implementation.
- Implementation does not stop with 'go-live': ensure ongoing monitoring, evaluation and adaptation of systems so that intended goals are being met and benefits realized. This also requires ongoing identification of barriers to effective use, along with strategies to overcome these barriers.

Strengthening and enabling the redesign of services at the different tiers of the system

In order to move to a person-centred system that takes a broad approach we need to better understand what matters to people and whether and how they would like to be involved at the different tiers of decision-making. A first step is to support the development and advancement of health literacy responsive organizations, as discussed above, but this needs to be informed by the systematic assessment of people's experiences, goals and preferences. We also need to better understand and develop further how those who are meant to organize, finance, govern and deliver services have to be supported if we want them to take people's views seriously and incorporate these into service (re)design and delivery. We briefly discuss these issues in turn.

Measuring what matters to people
Arguably, the science of measuring patient-centred outcomes is growing, yet metrics of 'success' continue to be defined by providers and payers

(Batalden et al., 2016). Coulter, Paparella & McCulloch in Chapter 7 have highlighted the need, at the level of the clinical encounter, for measurement to go beyond individual episodes or services and the prevailing biomedical paradigm. Instead, what is required is the development of measurement tools that reveal people's experiences across clinical pathways and service boundaries, as well as broader indicators that better reflect service users' goals and outcome preferences, along with better measures of concepts such as empowerment, autonomy, care coordination and self-management capabilities. In short, there is a need for novel or adapted measures that recognize the role of the person at the centre and reflect 'what matters to people'. Narrative accounts that describe encounters with clinicians in patients' own words can usefully complement statistical reports of survey data by providing insights into why current practices may not be working well, so informing quality improvement strategies (Schlesinger, Grob & Shaller, 2015).

At the meso and macro levels, new social media platforms have been proposed as a way to share information and narratives about health experiences and public views more broadly, adapting methods used in commercial sectors to better understand and respond to consumers (Rozenblum, Greaves & Bates, 2017). Monitoring social media may give providers insight into the drivers of a service user's assessment of their experience during an encounter with the service. Rozenblum, Greaves & Bates (2017) further highlighted the potential of social media to engage service users in ways that can directly impact behaviours and promote positive health outcomes, patient satisfaction, care delivery efficiency and improved quality of care. They also offer providers with a 'new set of information' suitable to inform the design and improve the delivery and evaluation of care. However, wider use of social media for the purpose of monitoring people's experiences and engaging them in the health service needs to carefully consider population groups that are least likely to use this format but whose voices may be most important to be heard; thus there remains a continued bias towards the young, wealthy and technologically savvy. There also remain concerns regarding privacy, stigma and patient consent, along with broader ethical concerns around online monitoring of social media platforms by providers (Rozenblum, Greaves & Bates, 2017), requiring careful attention to be given ways to protect privacy.

Importantly, as Coulter, Paparella & McCulloch note, if people's views and experiences are to be usefully incorporated into efforts to improve equitable and responsive delivery of health care, those measuring and monitoring these perspectives will need to be clear about the purpose of collecting related data. For example, whether data are being used for external reasons such as the provision of information for consumer choice, public accountability or pay-for-performance, or for internal use by providers as part of quality improvement schemes (Box 4.8). Each goal may be legitimate but requires the design of approaches that are appropriate for this purpose. Crucially, any such measurement will require service user and wider public input to ensure that we capture what matters to people. There is considerable potential for countries to collaborate and develop and test methods for ensuring that people's views and experiences are taken seriously and inform the (re)design of service organization and delivery at the different tiers of the system.

Box 4.8 Measuring and reporting the performance of institutions and practitioners in health care

The public release of information on the quality of health (and social) care delivered by identified providers can be seen to be located within broader concerns about accountability of health and social care systems. Reporting on provider performance aims to help hold the various actors in a given system to account by informing stakeholders and so enable them to make decisions, to facilitate the selection and choice of providers by service users and purchasers of care, to influence provider behaviour to enhance the quality of care, and to strengthen transparency of the system as a whole (Smith et al., 2009). Much of the published work on public reporting centres on the reporting of performance data of hospitals (Cacace et al., 2010), including, in the USA and the UK, individual surgeons (Behrendt & Groene, 2016), and, more recently, long-term care, while similar efforts within primary care are only emerging (Rechel et al., 2016).

One of the key objectives of public reporting systems is to support service user choice, yet available evidence suggests that people rarely search out information about the quality of care delivered by providers (Hussey et al., 2015). Low uptake of published information suggests that the available data do not sufficiently meet patients' information needs (Damman et al., 2009). Public reports

Box 4.8 (cont.)

vary widely in their accessibility, data transparency, appropriateness and timeliness. Variability of results can be confusing for users searching more than one website and it provides a potential source of bias and unfairness towards providers when used by regulators, purchasers or, indeed, service users (Austin et al., 2015). Further, few systems systematically involve service users or the wider public in the design of systems, including the selection of information to be reported on.

Lack of evidence does not imply lack of impact, however. There remains a shortage of rigorous evaluations of many major public reporting systems and there are also serious measurement problems. The effects of information systems on quality of care are difficult to isolate as these are frequently part of broader quality initiatives. Several authors have highlighted the risk of unintended consequences of the systematic reporting of information on quality of care delivered by identified providers. One example includes providers avoiding high-risk cases in an attempt to improve their quality ranking. Also, public reporting may result in providers focusing on improving those indicators that are reported on, such as waiting times, while diverting attention away from other, non-reported areas (Smith et al., 2009).

Investing in education and training

The move to person-centred care has considerable implications for the training of health and care professionals and how this needs to be adapted to enable professionals, organizations and systems engaging in a true partnership with individuals as service users and the wider public to provide the support appropriate to their preferences and needs. The delivery of person-centred care will require a new range of knowledge, skills and competences for professionals, managers and decision-makers but, as we noted in the context of health literacy above, our understanding of how to develop the workforce to put person-centred approaches into practice remains patchy (Box 4.9).

Box 4.9 Skills education and training framework for person-centred care in England

In England the national agency responsible for coordinating education and training within the health and public health workforce, Health Education England, published a skills education and training framework for person-centred care in 2017 (Health Education England, 2017). The framework is aimed at workforce leads to help them understand the knowledge, skills and capabilities of a person-centred workforce. It places communication and relationship-building skills at the core, setting out the underlying values and behaviours, juxtaposing desirable (what people receiving care and their carers would like to see in practice) and undesirable practices, along with learning outcomes that would be expected from education and training for staff to realize person-centred approaches. Importantly, the framework recognizes that developing new skills and knowledge on their own will not be sufficient to realize person-centred approaches and it highlights the need for a supportive system and culture within organizations that encourages and fosters behaviour change. It considers system levers for embedding person-centred communication and support in daily practice, including leaders and managers in organizations, human resources and organizational development, commissioners of services, education and training providers and the wider system, including regulators and professional bodies.

Managers need to consider approaches of how to best support their staff in implementing person-centred approaches. This will involve making relevant activities a priority, which in turn requires the ability of organizations to do so against the background of demands placed upon them by the wider system context. This also highlights the need for the wider policy framework to be alert to the potential tensions and unintended consequences of policies, and to create a policy environment that provides the means for those who are asked to implement change to acquire the actual capacity and competence to do so.

Health(care) system redesign

Our exploratory review of the evolution of person-centredness (Chapter 2) highlighted that much of the evidence on person-centredness has tended to focus on the interpersonal level between the care provider and the individual service user, while wider contextual issues at organizational level, let alone the systems level, have only rarely been addressed explicitly. These are heavily influenced by the relationships between different actors and institutions, and the wider regulatory, economic and cultural framework within which organizations and systems are embedded. This will make it difficult to identify specific levers and strategies for how to support and enable redesign that will fit all contexts. However, the available evidence does provide some important pointers that should be useful for all stakeholders involved, irrespective of health system characteristics. One source of evidence is Liberati et al. (2015), who reported a narrative review of studies examining organizational facilitators and barriers for achieving person-centred care. We summarize the findings of selected studies included in the review in Table 4.1. Identified levers for the implementation of person-centred care include a committed senior leadership as well as engagement of staff, service users and the wider community at all levels. This requires systematic measurement and feedback to continuously monitor people's experiences and a culture supportive of change and learning. Such an approach needs to be embedded in a wider policy framework, which ensures that there are clear incentives and lines of accountability that are supportive and aligned with the strategic vision of person-centredness.

The organizational levers described in these and related studies (e.g. Frampton et al., 2008) resemble in many ways the mechanisms and processes that were identified as the key drivers of large-system transformation in health care more broadly (Best et al., 2012) (Box 4.10).

Similar observations were reported by Hobbs (2009) in her review of concepts of patient-centred care. This highlighted the importance of the organizational and institutional context, with the distribution of authority and interaction of systems found to be of particular relevance. Thus, organizations that relied primarily on a command-and-control style of leadership were less likely to provide person-centred care compared to those with shared governance.

Table 4.1 *Levers for the implementation of person-centred care innovations in health care organizations*

	Shaller (2007)	Luxford, Sanfran & Delbanco (2011)	Hernandez et al. (2013)
Levers identified	– senior leadership, sufficiently committed and engaged to unify and sustain the organization in a common mission – strategic vision that is clearly and constantly communicated to every member of the organization – involvement of patients and families throughout the organization – supportive and respectful work environment that engages employees in all aspects of process design – systematic measurement and feedback to continuously monitor the impact of specific interventions and change strategies – built environment providing supportive and nurturing physical space and design for patients, families and employees alike – supportive technology that facilitates information access and communication between patients and caregivers	– strong, committed senior leadership – clear communication of strategic vision – active engagement of patient and families throughout the institution – sustained focus on staff satisfaction – active measurement and feedback reporting of patient experiences – adequate resourcing of care delivery redesign – staff capacity building – accountability and incentives – a culture strongly supportive of change and learning	– effective leadership, with the necessary technical and professional expertise and creative skills – strong internal and external motivation to change – clear and internally consistent organizational mission – aligned organizational strategy – robust organizational capability – continuous feedback and organizational learning

---

Box 4.10 Key factors that are likely to enhance the success of large-system transformation initiatives in health care

Best et al. (2012), in a realist review of examples of successful and less successful large-system transformations initiatives in health care, identified five factors or 'simple rules' that are likely to enhance the success of large-system transformation initiatives in health care:

- *Engage individuals at all levels in leading the change effort* through an explicit alignment of the formal vision and goals by top and middle-managers; an active management of the change strategy; small-scale pilot projects (to demonstrate to actors that change is worthwhile and possible); and assurance that people will not be penalized for taking actions that are part of the transformation.
- *Establish feedback loops* through active participation of all relevant stakeholder groups to determine the nature and range of measures to be used; ensuring actors' confidence in the validity of the measures, their understanding of what these mean and their ability to influence and revise the measures; and the inclusion of incentives (or penalties) for (not) acting upon feedback from reported measures.
- *Attend to history* through educating the leadership throughout the system about previous change efforts and their outcomes, along with factors that influenced outcomes in those efforts; and building on familiar and valued ideas and activities.
- *Engage physicians* through the alignment of professional and regulatory drivers; of the incentive structure; facilitation and guidance through the process; and professional examples through engaging physician leaders.
- *Involve patients and families* through increasing awareness among policy-makers and change agents of people's perspectives and priorities; increasing awareness that metrics reflect users' priorities; and increasing sense of equity that changes are inclusive and equitable.

Hernandez et al. (2013), in their assessment of person-centred innovation in health care organizations, highlighted the role of internal hierarchies in shaping person-centred care. They drew attention to the importance of external financial incentives and government regulations.

The role of incentive schemes in driving more person-centred care has been emphasized by a number of commentators. It has been argued that incentive schemes that focus on vertical, disease-specific biomedical outcome measures are likely to hinder the implementation of more horizontal and person-centred strategies that take account of the wider context within which people live (Heath et al., 2009) and which, as we have shown, will be important to support people living with their conditions (Reidy et al., 2016). Furthermore, as Schlesinger, Grob & Shaller (2015) have pointed out, strong financial incentives for biomedical or clinical outcomes risk undermining valued aspects of the service user–provider relationship. This implies that unless public policies, which have historically undervalued service user experience, are attentive to people's views more broadly, strong financial incentives for clinicians can threaten aspects of care that users most value. This in turn suggests that integrating user feedback with financial incentives and implementing these in ways that recognize the importance of non-financial incentives for quality improvement may help protect and promote user-valued outcomes. As with any scheme that involves financial incentives, the development and implementation would require a coherent strategic vision (Schlesinger, Grob & Shaller, 2015).

We have also noted earlier that person-centred approaches inevitably challenge standardization, with the latter having played an important role in reducing unintended variation in health services and contributed to improved quality and safety (Batalden et al., 2016). This too would caution any financial incentives linked directly to treatment measures. What is needed is flexibility to allow for 'intended' variation, with service providers responding to the needs and preferences of individuals and communities through active engagement and partnership while also offering the option of not being involved or not needing to choose if people prefer not to. As mentioned by Luxford, Safran & Delbanco (2011), such flexibility also stresses the importance of time needed for transforming service delivery towards person-centred care.

While financial and non-financial incentives that incorporate person-centredness may support incremental change, more efforts by those who organize, finance and govern health care are likely needed to support more fundamental redesign of service delivery. This view was recognized by Luxford, Safran & Delbanco (2011), who identified adequate resourcing of care delivery redesign as a lever for implementation of person-centred care. More fundamental or radical changes will likely need to be developed separately and tested against regular care before they are implemented more generally. Although such steps and practices are perhaps novel at the organizational and systems levels, they are fully accepted at the clinical level. This also suggests that adoption of similar steps and a systematic approach of exploration, evaluation and organizational learning may be an important lever towards real change. However, core to any of these moves will be the systematic and serious inclusion of the perspective of 'the public', as service user, carer, community, taxpayer or citizen, in the redesign of services at the different tiers. While it is encouraging to see that person-centredness has become a key priority for policy-makers nationally and internationally, those involved in service and system design would do well to recognize that the public voice still remains pretty much absent in many of the local strategies that are being considered to achieve this. This is a fundamental shortcoming and should be addressed by leaders at the organizational and system levels as a matter of priority. We hope that this book will help to support this process.

References

Allen C et al. (2016). Long-term condition self-management support in online communities: a meta-synthesis of qualitative papers. *Journal of Medical Internet Research*, 18:e61.

Anderson M, Perrin A (2017). Tech adoption climbs among older adults. Washington, DC: Pew Research Center.

Austin M et al. (2015). National hospital ratings systems share few common scores and may generate confusion instead of clarity. *Health Affairs*, 34:423–30.

Batalden M et al. (2016). Coproduction of healthcare service. *BMJ Quality & Safety*, 25:509–17.

Beauchamp A et al. (2017). Systematic development and implementation of interventions to OPtimise Health Literacy and Access (Ophelia). *BMC Public Health*, 17:230.

Behrendt K, Groene O (2016). Mechanisms and effects of public reporting of surgeon outcomes: a systematic review of the literature. *Health Policy*, 120:1151–61.

Berkman N et al. (2011). *Health literacy interventions and outcomes: an updated systematic review*. Rockville (MD): Agency for Healthcare Research and Quality.

Best A et al. (2012). Large-system transformation in health care: a realist review. *Milbank Quarterly*, 90:421–56.

Brach C et al. (2012). Ten attributes of health literate health care organizations. Available at: https://nam.edu/wp-content/uploads/2015/06/BPH_Ten_HLit_Attributes.pdf (accessed 2 February 2017).

Bundesministerium für Gesundheit und Frauen (2017). Gesundheitsziele Österreich. Richtungsweisende Vorschläge für ein gesünderes Österreich – Kurzfassung. Available at: https://gesundheitsziele-oesterreich.at/website2017/wp-content/uploads/2017/06/gz_kurzfassung_de_20170626.pdf (accessed 15 December 2017).

Cacace M et al. (2010). How health systems make available information on service providers: Experience in seven countries. Santa Monica: RAND and London School of Hygiene & Tropical Medicine. Available at: http://www.rand.org/content/dam/rand/pubs/technical_reports/2011/RAND_TR887.pdf (accessed 20 December 2017).

Carr S et al. (2014). Looking after yourself: Clinical understandings of chronic-care self-management strategies in rural and urban contexts of the United Kingdom and Australia. *SAGE Open Medicine*, 2:2050312114532636.

Castle-Clarke S, Imison C (2016). *The digital patient: transforming primary care*. London: The Nuffield Trust.

Coulter A, Jenkinson C (2005). European patients' views on the responsiveness of health systems and healthcare providers. *European Journal of Public Health*, 15:355–60.

Crowe S et al. (2015). Patients', clinicians' and the research communities' priorities for treatment research: there is an important mismatch. *Research Involvement and Engagement*, 1:2.

Damman OC et al. (2009). How do healthcare consumers process and evaluate comparative healthcare information? A qualitative study using cognitive interviews. *BMC Public Health*, 9:423.

Deber R et al. (2007). Do people want to be autonomous patients? Preferred roles in treatment decision-making in several patient populations. *Health Expectations*, 10:248–58.

Demain S et al. (2015). Living with, managing and minimising treatment burden in long term conditions: a systematic review of qualitative research. *PLoS One*, 10:e0125457.

Dodson S, Good S, Osborne R (2015). Health literacy toolkit for low- and middle-income countries: a series of information sheets to empower communities and strengthen health systems. New Delhi: World Health Organization, Regional Office for South-East Asia.

European Commission (2012). Redesigning health in Europe for 2020. eHealth Task Force Report. Luxembourg: Publications Office of the European Union.

European Commission (2017). The Digital Economy and Society Index (DESI). Available at: https://ec.europa.eu/digital-single-market/desi (accessed 19 August 2017).

European Parliament (2015). Bridging the digital divide in the EU. Available at: http://www.europarl.europa.eu/RegData/etudes/BRIE/2015/573884/ EPRS_BRI(2015)573884_EN.pdf (accessed 19 August 2017).

Foss C et al. (2016). Connectivity, contest and the ties of self-management support for type 2 diabetes: a meta-synthesis of qualitative literature. *Health and Social Care in the Community*, 24:672–86.

Frampton SB et al. (2008). Patient centered care, improvement guide. Derby, CT; Camden, ME: Planetree, Inc. and Picker Institute.

Fredriksson M, Eriksson M, Tritter J (2017). Who wants to be involved in health care decisions? Comparing preferences for individual and collective involvement in England and Sweden. *BMC Public Health*, 18:18.

Freidson E (1970). *Professions of medicine*. New York: Dodd Meads.

Gillespie R, Florin D, Gillam S (2004). How is patient-centred care understood by the clinical, managerial and lay stakeholders responsible for promoting this agenda? *Health Expectations*, 7:142–8.

Greenhalgh T (2015). Health literacy: towards system level solutions. *BMJ*, 350:h1026.

Greenhalgh T et al. (2015). Six 'biases' against patients and carers in evidence-based medicine. *BMC Medical Informatics and Decision Making*, 13:200.

Groene O et al. (2017). The health literacy dyad: the contribution of future GPs in England. *Education for Primary Care*, 28: 274–81.

Gutknecht-Gmeiner M, Capellaro M (2016). Evaluation der Österreichischen Plattform Gesundheitskompetenz (ÖPGK). Endbericht. Available at: https://oepgk.at/wp-content/uploads/2016/02/Evaluationsbericht-der-%C3%96PGK-2016.pdf (accessed 15 December 2017).

Guzys D et al. (2015). A critical review of population health literacy assessment. *BMC Public Health*, 15:215.

Hamilton J et al. (2017). What is a good medical decision? A research agenda guided by perspectives from multiple stakeholders. *Journal of Behavioral Medicine*, 40:52–68.

Health Education England, Skills for Health & Skills for Care (2017). Person-Centred Approaches: Empowering people in their lives and communities to enable an upgrade in prevention, wellbeing, health, care and support. A core skills education and training framework. Available at: http://www

.skillsforhealth.org.uk/services/item/575-person-centred-approaches-cstf-download (accessed 20 August 2017).

Heath I et al. (2009). Quality in primary health care: a multidimensional approach to complexity. *BMJ*, 338:b1242.

Heijmans M et al. (2015). *Study on sound evidence for a better understanding of health literacy in the European Union. Final report.* Brussels: European Commission.

Hernandez S et al. (2013). Patient-centered innovation in health care organizations: a conceptual framework and case study application. *Health Care Management Review*, 38:166–75.

Hilton S (2008). Education and the changing face of medical professionalism: from priest to mountain guide? *British Journal of General Practice*, 58:353–61.

Hobbs JL (2009). A dimensional analysis of patient-centered care. *Nursing Research*, 58:52–62.

Hussey P, Luft H, McNamara P (2015). Public reporting of provider performance at a crossroads in the United States: Summary of current barriers and recommendations on how to move forward. *Medical Care Research and Review*, 71:5S–16S.

Institute of Medicine (2001). *Crossing the quality chasm: a new health system for the 21st century.* Washington, DC: National Academies Press.

Iribarren S et al. (2017). What is the economic evidence for mHealth? A systematic review of economic evaluations of mHealth solutions. *PLoS One*, 12:e0170581.

Irvine D (1999). The performance of doctors: the new professionalism. *Lancet*, 353:1174–7.

Kickbusch I et al. (2013). *Health literacy. The solid facts.* Copenhagen: World Health Organization Regional Office for Europe.

Nolte E, Knai C, Saltman R (eds.) (2014). *Assessing chronic disease management in European health systems. Concepts and approaches.* Copenhagen: WHO Regional Office for Europe on behalf of the European Observatory on Health Systems and Policies.

Kraetschmer N et al. (2004). How does trust affect patient preferences for participation in decision-making? *Health Expectations*, 7:317–26.

Latulippe K, Hamel C, Giroux D (2017). Social health inequalities and eHealth: a literature review with qualitative synthesis of theoretical and empirical studies. *Journal of Medical Internet Research*, 19:e136.

Lennon M et al. (2017). Readiness for delivering digital health at scale: Lessons from a longitudinal qualitative evaluation of a national digital health innovation program in the United Kingdom. *Journal of Medical Internet Research*, 19:e42.

Levine D, Lipsitz S, Linder J (2017). Changes in Everyday and Digital Health Technology Use among Seniors in Declining Health. *Journals of Gerontology. Series A, Biological Sciences and Medical Sciences* [Epub ahead of print].

Liberati E et al. (2015). Exploring the practice of patient centered care: the role of ethnography and reflexivity. *Social Science & Medicine*, 133:45–52.

Lopes E, Carter D, Street J (2015). Power relations and contrasting conceptions of evidence in patient-involvement processes used to inform health funding decisions in Australia. *Social Science & Medicine*, 135:84–91.

Luxford K, Safran D, Delbanco T (2011). Promoting patient-centered care: a qualitative study of facilitators and barriers in healthcare organizations with a reputation for improving the patient experience. *International Journal for Quality in Health Care*, 23:510–15.

McMullan M (2006). Patients using the Internet to obtain health information: how this affects the patient–health professional relationship. *Patient Education and Counseling*, 63:24–8.

Mair F et al. (2012). Factors that promote or inhibit the implementation of e-health systems: an explanatory systematic review. *Bulletin of the World Health Organization*, 90:357–64.

Martin G (2008). 'Ordinary people only': knowledge, representativeness, and the publics of public participation in healthcare. *Sociology of Health & Illness*, 30:35–54.

May C, Montori V, Mair F (2009). We need minimally disruptive medicine. *BMJ*, 339:485–7.

May C et al. (2014). Rethinking the patient: using Burden of Treatment Theory to understand the changing dynamics of illness. *BMC Health Services Research*, 14:281.

Medical Professionalism Project (2002). Medical professionalism in the new millennium: a physicians' charter. *Lancet*, 359:520–2.

Nef T et al. (2013). Social networking sites and older users – a systematic review. *International Psychogeriatrics*, 25:1041–53.

NHS Scotland (2017). Making it easier. A health literacy action plan for Scotland. Available at: http://www.gov.scot/Resource/0052/00528139.pdf (accessed 15 December 2017).

Nøhr C et al. (2017). Nationwide citizen access to their health data: analysing and comparing experiences in Denmark, Estonia and Australia. *BMC Health Services Research*, 17:534.

Nolte E, Knai C, Saltman R (eds.) (2014). *Assessing chronic disease management in European health systems. Concepts and approaches.* Copenhagen: World Health Organization (acting as the host organization for, and secretariat of, the European Observatory on Health Systems and Policies).

Nutbeam D (2000). Health literacy as a public health goal: a challenge for contemporary health education and communication strategies into the 21st century. *Health Promotion International*, 5:259–67.

O'Connor S et al. (2016). Understanding factors affecting patient and public engagement and recruitment to digital health interventions: a systematic review of qualitative studies. *BMC Medical Informatics and Decision Making*, 16:120.

Österreichische Plattform Gesundheitskompetenz (2017). Österreichische Plattform Gesundheitskompetenz. Available at: https://oepgk.at/ (accessed 15 December 2017).

Parsons T (1951). *The social system.* London, Routledge.

Peek S et al. (2017). Origins and consequences of technology acquirement by independent-living seniors: towards an integrative model. *BMC Geriatrics*, 17:189.

Pope C (2003). Resisting evidence: the study of evidence-based medicine as a contemporary social movement. *Health (London)*, 7:267–82.

Rechel B et al. (2016). Public reporting on quality, waiting times and patient experience in 11 high-income countries. *Health Policy*, 120:377–83.

Reidy C et al. (2016). Commissioning of self-management support for people with long-term conditions: an exploration of commissioning aspirations and processes. *BMJ Open*, 6:e010853.

Renedo A, Komporozos-Athanasiou A, Marston C (2017). Experience as evidence: the dialogic construction of health professional knowledge through patient involvement. *Sociology*, Article first published online: 16 January 2017.

Ross J et al. (2016). Factors that influence the implementation of e-health: a systematic review of systematic reviews (an update). *Implementation Science*, 11:146.

Rowlands G et al. (2015). A mismatch between population health literacy and the complexity of health information: an observational study. *British Journal of General Practice*, 65:e379–86.

Rowlands G et al. (2017). Global health systems and policy development: implications for health literacy research, theory and practice. In: Logan R, Siegel E (eds.), *Health literacy. New directions in research, theory and practice.* Amsterdam: IOS Press.

Rozenblum R, Greaves F, Bates D (2017). The role of social media around patient experience and engagement. *BMJ Quality & Safety*, 26(10):845–8.

Schlesinger M, Grob R, Shaller D (2015). Using patient-reported information to improve clinical practice. *Health Services Research*, 50:2116–54.

Shaller D (2007). *Patient-centered care: what does it take?* New York.

Shilling C (2002). Culture, the 'sick role' and the consumption of health. *British Journal of Sociology*, 53:621–38.

Shippee N et al. (2012). Cumulative complexity: a functional, patient-centered model of patient complexity can improve research and practice. *Journal of Clinical Epidemiology*, 65:1041–51.

Sims T, Reed A, Carr D (2017). Information and communication technology use is related to higher well-being among the oldest-old. *Journals of Gerontology. Series B, Psychological Sciences and Social Sciences*, 72:761–70.

Smith P et al. (eds.) (2009). *Performance measurement for health system improvement. Experiences, challenges and prospects.* Cambridge: Cambridge University Press.

Sørensen K et al. (2012). Health literacy and public health: a systematic review and integration of definitions and models. *BMC Public Health*, 12:80.

Sørensen K et al. (2015). Health literacy in Europe: comparative results of the European health literacy survey (HLS-EU). *European Journal of Public Health*, 25:1053–8.

Tan S, Goonawardene N (2017). Internet health information seeking and the patient–physician relationship: a systematic review. *Journal of Medical Internet Research*, 19:e9.

TNS Opinion & Social (2017). Attitudes towards the impact of digitisation and automation on daily life. Special Eurobarometer 460. Brussels: European Union.

TNS Political & Social (2014). European citizens' digital health literacy. Flash Eurobarometer 404. Available at: http://ec.europa.eu/commfrontoffice/publicopinion/flash/fl_404_en.pdf (accessed 18 August 2017).

Trezona A, Dodson S, Osborne R (2017). Development of the organisational health literacy responsiveness (Org-HLR) framework in collaboration with health and social services professionals. *BMC Health Services Research*, 17:513.

Vassilev I et al. (2016). Social network type and long-term condition management support: a cross-sectional study in six European countries. *PLoS One*, 11:e0161027.

Wiering B, De Boer D, Delnoij D (2017). Patient involvement in the development of patient-reported outcome measures: a scoping review. *Health Expectations*, 20:11–23.

World Health Organization (2016). Framework on integrated, people-centred health services. Report by the Secretariat. Available at: http://apps.who.int/gb/ebwha/pdf_files/WHA69/A69_39-en.pdf?ua=1 (accessed 15 June 2017).

World Health Organization Regional Office for Europe (2013). *Health 2020. A European policy framework and strategy for the 21st century.* Copenhagen: WHO Regional Office for Europe.

World Health Organization Regional Office for Europe (2015). Priorities for health systems strengthening in the WHO European Region 2015–2020: walking the talk on people centredness. Available at: http://www.euro.who.int/__data/assets/pdf_file/0003/282963/65wd13e_HealthSystemsStrengthening_150494.pdf (accessed 15 June 2017).

Ziebland S, Wyke S (2012). Health and illness in a connected world: how might sharing experiences on the internet affect people's health? *Milbank Quarterly*, 90:219–49.

5 | Community participation in health system development

ALIZON K. DRAPER, SUSAN B. RIFKIN

Introduction

Much of the global dialogue around policies for health today focuses on the need for community participation in health systems to ultimately improve health among populations. Participation is not only promoted in the context of provision and utilization of health services but also as a key factor in the wider context of social determinants of health and health as a human right (World Health Organization, 2008a). Despite the growing interest in the role of participation, the evidence that links participation directly to better health remains weak (Rifkin, 2014), which creates barriers to gaining full support of governments, funding agencies and health professionals to promote this concept (Atkinson et al., 2011).

This chapter suggests important lessons for policy-makers, planners, managers and service providers who wish to enhance and promote community participation in health systems. It examines important underlying assumptions and different theoretical perspectives that provide the foundation to advocate for the benefits of community participation in health systems. Furthermore, it presents empirical evidence from a series of recent reviews and studies and identifies challenges to assessing the contribution of community participation to health systems and people's health.

The evolution of community participation in health systems

Early experiences of community participation in health systems can be traced to the early 20th century, with experiments in China using local lay people to help provide health services in poor rural areas. Local residents were trained to provide basic health care to their communities and this experiment expanded in countries in Asia and Africa under the banner of the International Institute of Rural Reconstruction (Taylor-Ide

& Taylor, 2002). Other examples include experiences in Africa, with King (1966) describing the involvement of local people assisting doctors in surgery and other interventions as part of their missionary work. The value of these approaches was seen in not merely having 'another pair of hands' but also of bringing skills and awareness to communities of the contribution of modern medicine to open their understanding of the link between science and behaviour for health improvements.

However, it was only the Alma Ata Declaration of 1978 that placed community participation on the global health agenda as part of a commitment to primary health care for World Health Organization member countries. The declaration identified health as a fundamental human right and stated that inequalities in health are "politically, socially and economically unacceptable" and that health care must be made "universally accessible to individuals and families in the community through their full participation" (World Health Organization, 1978, p. 1). The document highlighted equity and participation as key principles of national health policy, noting that "the people have the right and duty to participate individually and collectively in the planning and implementation of their health care". However, while the evidence to support policies addressing equity successively strengthened, gaining momentum with the World Health Organization's publication on the social determinants of health (World Health Organization, 2008a), policies to promote community participation have struggled to find strong evidence and direction.

Alma Ata helped to promote the creation of a core of community health workers inspired by the 'barefoot doctor' scheme in China that scaled up earlier experiments of the 1920s. Like their predecessors, barefoot doctors (subsequently village doctors) were local people who received medical training to provide first-line medical care and public health services to mobilize communities to focus on sanitation and the eradication of infectious disease (Cui, 2008). They were considered 'change agents' and seen to play an important part in modernizing health care in rural China. Elsewhere, similar national experiments in countries such as Columbia, Botswana and Sri Lanka were less successful, however, mainly because of conceptual and implementation problems, which failed to reap the wider benefits to be gained by developing community workers as change agents (Walt, 1990).

A different form of community participation in the health system was promoted by the Bamako Initiative, a joint WHO/UNICEF initiative that was implemented to varying degrees in countries in sub-Saharan Africa from the late 1980s (Mehrotra & Jarrett, 2002). The Initiative sought to decentralize health decision-making to the district level, and to involve the community by contributing financial resources and giving them a 'voice' in the management of the services. While seen to be successful in terms of community action as such, it was noted that community participation had not been as well-defined as originally thought; also, there was a lack of significant community empowerment. The overall acceptance of the Initiative was found to have been less than hoped for, because of poor local infrastructure, corruption and variable government support (McPake, Hanson & Mills, 1993).

Decentralization of decision-making to promote community participation gained wider traction during the 1990s, with the creation of committees composed of local people to make decisions about financial allocations to health, education and community development (Zakus & Lysack, 1998). Still, this approach to governance failed to gain universal acceptance. Challenges have been contextual, with for example resistance of governments to allow central authority to be reduced (Bossert & Beauvais, 2002). And although there have been examples of positive impacts, such as participatory budgeting as a format for community participation in countries such as Brazil, securing government support has not been always possible, especially in low resource settings (Boulding & Wampler, 2010).

The policy push for promoting community participation was further strengthened in the context of the Millennium Development Goals (UN General Assembly, 2001), along with subsequent calls for people-centred health systems (World Health Organization, 2008b) and the concurrent report on the social determinants of health (World Health Organization, 2008a). These documents promote an active role for individuals, families and communities as the intended beneficiaries of health systems in decision-making about planning and implementing health services and policies. Most recently, the Sustainable Development Goals highlight the importance of responsive, inclusive, participatory and representative decision-making at all levels (UN Sustainable Development Goals, 2015).

What we know about the contribution of community participation in health systems

The understanding and value of involving communities in health services and systems has greatly increased (World Health Organization, 2008b). In countries at all levels of development, governments, non-governmental organizations and private groups are recognizing the importance of including those who need and demand their services in decisions about how those services are delivered. However, it remains challenging for policy-makers, planners, managers and service providers to define outcomes and the factors that influence these outcomes (Milton et al., 2012; Popay, 2006; Preston et al., 2010; Rifkin, 2014; Wallerstein, 2006). This challenge is not restricted to the health field.

Reviewing the evidence of the value of community participation in development programmes, Mansuri & Rao (2013) found that community participation had made beneficial contributions to improving people's lives, but impacts varied by the nature of programmes. For example, they found that community-based development efforts have had limited impacts on income poverty, while participation in health service and education showed modestly positive results overall. However, at the same time it showed that people who benefit (most) tend to be the most literate, the least geographically isolated, and the most connected to wealthy and powerful people. The authors concluded that the overall evidence base remains thin, highlighting concerns about lack of effective systems of monitoring and evaluation and of attention to context in programme design. As a result, they argued, participatory development projects are likely to continue to be "driven more by ideology and optimism than by systematic analysis, either theoretical or empirical" (p. 3) and struggle to make a difference.

Assumptions underlying the contribution of community participation in health

One major reason for the relative lack of robust evidence around the contribution of community participation to health improvements is that relevant strategies tend to rest on a number of assumptions regarding the nature, role and outcomes of community participation. Rifkin (2012), in a review of community participation in health policy, found that these assumptions are rarely formally articulated or considered in the design and evaluation of initiatives to involve local people who are the intended beneficiaries in health services and systems. Yet despite the growing interest in community participation there has been little attempt to validate these assumptions. Rifkin (2009; 2012) has identified four key assumptions, which we discuss in the form of key lessons that have been learned so far.

There is a need to define 'community participation' at the outset of an intervention

Preston et al. (2010) carried out a research synthesis of empirical studies that sought to link rural community participation and outcomes. They found that only a few studies presented robust evidence of the benefit of community participation in terms of health outcomes. They noted that programmes had frequently failed to formulate realistic outcomes of what could be achieved and that without such clarity it would be challenging to measure whether they had met their goals. They further showed that even in those cases where the terms had been clarified at the beginning of an intervention, the outcomes tended to be context specific and not generalizable. There have been many different approaches to involving communities and the term community participation has been defined and theorized in many different ways (Kenny et al., 2013); we will come back to this issue below.

It cannot be assumed that people have the desire to be involved in decisions about their own health care

One driving force behind the Alma Ata Declaration was the assumption that people have the desire to be involved in decisions about the planning and implementation of their health care. Yet available evidence suggests that people, individuals and communities do not prioritize health care unless they have health problems. For example, McCoy, Hall & Ridge (2012), in a systematic review of health facility committees with community representation in low- and middle-income countries, concluded that members of the community did not want to be involved in decision-making about health care as such but rather they wanted access to care when they needed it. Priorities may be on more immediate needs such as food production, education or income generation, especially in low-resource settings, and there are often unrealistic expectations about the ability of the poor and marginalized to participate (Rifkin, 1985; Brett, 2003). Encouraging people to get involved in the planning or oversight of the delivery of services that are outside their personal health concerns has been shown to be difficult in both low- and middle-income countries (McCoy, Hall & Ridge, 2012; Rifkin, 2012) as well as in high-income settings (Carter, Tregear & Lachance, 2015; Farmer et al., 2015). For example, a recent cross-sectional study of the general population's desire to be involved in health care decisions in Sweden and England found that among those surveyed, only 44% reported wanting to be involved in local decisions about the organization and provision of services (Fredricksson & Tritter, 2017). Importantly, the study also found that individuals who wanted to make their own treatment decisions were also more likely to want to be involved in organizational decision-making. Available evidence has also highlighted the complexity of involving community people in activities dominated by health professionals. These complexities most often include dealing with local politics and ultimately power relationships.

It cannot be assumed that providing information to people about how to improve their health will result in positive behaviour change

There has been a long-standing assumption that providing health education and information will help people to change behaviour towards improved health. Examples include mass campaigns that historically were often focused on the control of disease and led by health professionals with little or no contribution from the intended beneficiaries (Gonzales, 1965). Mobilization efforts expanded following the 1978 Alma Ata Declaration, promoting 'community participation' in, for example, immunization uptake and acceptance of family planning. This largely profession-led approach was, however, challenged by the 1986 Ottawa Declaration (World Health Organization, 1986), which recognized that to ensure sustainable change, people needed to be empowered to engage in critical thinking and gain confidence through making their own decisions on actions and commitment. Defined as 'providing opportunities for those without power to gain knowledge, skills and confidence to make choices about their own lives' (Rifkin & Pridmore, 2001), the term 'empowerment' has come to replace 'participation', drawing attention to the need for active participation and transformation of thinking in order to create sustainable health changes (DeVos et al., 2009)

It cannot be assumed that once empowered, people will act the way professionals think they should

Experience not only in the field of health suggests that although empowerment is recognized as important, once communities are empowered they do not necessarily follow the expectations of those who facilitated this process. Whether the expected results are achieved depends on a number of factors, including leadership, trust, bonding with facilitators, compassion and building of partnerships (Rifkin, 2009), among others. This can be illustrated by the example of village health (or development) committees in low-income countries (McCoy, Hall & Ridge, 2012). There is an assumption that these committees would give the local population a 'voice' in decisions about health care delivery. However, available evidence suggests that these committees have had difficulty in fulfilling this role. For example, analysing community participation through facility boards and committees in the development and implementation of council health plans in Tanzania, Kilewo & Frumence (2015) identified several challenges, including lack of experience of committee members, lack of awareness about the role of the committee in the wider population, poor communication among committee members and officials, and lack of finances to carry out chosen projects. This highlights that it can be difficult to ensure that the desired results of empowerment actually lead to the expected outcomes. Power is about control and it is challenging in all circumstances.

Table 5.1 summarizes the key assumptions underlying the contribution of community participation in health as identified by Rifkin (2012). Taken together, this points to an overarching assumption about the nature of human agency, which conceives of human action to be uniform and predictable and that the provision of information will lead to behaviour change. Commonly referred to as the 'rational choice' model, this understanding of human action has, however, been shown not to be very effective in achieving sustained behaviour change (see, for example, National Institute for Health and Care Excellence, 2007). A large body of social science literature attests to the complexity of human actions and the ways in which not only agency, but also community participation and decision-making are embedded in particular social

Table 5.1 *Assumptions underlying the contribution of community participation in health: a summary*

Assumption	Experiences
Communities It is not necessary to define 'community' and/ or 'participation' before a participation process begins	Without clarification of underlying concepts and expectations, programmes will have difficulty in clearly stating objectives and thus have been unable to make rigorous evaluations. There have been many different approaches to involving communities and the term has been defined and theorized in many different ways.
Motivation People want to be involved in decisions relating to their health care	People's motivations are complex and often context specific.
Behaviour Giving people information will change their actions	Available evidence shows that the provision of information alone has limited impact and that any change achieved is rarely sustained over time.
Empowerment	Once given a role in decision-making about health care, people often do not act the way professionals think they should.

Source: based on Rifkin, 2012

and political contexts. Even apparently small differences in local contexts can influence both the process and the outcomes of participatory interventions (Derges et al., 2014). In the following section we discuss examples that illustrate the complexity and unpredictability of public participation in health systems development.

Constructs and rationales for community participation

"Community engagement [aka participation] is an umbrella term that encompasses a range of different approaches to involving communities of place and/or interest in activities aiming to improve health and/or reduce health inequalities. It therefore refers to an eclectic arena of

*activity with no single defining value base and no specific formal qual-
ifications for practitioners."*

(Popay, 2006, p. 2)

There are no standard definitions of 'community' or 'participation'. While in health promotion there is a broad acceptance that communities often constitute groups of people with common interests and/or identities, such as people with disabilities or the LGBT (lesbian, gay, bisexual and transgender) community, elsewhere community is most often defined in terms of people living within a given geographic area (MacQueen et al., 2001). Participation too has many definitions and as Popay (2006) stresses, it is important to recognize that the broad rubric of 'community participation' covers many different ways in which communities can be involved in health systems development, which are underpinned by differing sets of values and theoretical constructs. There is a vast literature on community participation, with contributions from many different academic disciplines including political science, sociology, anthropology development studies, psychology, public administration, communication studies and so forth, each of which conceptualizes participation in a different way.

Rifkin (1985), in an early analysis of community participation models in South-East Asia, and taking the perspective of planners, described different approaches to help understand how community participation has been implemented (Table 5.2). Importantly, her work highlighted early on that community participation is a process and not an intervention (Rifkin, 1996), which is core to identifying the challenges related to establishing a direct link between community participation and improved health outcomes. These challenges have been theorized in a number of ways. For example, Marent, Forster & Nowak (2012), in a review of community participation in the field of health promotion, identified seven social theories that have been used in the literature to articulate the function and process of community participation (critical theory, critical pedagogy, post-structuralism, social theory, political philosophy, critiques of modernity, and actor network theory). They found that the different theories provide different answers to and perspectives on key questions of participation in terms of the function of participation within specific social and political contexts, how lay actors are constituted as agents, and how the process of participation itself is understood.

Table 5.2 *Conceptual approaches to community participation in health*

Approach	Interpretation	Underlying rationale
Medical approach	Defines health as the absence of disease and participation as 'having people do what professionals ask'; often referred to as community mobilization	Utilitarian
Health service approach	Defines health as "the physical, mental and social well-being of the individual" (World Health Organization, 1948) and participation as community contribution in the form of time, materials and money to a project as defined by professionals	Combination of utilitarian and normative/ empowerment
Community development approach	Defines health as a human condition and participation as the planning and managing of activities by the community with professionals providing resources and facilitation	Normative/ empowerment

Source: Rifkin, 1985

Embedded within these different theoretical constructs of community participation are also differing rationales in terms of what are seen as the reasons for and benefits of community participation. Morgan (2001) identified two dominant rationales, the utilitarian model and the empowerment model. The utilitarian model argues that the reason for involving communities in the design of health services is that there is some demonstrable gain in efficiency and/or cost reduction. Others have referred to this as the substantive rationale, that is, participation will lead to better decision-making and to more effective health services by incorporating public or community views, and the instrumental rationale, namely people are more likely to accept decisions if they have had a role in making them (Fiorino, 1990). Alternatively, the empowerment rationale is based on the normative assumption that people and communities have the right to be involved in those decisions that affect them and their lives irrespective of demonstrable gains, and further that this process will empower them. It broadly equates to the democratic rationale that emphasizes the importance of equity and empowerment and their value in society (Wait & Nolte, 2006). There is also a consumerist perspective, which draws upon economic theory and the importance of consumer choice in enhancing not only markets, but service provision (Wait & Nolte, 2006). It is not possible to reconcile these different models of participation because they are based on different sets of values, but it illustrates the complex and contested nature of participation.

Most policy documents advocating community participation contain a mix of these different rationales, but differing approaches to and rationales for participation can give rise to tensions. These tensions in part derive from contrasting ideological and political values and also from concepts of citizenship (Martin, 2008). For instance, is the purpose and value of community participation only to improve the efficiency of service delivery by improving uptake of interventions, or should it be linked with broader concerns, such as equity, the reduction of health inequalities, governance and citizenship (Cornwall & Gaventa, 2001; Rifkin, 2003; Sen, 1999)? Another recurring source of tension is the issue of power, and specifically the extent to which it is or should be devolved to community members (Morgan, 2001; Nelson & Wright, 1995). This issue has been the focus of much critical commentary, particularly the backlash against participatory development as promoted by agencies such as the World Bank, in which, it was argued, participation had been co-opted as a technocratic solution that excluded the wider issues of poverty and inequality (see, for example, Cooke & Kothari, 2001). Others also point to unrealistic expectations regarding the ability of the poor and socially marginalized to participate in such programmes (Brett, 2003).

However, there is not merely the challenge of providing a standard definition of community participation and a standard theoretical approach within the context of health systems. Members of the public (community) may occupy very different roles, possibly simultaneously, as users, patients, consumers or citizens including community leaders and professionals themselves. Each of these roles carries with it different reasons for involvement, with implications for the mechanisms of involvement and their impact on decision-making (Callaghan & Wistow, 2006; Fredricksson & Tritter, 2017). We have highlighted earlier the common assumption that there is a desire among people to get involved in decision-making, but this cannot be taken for granted. Motives for wanting to be involved are also complex and can be conceptualized in different ways.

Experiences of community participation in health system design and development

As we have noted in earlier sections of this chapter, there is renewed interest in community participation internationally and within Europe. The World Health Organization has placed community participation as central to the improvement of primary health care (World Health Organization, 2008b) and integrated health services (World Health Organization, 2015), as well as to reducing inequalities in health (World Health Organization, 2008a). Within the context of Europe, the Council of Europe (2000) recommended that all member states should ensure citizen participation in all aspects of the health care systems from local to national levels and create structures to ensure this goal is achieved. To facilitate this, World Health Organization Europe has also produced a number of manuals on how to achieve community participation in health services (see, for example, World Health Organization Europe, 2002; Ferrer, 2015).

In this section, we explore a range of experiences in European settings that illustrate the different conceptualizations and rationales for community participation in health system design and development as described above. It is beyond the scope of this chapter to provide a comprehensive overview of the entire spectrum of experiences of community participation in health service design across European countries. Many experiences, particularly those at local level, are not formally documented and/or available in languages other than English. For these reasons, we mainly draw upon a number of recent systematic reviews of participation and related concepts: Conklin, Morris & Nolte (2015); Crawford et al. (2002); Dalton et al. (2016); Milton et al. (2012); Mockford et al. (2012); Ocloo & Matthews (2016); Tempfer & Nowak (2011). We also consider comparative overviews of approaches from a range of European countries as for example provided by the World Health Organization (World Health Organization Europe, 2006; World Health Organization, 2015) and the European Institute for Public Participation (European Institute for Public Participation, 2009).

It should be noted that within the published literature of studies on European experiences, examples from the United Kingdom dominate, perhaps reflecting the policy emphasis on public involvement in service delivery especially under the Labour government of 1997–2010 and its programme of public sector reform, which is perhaps best typified by the 2002 Wanless Report on the NHS that stressed the importance of increasing public engagement (Wanless, 2002). In addition, as indicated, there is a bias towards English-speaking countries generally, including the United States, Canada and Australia.

At the outset it is important to note that community participation in the context of health service design and delivery is very variable in terms of who is engaged, for what, how and why, and we examine these issues in turn.

Who is involved?

The majority of approaches to community participation that are documented in the literature focus on groups with shared health concerns. Groups whose participation has been sought include patients' groups who share a common illness (for instance, those with cancer or those who are HIV positive), users of specific services (for instance, primary care and maternity services), social groups who are seen as vulnerable (for instance, older people and those with mental illnesses), and hard-to-reach or disenfranchised groups (for instance, the LGBT community and the Roma). Participants are variously described as users, clients, consumers, citizens, patients, lay and/or community members, and these terms are often used interchangeably. The reasons for which involvement is sought are similarly varied and range from the narrow (for instance, how to improve the access to particular services) through to involvement in wider decision-making (for instance, regarding service reorganizations, budget allocations and possible hospital closures).

Why are people involved?

A wide range of methods or activities is used to involve people: focus groups, interviews, consultation meetings and workshops, citizens' juries/panels, and membership of boards or committees. Running through these experiences is a mix of the differing rationales that were described above. The utilitarian rationale appears to dominate, with the expectation that community participation will make things 'work better' in some way, but also the normative rationale that people have a right to be involved and the instrumental rationale that communities are more likely to accept decisions they have been involved in. In contrast, the empowerment rationale is less often mentioned, although in England patient empowerment has been a key element of the NHS Realising the Value Programme launched in 2014 (Wood et al., 2016).

What approaches are being used to involve communities?

The reviews considered in this chapter also show a mix of the approaches as defined by Rifkin (1985) (Table 5.2), and we illustrate these with three examples. Box 5.1 describes a community mobilization programme for mental health promotion among Cape Verdean immigrants in the Netherlands. This example can be seen to represent a medical approach to community participation (*see* Table 5.2), as it set out to mobilize the Cape Verdean community to engage with services as thought appropriate, but it also incorporated elements of the health service and community development approach as community members became involved in decision-making.

Box 5.2 describes a general approach to citizen participation in the Italian health care system, which illustrates a form of health services approach to community participation in which community members, as representatives of service users, were consulted and to some extent engaged as collaborators in local decision-making processes.

Box 5.1 The medical approach: community mobilization for mental health promotion among Cape Verdean immigrants in the Netherlands

Project Apoio was established in Rotterdam in 2000 to address the high rate of psychosocial problems among the small Cape Verdean community, who, while reporting a high rate of problems, were not utilizing the mental health care services available to them. The aim of the project was to engage this minority group and gain their views and insights in defining problems, designing solutions and also in decision-making. To this end, a user committee was established that included both community members and experts. The committee planned and executed various activities, such as

---

Box 5.1 (cont.)

home visits, radio programmes and organizing events to disseminate information. The project commenced as a form of mobilization in seeking the Cape Verdean community to engage with services as thought appropriate, but it also incorporated elements of the health service and community development approach as community members became involved in decision-making.

The project was deemed very successful and one of the outcomes was the creation of a therapeutic group in mental health care services designed specifically for the Cape Verdeans. Community members of the user committee also described the experience as empowering in that they felt more confident to act to improve their own lives and those of other community members. However, the project ended in 2009 due to lack of continued funding.

Source: De Freitas et al., 2014

Box 5.2 The health service approach: citizen participation in the Italian health care system

In 1994 the northern Italian region of Emilia-Romagna established mixed advisory committees in order to monitor and improve the quality of health care delivery by incorporating user perspectives. The principal membership of the committees included representatives of patients and service user associations, who were also responsible for coordinating the committees. The committees also included a minority membership of service delivery representatives (managers and health professionals). The purpose of the committees was to monitor and assess the quality of existing services from a user perspective. This approach can be considered as a health service approach in which community members, in this case representatives of service users, were consulted and to some extent engaged as collaborators.

An evaluation of the advisory committees used interviews and observations to examine the experiences of committee members and the impact of the committees in influencing the decisions of

---

Box 5.2 (cont.)

the health professionals. It found that in terms of providing a decision-space that brought together different actors, the committees were seen as successful in achieving participation and bringing together different perspectives and cultures and some successes in service delivery were achieved (e.g. reduction in waiting lists, better organization). Overall, however, most of the user and patient representatives felt that their influence on decision-making was limited. A number of constraints were identified including the unwillingness of health services managers to cede control and the commitments required of the user representatives, whose participation decreased over time.

Source: Serapioni & Duxbury, 2014

Box 5.3 illustrates what Rifkin (1985) (Table 5.2) described as the community development approach, using the example of community participation in the design of rural primary care services in Scotland, in which the responsibility for decisions regarding new service plans was delegated to the community members themselves.

Box 5.3 The community development approach: community participation in the design of rural primary care services in Scotland

This study examined a community participation process in four rural Scottish communities, the Remote Services Futures, conducted in 2008–2010 to identify local health needs and to plan new services to meet these needs. A participatory action research approach was explicitly used with the aim of not only consulting but also empowering community members. In each community, four workshops were held that moved from examining what the community considered their current and future health needs to the identification of priorities and services to meet these needs within a designated budget. Health professionals also attended some of the workshops to share information with community members,

Box 5.3 (cont.)

but the responsibility for decisions regarding new service plans was delegated to the community members themselves as in the community development or empowerment model of participation.

While the health delivery priorities in the early stages of the consultation process were very similar across all four communities, the communities engaged very differently and this led to different outcomes. Thus, one community decided to replicate their existing service as it met their needs, while two other communities developed new service plans to meet their local needs. The fourth community, however, withdrew from the final part of the process in which the new service models were designed and failed to develop a plan. The precise reasons for the withdrawal were unclear, with various external factors such as the weather and venue given as explanations, but it was also suggested that community members felt that participation represented a form of compliance or collusion with the health authority and the imposition of top-down changes. This example illustrates the need to understand local contexts and the complex reasons community members have to engage or to choose to not engage. It also shows that the process of community participation can be 'messy' and the outcomes unpredictable.

Source: Farmer & Nimegeer, 2014

How do different European countries approach 'community participation'?

The European Institute for Public Participation presented, in 2009, a review of European experiences in public participation with a focus on Germany, Italy and the UK. It found that while there were mechanisms for public participation in all countries and across a number of different sectors, including health system governance, the experiences and expectations varied greatly, reflecting different cultural contexts and political structures. This, and similar reviews, such as that by the Ninth Futures Forum (World Health Organization Europe, 2006), show that public participation, as it is practised, can be very variable in terms of the rationales and the approaches taken. For instance, in the UK many public policies relating to health care now set out a formal and legal requirement for people (described variously as patients, citizens, users, consumers and communities) to be involved and consulted in various aspects of health care delivery from all levels from national to local (Martin, Carter & Dent, 2018; NHS England, 2015). In comparison, public participation in the health system in France can be seen to be more limited, although patients and their representatives may participate in regional health conferences in defining public health priorities at the regional level, including development of the regional strategic health plan. The 2016 Health Reform Law has put in place mechanisms to further strengthen public involvement in health systems development (Chevreul et al., 2015).

As noted earlier in this chapter, the perceived value of community participation in health systems development is based on a series of assumptions, including an assumed desire of community members to be involved and how they will respond once engaged (Wait & Nolte, 2006). The process by which individuals participate, their motives and any benefits that may accrue to them remain largely unexamined[1], although a small number of empirical studies points to the complexity of people's reasons and subjective benefits gained. Fienig et al. (2012), in a study of citizen participation in the Netherlands, found that participants had multiple motives to take part in a health promotion programme, some of which related to personal benefits (achieving a sense of purposeful action, self-development and enhanced sense of status) and others that were more altruistic (making a contribution to others). In another European study, Van Eijk & Steen (2016) explored citizen participation in a number of different public service projects, including health service delivery, which comprised client councils in health care for older people in the Netherlands, and user councils for the health care of people with disabilities in Belgium. The authors found that people's reasons for participating combined a mix of self-interest and altruism. They argued for the need to understand the interplay between personal characteristics, including feelings of self-efficacy, and characteristics of the wider community, such as social capital, with high levels of social connectedness providing both opportunities and constraints to

---

1 There is a large body of literature on volunteerism, however, which shows the complexity of people's reasons for volunteering, the benefits that accrue to people from volunteering and factors that might influence this. See for example, Haddad (2004), Jenkinson et al. (2013) and Weng & Lee (2016).

participation. While positive benefits may be gained for individuals, a rapid review by Attree et al. (2011) of the experiences of community participation for individuals found that there were also some unintended negative consequences, such as stress and tiredness caused by demands placed upon people. These findings echo the argument of Brett (2003) that some community participation programmes fail because of unrealistic and sometimes excessive demands on the ability of the poor and marginalized in particular to participate.

The multiple definitions of and differing approaches to community participation make it challenging to draw any robust conclusions on the outcomes of community participation. A major reason is that most examples do not clearly specify the type of participation achieved and who participated (e.g. representatives of health care users or ordinary citizens), which makes it difficult to link participation with the intended outcomes (Conklin, Morris & Nolte, 2015). Also, few experiences are formally evaluated and documented. That said, one broad finding which is consistent across all of the reviews cited here is that community participation can make a difference, but not always. Findings are not sufficiently consistent to suggest that any particular approach is more or less successful. Indeed, Milton et al. (2012) concluded that while some studies show positive impacts on some elements of service delivery, such as planning, the evidence is not conclusive, in part due to the multiple influences on service delivery. Tempfer & Nowak (2011) also advised caution, but they identified a number of factors that can be associated with positive outcomes, including appropriate financing of the initiative, logistics, and systems of communication, and partnerships with relevant organizations. Importantly, while there is lack of clear empirical evidence on the outcomes of participation, as Conklin, Morris & Nolte (2015) pointed out, we must not lose sight of the other reasons for public participation, namely the democratic, empowerment and normative rationales that people have a right to be involved and that the process of participation can have its own benefits and intrinsic value.

Lessons from experiences of community participation in health systems development

Experiences of community participation in health systems development as described in the preceding sections mirror the observations discussed in earlier parts of this chapter, which are relevant to policy-makers, planners, managers and service providers who wish to strengthen community participation in health systems.

First, community participation in health systems development has been interpreted differently in different system contexts. Much of the early work around community participation originates from low- and middle-income countries as we have highlighted in earlier sections of this chapter, whereas in high-income settings the discussion has focused more on the involvement of people in the decision-making processes at levels ranging from the local to the national depending on the national context. There are a number of rationales behind pursuing participation as noted, but it is not always recognized that differing rationales have consequences for how a participation process might be designed and implemented and how the outcomes (if any) are used (or not). Similarly, the terms patient, user, consumer, citizen, community and public are often used interchangeably without recognizing that each of these framings implies different roles and reasons for their engagement (*see also* Chapter 3). Especially in the context of low-resource settings, much emphasis for participation is seen in specific health service programmes, such as universal health care, although there is also concern on the broader issue of health as a human right (DeVos et al., 2009).

Second, viewing community participation as a process rather than an intervention demands a better understanding of this process. Understanding community participation as a means to move from information sharing to empowerment needs to be documented in specific situations and on a national scale. At present, much of the literature focuses on the success of programmes and does not document failures. As a result, important lessons about the process and its challenges are missing.

Third, the utilitarian rationale to community participation is promoted by the neo-liberal environment that has dominated many countries over recent decades. It is based on the assumption that enhancing participation will lead to more (cost-)effective services and systems. Yet as we have seen, the evidence that community participation will lead to, say, more effective service delivery remains, at best, patchy. There is thus a need to be explicit, from the outset, as to what a given strategy is seeking to achieve and, importantly, the approach that will be most suited to achieve the objectives. We have found that the medical approach and health service approach tend to dominate practice while the community development approach often dominates the rhetoric. As a result, not only is the process top-down rather than bottom-up but it is also controlled by professionals rather than communities challenging empowerment goals.

Fourth, a continued lack of conceptual clarity regarding both the nature and the purpose of community participation makes it hard to draw any firm conclusions regarding its role in achieving improved health outcomes or in improving health service design and development. Much of the writing on the contribution of community participation in low- and middle-income countries has sought to use the randomized controlled trial design as the evaluation framework (Rifkin, 2014). This approach has been criticized because it is difficult to meet the criteria of reliability and replicability of outcomes as standard definitions of 'community' and 'participation' do not exist. It remains difficult to reconcile the demands of scientific rigour with evidence from case studies and systematic reviews. There is the tension between documenting a process that is context specific and one which is seeking to identify generalizations that can be used to scale up programmes. This dilemma is one which is found in complex interventions in health.

A way forward

As this chapter shows, identifying, understanding and replicating the outcomes of community participation in health systems development are not simple. Mansuri & Rao (2013) noted, in the context of low- and middle-income countries, that the evidence for benefits of participation in public service programmes are mainly based on optimism and ideology, and they highlighted the need for more robust evidence on the outcomes and impacts of participation. The reviewed experiences provide pointers to ways to evaluate and implement the loosely documented but clearly perceived benefits of community participation for improved outcomes in people's health. The following suggests a way forward.

First, there is a need to understand the context, history and culture of those who are meant to benefit from participation. Available evidence does not allow for generalizations about the contribution of community participation to health improvements particularly in service development, design, implementation and evaluation. There is a need for policy-makers, programme managers and community people to agree on a definition of community and participation and on theoretical concepts and approaches to inform the design and implementation of community participation in health programmes. Because of the difficulty in providing a standard definition of these terms and a common theoretical context, this agreement might be best done in the context of a specific programme. While there is no blueprint to ensure that community participation will produce predictable and positive successes, it is possible to learn from the various experiences that we have illustrated here to create a programme-specific definition of terms to identify programme objectives, processes and outcomes.

Second, there is a need to promote empowerment by involving people and to recognize the role of power and control. An often not stated but implicit goal of participation is to ensure changes are sustainable. This requires ownership of the intervention by the community (targeted or inclusive) rather than imposition by policy-makers or professionals. For this reason, it is imperative to examine questions about power and control to ensure that participatory interventions do not unintentionally reinforce potentially harmful social structures and actions that are inherent in community participation (George et al., 2015). Marston et al. (2016) explicitly identified power-sharing as key to enable a transformation of community action to foster new relationships and systems capable of identifying, acting upon and sustaining health improvements envisioned by those promoting community participation. There is thus a need for better documentation of successes and failures of community participation in health systems development to help inform the design and implementation of community participation approaches.

Third, there is a need to view participation as a process and not as an intervention. The medical approach to community participation as discussed in this chapter is largely rooted in the biomedical model and tends to view community participation as an intervention. This is problematic because if community participation is aimed at truly empowering the community through community development, there is a need to consider the wider context beyond the medical model to understand community dynamics. Otherwise there is a risk that approaches to participation continue to reproduce unsuccessful experiences that view communities as a single entity that acts in accordance and consents to health inventions proposed by professionals.

Fourth, there is a need to use evaluation procedures that examine the process and identify both intended and unintended outcomes. Existing evaluations rarely identify the importance of context, history, and intended and unintended outcomes of community participation in programmes. This has changed more recently, with approaches increasingly using realist-approaches in order to assess the outcomes of health interventions in community-based services (Greenhalgh et al., 2015; Prashanth et al., 2012; Vareilles et al., 2015). However, such approaches have rarely been applied to assessing the role of community participation in health systems development.

Conclusion

This chapter has examined some of the key underlying assumptions of and different theoretical perspectives for the benefits of community participation in health systems, reviewed empirical evidence and identified challenges to assessing the contribution of community participation to health systems and people's health. It found that there is some evidence to suggest that community participation in health systems development in different settings can make beneficial contributions to health improvements (Mansuri & Rao, 2013; World Health Organization, 2015). However, there is no linear association between community participation and sustained improved health of local people and we have described a number of reasons for this.

We have shown that there is a need now to more systematically address the underlying definitional, conceptual and methodological challenges and to use frameworks that are more suited to explore participation as a complex and dynamic process and that considers the 'community' as a complex and dynamic process in itself while also taking full account of the intended beneficiaries' (i.e. the community's) ideas and preferences, including a potential choice of not wanting to be involved. The Alma Ata Declaration highlighted that the purpose of involving communities in health care and health systems development is to improve the lives of people, particularly those who have been marginalized by existing social developments. Health policy-makers, planners, managers and service providers who seek generalizable approaches can easily overlook this aim and fail to respond to the basic goals of equity and participation.

References

Atkinson JA et al. (2011). The architecture and effect of participation: a systematic review of community participation for communicable disease control and elimination. Implications for malaria. *Malaria Journal*, 10:225. Available at: http://malariajournal.com/content/10/1/225 (accessed 27 June 2017).

Attree P et al. (2011). The experience of community engagement for individuals: rapid review of evidence. *Health and Social Care in the Community*, 19(3):250–60.

Bossert TJ, Beauvais JC (2002). Decentralization of health services in Ghana, Zambia, Uganda and the Philippines: a comparative analysis of decision space. *Health Policy and Planning*, 17(1):14–31.

Boulding C, Wampler B (2010), Voice, Votes, and Resources: Evaluating the Effect of Participatory Democracy on Well-being. *World Development*, 38(1):125–35.

Brett EA (2003). Participation and accountability in development management. *Journal of Development Studies*, 40:1–29.

Callaghan GD, Wistow G (2006). Public, patients, citizens, consumers? Power and decision making in primary health care. *Public Administration*, 84(3):583–601.

Carter MW, Tregear ML, Lachance CR (2015). Community engagement in family planning in the U.S.: a systematic review. *American Journal of Preventive Medicine*, 49(2 Suppl 1):S116–23.

Chevreul K et al. (2015). France: Health system review. *Health Systems in Transition*, 17(3):1–218.

Conklin A, Morris Z, Nolte E (2015). What is the evidence base for public involvement in health-care policy: results of a systematic review. *Health Expectations*, 18(2):153–65.

Cooke B, Kothari U (2001). *The tyranny of participation*. London: Zed Books.

Cornwall A, Gaventa J (2001). From users and choosers, to makers and shapers: repositioning participation in social policy. *IDS Working Paper* 127, Brighton: IDS.

Council of Europe (2000). *Recommendation no. 5 of the committee of ministers on the development of structures for citizen and patient participation*. Strasbourg: Council of Europe Committee of Ministers.

Crawford MJ et al. (2002). Systematic review of involving patients in the planning and development of health care. *BMJ*, 325(7375):126.

Cui WY (2008). China's village doctors take great strides. *Bulletin of the World Health Organization*, 86(2):909–88.

Dalton J et al. (2016). Service user engagement in health service reconfiguration: a rapid evidence synthesis. *Journal of Health Service Research and Policy*, 21(3):195–205.

De Freitas C et al. (2014). Transforming health policies through migrant use involvement: lessons learnt from three European countries. *Psychosocial Intervention*, 23:105–13.

Derges J et al. (2014). 'Well London' and the benefits of participation: results of a qualitative study nested in a cluster randomised trial. *BMJ Open*, 4:e003596.

DeVos P et al. (2009). Health through people's empowerment: a rights-based approach to participation. *Health and Human Rights*, 11(1):23–35.

European Institute for Public Participation (2009). *Public participation in Europe: an international perspective*. Bremen: EIPP.

Farmer J, Nimegeer A (2014). Community participation to design rural primary healthcare services. *BMC Health Services Research*, 14:130–40.

Farmer J et al. (2015). An exploration of the longer-term impacts of community participation in rural health services design. *Social Science & Medicine*, 141:64–71.

Ferrer L (2015). *Engaging patients, carers and communities for the provision of coordinated/integrated health services: strategies and tools*. Copenhagen: WHO Europe.

Fienieg B et al. (2012). Why play an active role? A qualitative examination of lay citizens' main motives for participation in health promotion. *Health Promotion International*, 27:416–26.

Fiorino DJ (1990). Citizen participation and environmental risk: a survey of institutional mechanisms. *Science, Technology, & Human Values*, 15(2):226–43.

Fredricksson M, Tritter J (2017). Disentangling patient and public involvement in health care decisions: why the difference matters. *Sociology of Health & Illness*, 39(1):95–111.

George A et al. (2015). Community participation in health systems research: a systematic review assessing the state of research: the nature of interventions involved and the features of engagement with communities. *PLoS ONE*, 10(10):e0141091.

Gonzales CL (1965). *Mass campaigns and general health services*. Geneva: World Health Organization.

Greenhalgh T et al. (2015). Protocol – the RAMESES II study: developing guidance and reporting standards for realist evaluation. *BMJ Open*, 5:e0088567.

Haddad MA (2004). Community determinates of volunteer participation and the promotion of civic health: the case of Japan. *Nonprofit and Voluntary Sector Quarterly*, 33(3):8S–31S.

Jenkinson CE et al. (2013). Is volunteering a public health intervention? A systematic review and meta-analysis of the health and survival of volunteers. *BMC Public Health*, 13.

Kenny A et al. (2013). Community participation in rural health: a scoping review. *BMC Health Services Research*, 13:64.

Kilewo EG, Frumence G (2015). Factors that hinder community participation in developing and implementing comprehensive council health plans in Manyoni District, Tanzania. *Global Health Action*, 8:10.3402/gha.v8.26461.

King M (1966). *Medical care in developing countries*. Nairobi: Oxford University Press.

McCoy D, Hall JA, Ridge M (2012). A systematic review of the literature for evidence on health facility committees in low and middle-income countries. *Health Policy and Planning*, 27:449–66.

McPake B, Hanson K, Mills A (1993). Community financing in Africa: an evaluation of the Bamako Initiative. *Social Science and Medicine*, 36(11):1383–95.

MacQueen KM et al. (2001). What is Community? An evidence-based definition for participatory public health. *American Journal of Public Health*, 91(12):1929–38.

Mansuri G, Rao V (2013). *Localizing development: does participation work?* Washington, DC: World Bank.

Marent B, Forster R, Nowak P (2012). Theorizing participation in health promotion: a literature review. *Social Theory & Health*, 10:188–207.

Marston C et al. (2016). Community participation for transformative action on women's, children's and adolescents' health. *Bulletin of the World Health Organization*, 94:376–82.

Martin GP (2008). 'Ordinary people only': knowledge, representativeness, and the publics of public participation in healthcare. *Sociology of Health and Illness*, 30:35–54.

Martin GP, Carter P, Dent M (2018). Major health service transformation and the public voice: conflict, challenge or complicity? *Journal of Health Services Research & Policy*, 23(1):28–35.

Mehrotra S, Jarrett S (2002). Improving basic health service delivery in low-income countries: 'voice' to the poor'. *Social Science and Medicine*, 54:1685–90.

Milton B et al. (2012). The impact of community engagement on health and social outcomes: a systematic review. *Community Development Journal*, 47:316–34.

Mockford C et al. (2012). The impact of patient and public involvement on UK NHS health care: a systematic review. *International Journal for Quality in Health Care*, 24(1):28–38.

Morgan L (2001). Community participation in health: perpetual allure, persistent challenge. *Health Policy and Planning*, 16:221–30.

National Institute for Health and Care Excellence (2007). *Behaviour change at population, community and individual levels*. London: NICE.

Nelson N, Wright S (eds.) (1995). *Power and participatory development: theory and practice*. London: Intermediate Technology Publication.

NHS England (2015). *Planning, assuring and delivering Service Change for Patients*. London: NHS England/Operations and Delivery.

Ocloo J, Matthews R (2016). From tokenism to empowerment: progressing patient and public involvement in healthcare improvement. *BMJ Quality Safety*, 25(8):626–32.

Popay J (2006). *Community engagement and community development and health improvement: a background paper for NICE*. London: NICE.

Prashanth N et al. (2012). How does capacity building of health managers work? A realist evaluation study protocol. *BMJ Open*, 2:e000882.

Preston R et al. (2010). Community participation in rural primary health care: intervention or approach? *Australian Journal of Primary Health*, 16(1):4–16.

Rifkin SB (1985). *Health planning and community participation: case studies in South-East Asia*. Dover, NH: Croom Helm.

Rifkin SB (1996). Paradigms Lost: Toward a new understanding of community participation in health programs. *Acta Tropica*, 61:79–92.

Rifkin SB (2003). A framework linking community empowerment and health equity: it is a matter of CHOICE. *Journal of Health, Population and Nutrition*, 21:168–80.

Rifkin SB (2009). Lessons from community participation in health programs: a review of the post Alma Ata experience. *International Health*, 1:31–6.

Rifkin SB (2012). Translating Rhetoric to Reality: a review of community participation in health policy over the last 60 years. Available at: http://www.wzb.eu/sites/default/files/u35/rifkin_2012_rhetoric_to_reality_a_review_of_cp_and_health_policy.pdf (accessed 1 August 2016).

Rifkin SB (2014). Examining the links between community participation and health outcomes: a review of the literature. *Health Policy & Planning*, 29:ii98–ii106.

Rifkin SB, Pridmore P (2001). *Partners in Planning. Information, Participation and Empowerment.* London: Macmillan Education Ltd.

Sen A (1999). *Development as Freedom.* Oxford: Oxford University Press.

Serapioni M, Duxbury N (2014). Citizens' participation in the Italian health-care system: the experience of the Mixed Advisory Committees. *Health Expectations*, 17(4):488–99.

Taylor-Ide D, Taylor CE (2002). *Just and lasting change: when communities own their futures.* Baltimore: Johns Hopkins University Press.

Tempfer CB, Nowak P (2011). Consumer participation and organizational development in health care: a systematic review. *Wiener klinische Wochenschrift*, 123(13–14):408–14.

UN General Assembly (2001). Road map towards the implementation of the United Nations Millennium Declaration. Report of the Secretary-General. Available at: http://www.un.org/millenniumgoals/sgreport2001 .pdf?OpenElement (accessed 7 November 2017).

UN Sustainable Development Goals (2015). Website. Available at: http://www .un.org/sustainabledevelopment/sustainable-development-goals/ (accessed 27 June 2017).

Van Eijk C, Steen T (2016). Why engage in co-production of public service? Mixing theory and empirical evidence. *International Review of Administrative Science*, 82(1):28–46.

Vareilles G et al. (2015). Understanding the motivation and performance of community health volunteers involved in the delivery of health programs: a realist evaluation protocol. *BMJ Open, 5.*

Wait S, Nolte E (2006). Public involvement policies in health: exploring their conceptual basis. *Health Economics, Policy and Law*, 1:149–62.

Wallerstein N (2006). *What is the evidence on effectiveness of empowerment to improve health?* Copenhagen: WHO Regional Office for Europe. Available at: http://www.euro.who.int/__data/assets/pdf_file/0010/74656/E88086.pdf (accessed 7 November 2017).

Walt G (ed.) (1990). *Community Health Workers in nation programmes: Just another pair of hands?* Milton Keynes: Open University Press.

Wanless D (2002). *Securing our future health: taking a long-term view. Final Report.* London: HM Treasury. Available at: https://www.yearofcare.co.uk/ sites/default/files/images/Wanless.pdf (accessed 22 August 2016).

Weng SS, Lee JS (2016). Why Do Immigrants and Refugees Give Back to Their Communities and What Can We Learn from Their Civic Engagement? *Voluntas*, 27:509–24.

Wood S et al. (2016). *At the heart of health: realising the value of people and communities.* London: Nesta.

World Health Organization (1948). *Constitution Basic Documents.* Amended forty-fifth edition, Supplement, October 2006. Available at: http://www .who.int/governance/eb/who_constitution_en.pdf (accessed 22 August 2016).

World Health Organization (1978). *Primary Health Care.* Geneva: World Health Organization.

World Health Organization (1986). *Ottawa Charter on Health Promotion.* Geneva: World Health Organization.

World Health Organization (2008a). *Commission on the Social Determinants of Health. Closing the gap in a generation.* Geneva: World Health Organization.

World Health Organization (2008b). *World Health Report 2008 – Primary Health Care. Now More Than Ever.* Geneva: World Health Organization.

World Health Organization (2015). *People-centred and integrated health services: an overview of the evidence.* Geneva: World Health Organization.

World Health Organization Europe (2002). *Community participation in local health and sustainable development: approaches and techniques.* Copenhagen: World Health Organization Europe.

World Health Organization Europe (2006). *Futures forum on health systems governance and public participation.* Copenhagen: World Health Organization Europe.

World Health Organization Europe (2015). *Engaging patients, carers and communities for the provision of coordinated/integrated health services: strategies and tools.* Copenhagen: World Health Organization Europe.

Zakus D, Lysack L (1998). Revisiting community participation. *Health Policy and Planning,* 13(1):1–12.

6 Patient and public involvement in research

PETER BERESFORD, JASNA RUSSO

Contextualizing patient and public involvement in research

The increased interest internationally in patient and public involvement (PPI) in health and social care research cannot adequately be understood in isolation. It needs to be seen in the context of broader social and political developments. Emergence of PPI in research reflects major changes in both national and supranational politics and in grassroots social movements. Putting it in context allows us to move on from the tendency to treat participation at all levels in warm terms as like 'mom and apple pie' (Beresford & Croft, 1993). However, the complexity and ambiguity of both the practice and the conceptualization of participation also make it essential to problematize it.

This is reflected in the most recent expression of participatory democracy at the time of writing this chapter: the public referendum decision for the United Kingdom to leave the European Union. It is difficult to see how this outcome of public participation is likely to serve the economic, political or social interests of most of those who voted for this option. We perceive PPI in research as inseparable from the larger societal context in which it emerges. PPI is closely inter-related with and no less problematic than participatory democracy, or as Madden & Speed (2017) put it:

> "The normative shift toward PPI has taken place within a neoliberal policy context, the implications of which need to be explicitly considered, particularly after the Brexit referendum which has left policy makers and researchers wondering how to better appeal to a distrustful public subjected to 'post-truth' and 'dog whistle' politics."

It is important to note that there has not been one single driving force behind PPI in research. Instead at least two key sources of interest can be identified: the state and its policy-makers on one side and service users and their organizations on the other. These have emerged at different times and with different underpinning ideologies and principles.

One of the obstacles to the development and implementation of PPI in research has been the tendency to confuse and conflate these main two drivers, which can be seen to have different aims and processes. Both are critically linked with political changes taking place in the latter part of the 20th century, that is, the shift away from post-war policies of state intervention, welfarism, statist service provision and aspirations to reduce social and economic inequality, towards a more neoliberal, market-driven, globalized and individualistic politics (Beresford, 2016).

It is impossible to approach the topic of PPI in research from any neutral perspective and one can only make one's own standpoint transparent. Our approach is greatly informed and influenced by our long-term engagement in the disabled people's movement including federal and international organizations of patients, mental health service users and psychiatric system survivors. Our efforts to understand and advance PPI in research originate much more from the experiences and lessons learned from being involved than from involving. We hope that our critical approach towards various activities termed as PPI will foster further analysis, rethinking and strengthening of PPI initiatives.

Competing approaches to involvement in research

The UK has played an important pioneering role in the development of both the democratic (Beresford, 2002) or rights-based (Madden & Speed, 2017) and the consumerist (Beresford, 2002) or pragmatic and outcome-oriented PPI (Madden & Speed, 2017). However this is not to say that these two developments have not blossomed much more internationally or indeed globally.

The first of these developments was the emergence in the UK during the 1970s of emancipatory disability research (Hunt, 1981; Campbell & Oliver, 1996; Barnes & Mercer, 1997). This grew out of disabled people's dissatisfaction with their treatment at the hands of state welfare policy; their rejection of their inferior status in society; and the barriers and discrimination they faced. It resulted in the creation of the disabled people's and then other welfare service users movements (Campbell & Oliver, 1996). It was also associated with their distrust of conventional research which they saw as on the side of service providers, advancing the existing research agendas, rather than service users being able to articulate and follow their own research priorities. This model was first advanced by the disabled people's movement and relates to feminist and community education models of research (Reason & Rowan, 1981; Roberts, 1981; Oliver, 1983; Maguire, 1987; Oliver, 1990). It has had three key concerns:

- to equalize the relationships of research production between researcher and researched;
- to support the empowerment of research 'subjects' shifting their role to that of participants; and
- to achieve broader social and political change in line with the rights, demands and interests of such groups and constituencies.

The second driver of public and patient involvement in health and social care research came much later, from mainstream researchers and the service system. A significant indicator of the emergence of this interest was the establishment in 1996 of the governmental National Institute for Health Research body INVOLVE, committed to this goal (INVOLVE, 2015). Originally it was called *Consumers In NHS Research*, a title that reflects the prevailing ideological origins of such state or service system interest in public involvement in research. This approach and its ideological basis have predominated in state- and service-led approaches to user involvement in research and other aspects of social work and social policies. It is not difficult to see also how this can be consistent with market-led and even neoliberal ideological approaches to politics and policy, with both sharing consumerist values.

The first ideological approach to user involvement in research can helpfully be described as an empowerment or democratic one, where the aim is the redistribution of power and authority, away from researchers and research funders, to serve a liberatory purpose for research participants. The second is appropriately understood as a consumerist/ managerialist one (Beresford, 2002). It tends to be based on the argument that it is important to include the perspectives of people on the receiving end of research to ensure that the consumer voice is included to ensure greater research efficiency and effectiveness and to gain the benefit of user views. So here the service user and their opinions serve as an additional helpful data source for shaping and undertaking research.

If the first approach is essentially about empowerment, the second is more concerned with extraction. But confusingly, both approaches use the same language, the same terminology, the same rhetoric. This may help explain why there are so many misunderstandings, damaged hopes and unfulfilled expectations in relation to PPI in research. The reality is that it is a very different matter to be involved in research in an advisory or consultative role than it is in a controlling one and betokens very different research ends and means.

Thus PPI may be seen to serve both regressive and progressive roles in population health improvement. So, for instance, pharmaceutical companies use individual patient testimonies to maintain a narrow emphasis on treatment with medication, while user-led organizations have highlighted holistic and social approaches. How these roles of PPI are understood is also conditional on the ideological and political perspective adopted. Consumerist user involvement research, with its emphasis on consultation, market research and intelligence gathering, readily serves the purposes of outsourcing, privatizing and choice agendas, with their commitment to audit, satisfaction surveys, outcome measures and regulatory frameworks (Simmons, Powell & Greener, 2009). The same is not necessarily true for user-controlled research. Its democratizing impulse and commitment to redistribute power can lead to conflict with prevailing policy and research agendas and a sense among its advocates of being tokenized rather than truly involved. This happens when service users are expected to serve pre-defined research purposes and acquire smaller technical roles within traditional research scenarios (Russo & Stastny, 2009). We will consider these issues in more depth when discussing different forms of PPI and efforts to understand and measure its impact.

Note on terminology

Public and patient involvement is an umbrella term for activities and efforts taking place under different frameworks such as civil society and service user/consumer involvement or participation in research. The term 'patient' is often not a term of preference among those attempting to acquire other roles in research than that of the research subject. Furthermore, different understandings and practices of PPI often find their expression in the terms used. In order to present and discuss those different approaches we decided to keep those different terms throughout this chapter rather than impose consistency. The terms involvement and participation are used interchangeably in this chapter to mean the same.

PPI initiatives in research: a summary overview of selected examples

The World Health Organization's Declaration of Alma Ata from 1978 appears to be one of the first international policy documents with an explicit statement that "[t]he people have the right and duty to participate individually and collectively in the planning and implementation of their health care" (World Health Organization, 1978). As described in Chapter 5 of this volume, the uptake of this idea has been very uneven across different countries and regions, not least because of the lack of service users' and patients' organizations in many parts of the world. In those countries where such representative organizations exist, the development of PPI can primarily be traced in the implementation and evaluation of health care and is far less present in research and knowledge production (World Health Organization, 2006). The degree of inclusion of civil society and in particular patient representatives in research also varies. While in some countries PPI remains a foreign concept, in others we can already talk in terms of the 'mainstreaming' or even 'institutionalizing' of PPI in research, and we illustrate this with selected examples below in order to provide a sense of how different structures or initiatives to foster PPI emerge and what their work can look like. We choose to describe briefly two national organizations, one international, academic initiative, one international research project led by a patient organization, and one value framework developed by a national service user organization. Later on we will refer to these examples and their different purposes and origins when discussing the overall impact and future of PPI.

NIHR INVOLVE, UK

The already mentioned organization NIHR INVOLVE is a national advisory body based in the UK (INVOLVE, 2015), although its future is uncertain. Funded by the National Institute for Health Research (NIHR), this governmental initiative is unique not only because it is almost certainly the longest-established organization of its kind (founded in 1996) but also because of its international visibility, expertise and number of resources produced over the years. INVOLVE's main goal is to "support active public involvement in social care and health research" (INVOLVE, 2015) and its webpages include a rich collection of publications, webinars and clips that speak to different audiences including researchers, research funders and commissioners as well as those interested to influence research as public or patient representatives. These various resources cover a broad spectrum of topics such as guidance on how to start PPI in research and how to create training and support packages, advice on payment and recognition of public involvement, debates on assessing the impact of PPI, and others. Use of accessible language and their free availability make INVOLVE materials a helpful starting point for individuals and organizations interested in PPI in the UK and beyond. The materials include briefings for researchers about how to work in participatory ways, a toolkit for planning the cost of involvement, issues around including black and minority service users in research, a jargon buster, explanations of user-controlled research and other resources. Additionally, INVOLVE provides a directory of organizations interested in PPI, including some based outside the UK; it organizes regular conferences and provides advice. The very existence of this unique organization continues to impact internationally. INVOLVE has, for example, had an important role in developing the framework for user involvement in research in Denmark (Hørder, 2012), where the Knowledge Center for User Involvement (ViBIS) was established in 2011. Materials produced by INVOLVE also supported and underpinned early claims of mental health service users in Germany for their involvement in research (Russo, 2004).

The Patient-Centered Outcomes Research Institute (PCORI), USA

The US-based Patient-Centered Outcomes Research Institute (PCORI, 2011–2017) is a federal, non-governmental initiative. Unlike NIHR INVOLVE, it has the aims of funding health research projects that are relevant to patients in terms of the initial research questions, engaging with public and patient representatives throughout the research process, and also ensuring that the relevant outcomes will be accessible to patients to help inform their decisions. Patient and carer representatives are involved in the studies' review process together with other experts; the funding decisions are made by the organization itself with limited patient involvement. PCORI supports patient-centred outcomes research and comparative clinical effectiveness research. The research studies within these two categories tend to be conventional in their methodology. They include randomized controlled trials, pragmatic clinical studies, and observational and methodology studies. Participatory approaches, community action and collaborative research are not explicitly mentioned. PCORI started funding research in 2012 and the full list of 570 projects that this Institute had funded by the end of 2016 can be found on their website (Patient-Centered Outcomes Research Institute, 2011–2017). One investigation of the projects that PCORI funded in its early years (2011–2014) has opened up significant dilemmas about whether the scope and the mission of this organization are actually reflected in its allocation of grants (Mazur, Bazemore & Merenstein, 2016).

PCORI has also provided funding to the US Cochrane Center's initiative, Consumers United for Evidence-Based Healthcare (CUE), to help building the PCORI community among other aims (Box 6.1) (CUE, 2017).

The *Governer Board* of PCORI is in part appointed directly by the Comptroller General of the United States. It has a total of 21 members, three of whom have to be patient/consumer representatives. Additionally, PCORI has a number of committees including, for example, the Methodology Committee which "defines methodological

---

Box 6.1 Consumers United for Evidence-Based Healthcare

CUE is a national coalition of health and consumer advocacy organizations, which was established in 2003 on the initiative of the US Cochrane Center. It comprises about 40 member organizations, which are not supposed to be dominated by pharmaceutical companies or any other commercial interest. CUE seeks to promote the health of populations and the quality of health care through "empowering consumers, public health policy makers, and healthcare providers to make informed decisions" (CUE, 2017), based on the best available evidence through research, education and advocacy.

CUE focuses on training and empowering patients and their organizations in order to foster their partnerships with policymakers. They offer a number of useful online resources such as free online courses, webinars, lectures, video summaries of Cochrane reviews, etc.

standards for PCORI-funded research and guides healthcare stakeholders towards the best methods for patient-centered outcomes research".
We were not able to identify any patient representatives on this or any
other committees, nor any related rule.

International Collaboration for Participatory Health Research (ICPHR)

The International Collaboration for Participatory Health Research
(ICPHR) started in 2009 with the goal of strengthening participatory
approaches to health research in terms of its definition, enhancing its
quality and reinforcing its impact (International Collaboration for
Participatory Health Research, 2014). Besides members from Europe,
Australia, Canada, New Zealand and the USA, it brings together academic researchers also from Bangladesh, Brazil, Ghana, Mexico, Peru
and Thailand. They all address health inequalities in their work, focus
on voicing the needs of disadvantaged communities, and work in a participatory manner. ICPHR has its head office in Berlin, Germany, and
holds annual working meetings and scientific seminars. Additionally,
it provides training in participatory health research. ICPHR collabora-
tively issues position papers on topics relating to defining participatory
research, its main ethical principles, and so on. The network is coordinated by a consortium of nine academics, none of whom represents
the marginalized communities that are its main concern.

Value+. Promoting Patients' Involvement in EU-supported Health-related Projects

Funded by the European Commission's Public Health Programme, this
two-year inquiry (2008–2010) coordinated by the European Patients'
Forum (2017) aimed to enhance understanding of what constitutes
meaningful involvement of patients' organizations in European Union-
supported health projects at EU and national levels. It started with the
mapping of patient involvement in such projects, but then evolved into a
broad consultation exercise with a variety of stakeholders that led to the
production of comprehensive resources specifically tailored to different
audiences, including patient organizations, health project leaders and
policy-makers (European Patients' Forum, 2010a; 2010b; 2010c). What
was unusual about this project, in relation to other EU-funded actions, was

the leadership of patient organizations, both in its consortium and among its various partners. The outputs of *Value+* not only make a strong case for patient involvement but also explain all the requirements and steps in such processes. This project produced a range of documents including a handbook for project leaders (European Patients' Forum, 2010a), a toolkit for patient organizations (European Patients' Forum, 2010c) and policy recommendations (European Patients' Forum, 2010b). It is unclear whether and how the main messages from this unique project have been followed up in the practice or distribution of European health research funds.

4PI National Involvement Standards, UK

This framework addresses different areas of user involvement in health and social care including research and evaluation. It was developed by a group of UK mental health service users and carers (Faulkner et al., 2015a; Faulkner et al., 2015b) as a part of the *National Involvement Partnership* project (NSUN). Funded by the Department of Health, this three-year project (2012–2015) also promotes the adoption of 4PI standards by a wide range of organizations as "a means to enable services, organisations and individuals to think about how to make involvement work well" (p. 5). Based on the vision 'Nothing about us without us', this simple five-point framework easily translates across disciplines and geographic areas while addressing core issues of involvement (Box 6.2). By 2017 more than 60 UK organizations had endorsed the standards (National Survivor User Network, 2017).

Concluding observations about reviewed PPI initiatives in research

As the initiatives described above illustrate, PPI in research can be based on different points of departure and have different scopes. A top-down character is typical for the largest and most influential of such initiatives, such as PCORI in the USA. Notably, despite their best intentions, the described initiatives sometimes fail to ensure sufficient inclusion in their own work of the voices and perspectives that they seek to strengthen. This is probably most obvious in purely academic efforts such as ICPHR. On the other hand, the rare PPI projects initiated by patient organizations themselves, such as *Value+*, tend to lack the means to formally influence the decision-making processes of

---

Box 6.2 4PI Involvement Standards (NSUN)

PRINCIPLES: Meaningful and inclusive involvement depends on a commitment to shared principles and values. This includes valuing the contribution of service users and carers equally to those of professionals.

PURPOSE: The purpose of involvement should be clear and clearly communicated to everyone involved in the activity as well as the wider organization.

PRESENCE: A diversity of service users and carers should be involved at all levels and all stages of an organization or project. The people who are involved should reflect the nature and purpose of the involvement. Service users and carers should have the opportunity to be involved separately as they may have different priorities.

PROCESS: The process of involvement needs to be carefully planned in terms of issues like recruitment, communications, being offered appropriate support and training and payment, so that service users and carers, including those from marginalized communities, can get involved easily and make the best possible contribution.

IMPACT: For involvement to be meaningful, it needs to make a difference to the lives or the experiences of service users and carers.

---

mainstream research (Beresford & Croft, 2012; ENUSP, 2009). The 4PI standards of involvement provide an example of a bottom-up approach to conceptualizing involvement, which demonstrates the relevance and the potential influence of user-led involvement projects when they are adequately supported. The differences in actual power to initiate and influence changes need to be considered when assessing the impact of PPI in research because regardless of the quality of the PPI process itself, not everybody is in a position to make a real impact.

Levels of PPI in research

NIHR INVOLVE has identified three levels of PPI in health and social care research, based on the formal role of service users/patients in the research process (Royle et al., 2001). These are:

- consultation, where the input of service users is optionally added to the existing structures of research;
- collaboration, where service users and their representative organizations jointly undertake research with researchers and their organizations; and
- control, where service users design and undertake research and it is under their control throughout the entire process.

These levels have often been seen as forming a continuum from less to total user control. However, this is open to question, given the different, conflicting values that can underpin each of these approaches to PPI. Sweeney & Morgan (2009) have highlighted the shortcomings of these categories in real collaborative scenarios and include 'contribution' as an additional category, which refers to "research where service users/survivors make a significant and meaningful contribution to research but with power and decision making still residing with traditional researchers" (p. 29). Their analysis was offered in the context of mental health research, but the unequal value and status of different sources of knowledge and the resulting hierarchies in research conduct are demonstrated in all health and social care research (Glasby & Beresford, 2006). The dominance of professional expertise is an important part of the dynamics of involvement at all these levels. This dominance also extends to user-controlled research, which was historically the first way in which former research 'subjects' started taking an active part in knowledge production (Russo, 2012). Even though consultation and collaboration emerged later on, user-controlled research projects are the most difficult to find because what started as user control was often subsequently channelled into lower degrees of involvement.

The different modalities of participatory health and social care research continue to be judged against traditional criteria of what constitutes good (natural) science (Rose, 2008). Within such a working context, which extends from applications for funding to academic dissemination of findings, the greater levels of participation are frequently granted less scientific value (Beresford, 2003; Rose, 2009).

Co-production has recently been introduced as an additional concept in the development of health and social care services in order to address the power imbalances of collaboration. Adopting principles of co-production is among the explicit recommendations from the independent strategic review of public involvement in the National

Institute for Health Research (National Institute for Health Research, 2015). Advocates say:

> "Co-production is not determined by what the professional or service wants but focuses on the equal contribution of service users and communities. To ensure full collaboration, the co-production process should be about achieving equality and parity between all those involved" (National Development Team for Inclusion, 2016, p. 1).

Co-production is a concept which is applicable to research, especially regarding its main principles, including a commitment to equality, diversity, accessibility and reciprocity, as for instance elaborated by the Social Care Institute of Excellence in the UK (2013/2015). At the time of writing this chapter, INVOLVE led a project that aims to "identify how the discourse, elements and principles of co-production could be used to evolve and improve patient and public involvement in research" (INVOLVE, 2016, p. 4).

PPI at different research stages and in research structures

We have seen that PPI can be of different intensity in terms of the level of involvement. In this section we look at PPI in different phases of the research process and in related structures. The potential reach of PPI is broad; it can extend through the whole process of research, from its initiation to the dissemination of its outcomes and beyond, including:

- Identifying the topic of research and research questions
- Commissioning research
- Seeking, obtaining and managing research funding
- Undertaking the research
- Organizing and managing the research
- Collating and analysing data
- Reporting findings
- Producing publications and other outputs
- Developing and carrying out dissemination activities
- Prioritizing the outcomes and undertaking follow-up actions.

There may be PPI in none, some, or all of these stages. There may also be different degrees of such involvement, ranging from low to high. Sweeney & Morgan (2009) developed a two-dimensional illustration of the different levels of involvement at particular research stages, which offers a comprehensive overview of how user involvement can be implemented in practice. Figure 6.1 shows an *abbreviated* version

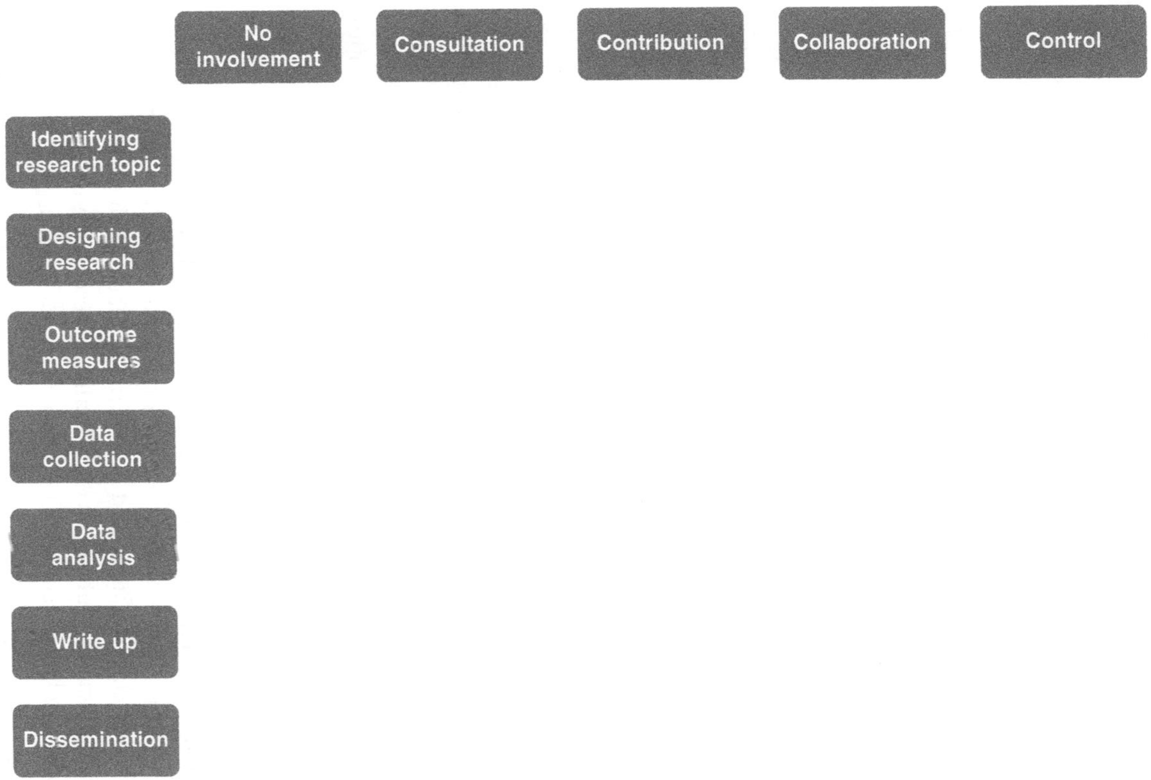

Figure 6.1 Levels and stages of service user involvement in research

Source: adapted from Sweeney & Morgan, 2009, pp. 32–3

of this model. The combinations between stages of research (vertical axis) and the intensity of user involvement (horizontal axis) may result in a multitude of research scenarios.

Public and patient involvement may not only take place in research projects, but also in the structures and institutions of research. Arguably, ensuring more of the latter is a key way of advancing the former. This can include ensuring PPI in the following research-related activities and structures:

- Identifying and setting research agendas and research priorities
- Developing research methods and methodologies
- Research funding organizations and funding decision-making processes
- Research organizations' governance
- Research training and education
- Recruitment, supervision and promotion of researchers
- Academic institutions' research strategy and research assessment
- Peer review and other selection processes for research publications/ outputs
- Editorial roles in research journals and other publications
- Organization of research events and conferences
- Speaking on research platforms.

Although examples of each of the above can be found, their occurrence is uneven. A 2015 study from England and Wales investigating PPI in different parts of the research process reported that the 'most common PPI activities' that were undertaken were being a member of the research project's advisory or steering committee and involvement in developing or reviewing patient information leaflets (Wilson et al., 2015). This suggests that PPI in research is still some distance away from being comprehensively and systematically in place, or that it represents an accepted feature of the research landscape.

With regard to different levels and stages of PPI, we wish to emphasize that none of these is more or less important than the others. If undertaken with due consideration and commitment, each of these PPI activities can significantly shift the overall quality of research both in terms of its process and its outcomes. Or as Staniszewska & Denegri (2013) put it:

> "It may be that real progress will only be marked when poor PPI is seen as a fatal flaw in a research study, something which fundamentally undermines research quality, as opposed to an optional extra" (p. 69).

Understanding the impact of patient and public involvement in research

Research impact ideally relates to changes perceived as positive in health or social care that result from research and it is usually understood as something that occurs (or does not occur) *after* a research project has been completed. In participatory research, impact additionally includes the impact of the *overall process* on those involved or as Wadsworth (1998) noted: "Change does not happen 'at the end' – it happens throughout". Generally, there is much more emphasis on positive impacts although it is known that some research can impact negatively or lead to retrograde developments in health and social care policies (Cotterell et al., 2011). The decisive question in the assessment of research, including the assessment of PPI, is about who defines the desirable impact of research. Another important aspect is the actual formal power of those in charge of research to inform and influence the practice of service delivery and enact change. Researchers frequently have little say or control in such areas.

There are opposing views on the overall impact of PPI in research. When articulated as a question whether PPI impacts the research process, the assessments are more positive. For example, the RAPPORT study of PPI in research identified "PPI related outcomes" in all of its eight case studies in different health fields, such as defining the research question, changes to study design, improvements to recruitment materials, and dissemination (Wilson et al., 2015). However, when placed in a broader context of growing health and other inequalities, the overall role and purpose of PPI is subject to growing criticism. Thus, commenting on recent developments in PPI in research in the UK, Madden & Speed (2017) noted that the range of PPI activities can be seen "as a form of busywork in which the politics of social movements are entirely displaced by technocratic discourses of managerialism" (p. 5). They concluded that PPI formed "part of a wider politics of knowledge in which patient groups, clinicians and universities are co-opted into a corporatized health research agenda [...]" (p. 5).

Different perspectives on the impact of PPI in research and its assessment are closely related to the overall approaches to participation and understanding of its scope. Perspectives range from equating impact with the number of publications in scientific journals to the issue of how empowering and transformative the overall process has been for all involved (Staley, 2009). Box 6.3 provides two examples that illustrate differences in understanding of what constitutes a good outcome of participation and collaborative research work.

Participation can be positioned within the conventional understanding of research as a primarily clinical enterprise and applied as a tool to improve specific aspects of conventional research conduct. Conversely, Oliver (1992) emphasized the social relations of research production and that these can have lasting transformative effects on everybody involved. It points to the understanding of impact as a less measurable phenomenon that can question and alter the entire research process.

Existing systematic reviews of the impact of participation in research are largely based on academic papers focusing on discussions of the impact of PPI. Although such systematic reviews can include service users in advisory roles (Brett et al., 2014b), the perspectives of those actually involved in studies within the review remain largely absent. This highlights that assessments of PPI impact tend to remain expert-dominated.

Box 6.3 Understanding the impact of research participation

Based on an analysis of patient involvement in 374 studies in mental health research in England, Ennis & Wykes (2013) highlighted the utility of patient involvement for the successful undertaking of research, noting that "[s]tudies that involved patients to a greater extent were more likely to have achieved recruitment targets ($\chi^2 = 4.58$, $P < 0.05$), defined as reaching at least 90% of the target" (p. 1).

In comparison, the disability theorist, activist and researcher Oliver (1997) emphasized the experiences of all participants as well as the broader social relations of research. His discussion of the emancipatory potential of research reminds us that impact is not a matter of easily identifiable aspects nor that there can be ready-made recipes of how to achieve research impact:

"[...] the question of doing emancipatory research is a false one, rather the issue is the role of research in the process of emancipation. Inevitably this means that research can only be judged emancipatory after the event; one cannot 'do' emancipatory research (nor write methodology cookbooks on how to do it), one can only engage as a researcher with those seeking to emancipate themselves" (p. 25).

The systematic review of PPI impact undertaken by Brett et al. (2014a) provided clear evidence that PPI impacts on all stages of the research process, from its initial stages all the way through to the implementation and dissemination stages. However, the review identified both 'beneficial' and 'challenging' impacts at all stages. In light of the above discussion about different perspectives on impact it seems notable that the review interpreted the finding that PPI "led to research findings being disseminated before the academic papers are published, thereby jeopardizing academic publication" (p. 644) as having a 'challenging' rather than a 'beneficial' impact. This takes us back to the question of whose perspective and ultimately whose interests are prioritized when assessing the impact of research. Judgements of the impact of PPI on a research process are normative.

A subsequent international systematic review of the impact of PPI focused for the first time on people involved in the research process (Brett et al., 2014b). It demonstrated that in reporting the impact of participatory research there was notably more emphasis on the personal benefits to service users directly involved in the research process than reports about how PPI might affect the larger communities that the research is about. The review highlighted the importance of both the process and the context within which PPI takes place, which may lead to positive as well as to negative impacts on people involved. These include the planning, training and adequate funding of PPI.

In this context, we wish to come back to the aforementioned framework for user involvement in health and social care including research and evaluation, the *4PI National Involvement Standards* (Faulkner et al., 2015). We find this framework helpful for the discussion of the impact of PPI not only because it centres on the perspectives of those involved but because it regards impact as part of involvement standards. As noted in Box 6.2, the framework comprises five elements or principles on which to "base standards for good practice, and to measure, monitor and evaluate involvement" (p. 8), which comprise shared values and principles; a clear purpose; the presence of service users from different backgrounds at all levels and in all aspects of the activity; carefully planned involvement process; and impact. With regard to the latter, the authors emphasize: "We are not interested in involvement for its own sake; for involvement to be meaningful, it must make a difference" (p. 11). Furthermore, the framework suggests that the impact of involvement can be continuously monitored throughout a given project, as well as assessed at the end. The framework can also helpfully be read in association with the findings on enabling fully inclusive and diverse involvement (both in research and in evaluating impact) offered by the UK Shaping Our Lives, *Beyond the Usual Suspects*, user-controlled research and development project (Beresford, 2013).

At the end of this brief overview of different understandings of PPI impact and its assessments, we wish to stress the importance of centring on the perspectives of those actually involved in the research and disrupting the dominance of solely academic and researchers' discourses on impact. The question of whether PPI will have impact or not is inseparable from the timely assessment of the entire approach to the research process, in regard to its structures and its context and the degree to which these can enable or inhibit such impact.

Methodological challenges posed by PPI in research

Neither user-controlled research nor other participatory approaches to research are narrowly associated with any particular research method. The position of the International Collaboration for Participatory Health Research (2013) is that "participatory health research is a research *approach*, not a research *method*" (emphasis in original). Participatory approaches are much better understood through their specific values and principles, which in consequence do have implications for research methods and guide the whole research process. These values and principles refer to transparency, democratizing research, equalizing research relationships and supporting change and empowerment.

As noted earlier, PPI in research has become more established in recent years. For example, in the UK many statutory and independent funders require evidence of PPI in grant proposals and research projects they support. However, there still seem to be unresolved tensions between conventional research values on one side and the idea inherent in all forms of user involvement in research on the other, namely that it is important to engage with service users'/research subjects' experience and knowledge. Traditionally research has been understood as the most systematic, rigorous, indeed scientific way of generating knowledge. It has been conceived of as an activity exclusively undertaken by people with professional expertise in the methods and methodology of research. Such research has been particularly associated with the values of neutrality, objectivity and distance from its subject (Beresford, 2003).

The 'unbiased value-free' position, based on the professional expertise of the researcher, is seen as a central tenet of such research. By claiming to eliminate the subjectivity of the researcher, the credibility of the research, and the rigour, reliability and replicability of its findings are seen to be maximized. The introduction of *experiential knowledge* into research that came about with PPI, to which traditional research principles grant less value and credibility, can be seen to be at odds with such thinking. Experiential knowledge is understood as knowledge that comes from lived experience rather than from professional training or research and experiment. This type of knowledge can take individual and collective forms. Its inclusion in research continues to be a major challenge to the acceptance of PPI in research, particularly user-controlled research, with its overtly political purposes of bringing about change in line with the rights and needs of research participants as law and the participants themselves define them.

At the same time, the devaluing of experiential knowledge in much traditional research has increasingly come to be seen as problematic. This issue of marginalizing the knowledge of particular vulnerable groups has begun to be talked about in terms of 'epistemic violence' (Liegghio, 2013) or 'epistemic injustice' (Fricker, 2010), meaning devaluing and marginalizing the knowledge of people who suffer abuse, discrimination and oppression. PPI in research thus raises the uncomfortable issue of including experiential knowledge centrally and on equal terms with other kinds of knowledge. It means working towards achieving epistemic justice and ensuring that everybody can contribute to creating a general knowledge base and that perspectives of entire social groups are no longer excluded from that process. We are beginning to see the real involvement of ordinary and disadvantaged people in research, for example people with learning difficulties, who communicate differently or experience dementia (Faulkner, 2004). There is also a growing body of, and discussion about, user-controlled research where people who have traditionally been the objects of research are now carrying out their own research and so restoring their epistemic existence (Beresford & Croft, 2012).

However, if PPI in research is to develop effectively as part of the mainstream, then it will need to be evaluated carefully and thoroughly and from different perspectives. It is only in this way that we are likely to receive a reliable picture of its strengths and weaknesses and potential impact. This needs to be a process of evaluation in which service users, their organizations, research participants and user researchers, alongside other stakeholders, are involved fully and equally drawing on their plural criteria. Such comprehensive assessment of participation should extend to exploring developments internationally, considering specific political, economic and cultural contexts.

Ensuring diverse involvement in research

One reason for the development of schemes for participation has been the realization that less powerful groups and groups facing discrimination are often excluded from conventional arrangements for political and policy decision-making. However, the evidence indicates that the same problem arises with arrangements for involvement. The aforementioned UK Shaping Our Lives project (Beresford, 2013) has highlighted just how many groups tend to remain excluded from participatory initiatives. Five key groups of service users were identified, excluded on the basis of:

- *equality issues*, for example, in relation to ethnicity, gender, age, sexuality, disability, culture, class or faith;
- *where they live*, for example, if homeless, in the penal system, without citizenship rights or in residential institutions;
- *communicating differently*, for example, non-verbally, through sign language or where the national language is not their first language;
- *the nature of their impairments*, if these are complex, multiple or seen as costly to ensure access; and
- *being seen as unwanted voices*, who may express critical or negative opinions.

In the context of research, there still seem to be major barriers in the way of some groups of service users undertaking or being involved in research, reflecting broader problems in user involvement. At the same time the argument that service users are not a homogeneous group and the issue of representativeness (Crepaz-Keay, 1996) continues to be used by critics of PPI research.

There is particularly a need for work on improving access to under-take such research with older people, ethnic service users from racialized groups, and refugees and asylum seekers. These are important gaps, first because older people are the largest and fastest growing group of health and social care service users and second, because people from black and minority ethnic communities are known to have poorer access to health and social care support and to be more likely to receive devalued and compulsory services than valued and highly regarded ones (Care Quality Commission, 2010; Centre for Social Justice, 2011). The use of the term 'hard to reach' has been thoroughly criticized in this context and in relation to public involvement more generally (Brackertz, 2007; Kalathil, 2013). Rather than focusing on factors that foster or inhibit involvement, identifying certain groups and communities as 'hard to reach' locates the problem within those groups and communities. Kalathil (2013) analyses such an approach and its ultimate implication that "they are the problem and not the ways in which the involvement is defined or undertaken" (p. 123). We agree with this author in her conclusion that

> "No communities are, by definition, 'hard to reach'. However, [...] there are practices, prejudices, belief systems and experiences that collude to create exclusion of some communities from involvement initiatives [...]" (p. 131).

Shifting the culture of participation – always thinking in terms of whose voices are absent or treated as if they are 'hard to hear', and what needs to be done in order to reach and include them on equal terms – remains one of the central tasks for the future of public and patient involvement in research.

Next steps for PPI in research

Public and patient involvement in research has emerged as a significant new research approach internationally in a relatively short time. It has pioneered research in new areas and resulted in a very diverse range of research projects, involving a wide range of citizen and service user groups (Faulkner, 2010). At the same time, it continues to face major practical, theoretical and philosophical challenges. Serious questions are still raised about both its quality and sustainability. Strategies will need to be developed to address issues of its current limited credibility, its inadequate and inferior funding and what have been described as 'incidents of direct discrimination during the course' of research projects (Beresford & Croft, 2012). A series of steps can be identified for placing PPI research on a firmer, better established and better evidenced basis. These include:

- *strengthening the theoretical basis of research with PPI* to better address criticisms of its principles and approach;

- *building research education and training,* both to support the development of PPI and user-controlled research and to help those likely to be affected by research more generally gain a better understanding of such participatory approaches;
- *rationalizing welfare benefits.* Although involvement in research can offer some service users routes into paid and unpaid work, the direction of travel of the benefits systems currently increasingly obstructs rather than supports this and requires reform;
- *equalizing access to funding.* At present, PPI research, particularly user-controlled research, receives a disproportionately low level of funding and this needs to be reviewed in the light of what it may have to offer;
- *comprehensively evaluating PPI in research and especially user-controlled research,* involving service users and their organizations in the process to gain a better understanding of these approaches, including in an international context;
- *addressing diversity.* There still seem to be barriers in the way of many groups of people becoming involved in research, reflecting broader problems in participation work. More needs to be done to improve access to undertake such research for older people, black and minority ethnic service users, and refugees and asylum seekers;
- *fostering user-controlled organizations.* User-controlled organizations provide a particularly supportive home for user-controlled research. At present they are under-developed, under-resourced and insecure. Creating policy to strengthen their position is key to securing the development and future of PPI and user-controlled research;
- *ensuring greater PPI in research structures.* Its proponents need to be ensured equal access to research publications, peer review processes, grant funding systems, and identifying barriers and ways of overcoming them; and
- *building alliances and sharing knowledge.* There is a need to improve the sharing of learning from PPI and user-controlled research. Building new networks and relationships and enhancing means of exchange across countries is likely to help with this.

Taken together, these proposals offer a set of building blocks for developing a strategy for critiquing, evaluating and advancing patient and user involvement in research, a strategy which must itself be fully and equally participatory.

References

Barnes C, Mercer G (eds.) (1997). *Doing Disability Research*. Leeds: Disability Press.

Beresford P (2002). User Involvement in Research and Evaluation: Liberation or Regulation. *Social Policy & Society*, 1:95–105.

Beresford P (2003). *It's Our Lives: a short theory of knowledge, distance and experience*. London: Citizen Press in association with Shaping Our Lives.

Beresford P (2013). Beyond the Usual Suspects: Towards inclusive User Involvement – Research Report. Available at: http://www.shapingourlives .org.uk/documents/BTUSReport.pdf (accessed 22 December 2016).

Beresford P (2016). *All Our Welfare: Towards Participatory Social Policy*. Bristol: Policy Press.

Beresford P, Croft S (1993). *Citizen Involvement: a practical guide For Change*. Basingstoke: Palgrave Macmillan.

Beresford P, Croft S (2012), User Controlled Research. Scoping review. Available at: http://sscr.nihr.ac.uk/PDF/ScopingReviews/SSCR-Scoping-Review_5_web.pdf (accessed 27 June 2018).

Brackertz N (2007). Who is hard to reach and why? ISR working paper. Available at: http://researchbank.swinburne.edu.au/vital/access/manager/ Repository/swin:6419 (accessed 14 September 2016).

Brett J et al. (2014a). A Systematic Review of the Impact of Patient and Public Involvement on Service Users, Researchers and Communities. *Patient*, 7:387–95.

Brett J et al. (2014b). Mapping the impact of patient and public involvement on health and social care research: a systematic review. *Health Expectations*, 17:637–50.

Campbell J, Oliver M (1996). *Disability Politics: Understanding Our Past, Changing Our Future*. London: Routledge.

Care Quality Commission (2010). Monitoring the use of the Mental Health Act in 2009/10. Available at: http://www.cqc.org.uk/sites/default/files/ documents/cqc_monitoring_the_use_of_the_mental_health_act_in_200910_ main_report_tagged.pdf (accessed 22 December 2016).

Centre for Social Justice (2011). Completing the Revolution: transforming mental health and tackling poverty. Available at: http://www .centreforsocialjustice.org.uk/library/completing-revolution-transforming-mental-health-tackling-poverty (accessed 22 December 2016).

Cotterell P et al. (2011). Service User Involvement in Cancer Care: the impact on service users. *Health Expectations*, 14:159–64.

Crepaz-Keay D (1996). Who do You represent? In: Read J, Reynolds J (eds.) *Speaking Our Minds. An anthology.* London: MacMillan Press Ltd.

Consumers United for Evidence-based Healthcare (CUE) (2017). *CUE Clearinghouse: Opportunities for Consumer Engagement* [Online]. Available at: http://us.cochrane.org/cue-clearinghouse-opportunities-consumer-engagement (accessed 27 June 2018).

Ennis L, Wykes T (2013). Impact of patient involvement in mental health research: longitudinal study. *British Journal of Psychiatry,* 203:381–6.

ENUSP (2009). Nothing about us without us. How to make this a reality? Report of the Empowerment Seminar, 13–14 March 2009 in Brussels. *Empowerment seminar jointly organised by Mental Health Europe and the European Network of (ex-)Users and Survivors of Psychiatry.* Available at: http://enusp.org/wp-content/uploads/2016/05/empow-seminar2009.pdf (accessed 13–14 March 2009).

European Patients' Forum (2010a). The Value+ Handbook for Project Co-ordinators, Leaders and Promoters on Meaningful Patient Involvement. Available at: http://www.eu-patient.eu/globalassets/projects/valueplus/doc_epf_handbook.pdf (accessed 22 December 2016).

European Patients' Forum (2010b). The Value+ Policy Recommendations. Patient Involvement in Health Programmes and Policy. Available at: http://www.eu-patient.eu/globalassets/projects/valueplus/doc_epf_policyrec.pdf (accessed 22 December 2016).

European Patients' Forum (2010c). The Value+ Toolkit for Patient Organisations on Meaningful Patient Involvement. Patients Adding Value To Policy, Projects and Services. Available at: http://www.eu-patient.eu/globalassets/projects/valueplus/value-toolkit.pdf (accessed 22 December 2016).

European Patients' Forum (2017). *European Patients Forum: Value +.* Available at: http://www.eu-patient.eu/whatwedo/Projects/ValuePlus/ (accessed 22 December 2016).

Faulkner A (2004). Capturing the experiences of those involved in the TRUE Project: a story of colliding worlds. Available at: http://www.invo.org.uk/wp-content/uploads/2012/01/CollidingWorlds2004.pdf (accessed 22 December 2016).

Faulkner A (2010). *Changing Our Worlds: examples of user-controlled research in action.* Eastleigh: INVOLVE.

Faulkner A et al. (2015a). 4PI National Involvement Standards. Executive Summary. London: National Survivor User Network. Available at: https://www.nsun.org.uk/Handlers/Download.ashx?IDMF=e1c3cfa4-c32e-47ff-8795-c45f523458c1 (accessed 27 June 2018).

Faulkner A et al. (2015b). 4PI National Involvement Standards. Involvement for Influence. Full report. London: National Survivor User Network. Available at: https://www.nationalvoices.org.uk/sites/default/files/public/4pinationalinvolvementstandardsfullreport20152.pdf (accessed 27 June 2018).

Fricker M (2010). *Epistemic Injustice. Power and the Ethics of Knowing.* New York: Oxford University Press.

Glasby J, Beresford P (2006). Who Knows Best?: Evidence-based practice and the service user contribution. *Critical Social Policy*, 26:268–84.

Hørder M (2012). The Role of INVOLVE for developing the Framework for User Involvement in Research in Denmark. Presentation at the 8th biennial INVOLVE conference in Nottingham, UK, 13–14 November 2012. Available at: http://www.invo.org.uk/wp-content/uploads/2013/01/2.7-Horder.pdf (accessed 27 June 2018).

Hunt P (1981). Settling Accounts With The Parasite People: a critique of 'A Life Apart' by E.J. Miller and G.V. Gwynne. *Disability Challenge*, 1:37–50.

International Collaboration for Participatory Health Research (ICPHR) (2013). Position Paper 1: What is Participatory Health Research? Version: May 2013. Available at: http://www.icphr.org/uploads/2/0/3/9/20399575/ichpr_position_paper_1_defintion_-_version_may_2013.pdf (accessed 27 June 2018).

International Collaboration for Participatory Health Research (ICPHR) (2014). Website. Available at: http://www.icphr.org/uploads/2/0/3/9/20399575/what_is_the_icphr_-_short_description_-_version_2014_10_20.pdf (accessed 27 June 2018).

INVOLVE (2015). Website. Available at: http://www.invo.org.uk/ (accessed 22 December 2016).

INVOLVE (2016). Co-production: old wine in new bottles or vintage PPI? *INVOLVE Newsletter*, Winter 2016/2017. Available at: http://www.invo.org.uk/wp-content/uploads/2017/02/INVOLVENewsletterwinter2016-17FINAL-1.pdf (accessed 22 February 2017).

Kalathil J (2013). "Hard to reach"? Racialised groups and mental health service user involvement. In: Staddon P (ed.) *Mental health service users in research: critical sociological perspectives.* Bristol: Policy Press.

Liegghio M (2013). A Denial of Being: Psychiatrization as Epistemic Violence. In: LeFrancois BA, Reaume G, Menzies RJ (eds.) *Mad Matters: A Critical Reader in Canadian Mad Studies.* Toronto: Canadian Scholars Press Inc.

Madden M, Speed E (2017). Beware Zombies and Unicorns: Toward Critical Patient and Public Involvement in Health Research in a Neoliberal Context. *Frontiers of Sociology*, 2:7.

Maguire P (1987). *Doing Participatory Research: a Feminist Approach.* Boston: Center for International Education, University of Massachusetts.

Mazur S, Bazemore A, Merenstein D (2016). Characteristics of Early Recipients of Patient-Centered Outcomes Research Institute Funding. *Academic Medicine*, 91:491–6.

National Development Team for Inclusion (NDTI) (2016). Position Paper: are mainstream mental health services ready to progress transformative co-production? Available at: http://www.ndti.org.uk/uploads/files/MH_Coproduction_position_paper.pdf (accessed 15 September 2016).

National Institute for Health Research (NIHR) (2015). Going the extra mile: improving the nation's health and wellbeing through public involvement in research. Available at: https://www.nihr.ac.uk/about-us/documents/Extra%20Mile2.pdf (accessed 27 July 2017).

National Survivor User Network (2017). 4Pi national involvement standards. Available at: https://www.nsun.org.uk/faqs/4pi-national-involvement-standards (accessed 20 November 2017)

Oliver M (1983). *Social Work and Disabled People.* Basingstoke: Macmillan.

Oliver M (1990). *The Politics of Disablement.* Basingstoke: Macmillan and St Martin's Press.

Oliver M (1992). Changing the Social Relations of Research Production? *Disability, Handicap & Society*, 7:101–14.

Oliver M (1997). Emancipatory Research: realistic goal or impossible dream? In: Barnes C, Mercer G (eds.) *Doing Disability Research.* Leeds: Disability Press.

Patient-Centered Outcomes Research Institute (PCORI) (2011–2017). Website. Available at: http://www.pcori.org/ (accessed 27 June 2018).

Reason P, Rowan J (1981). *Human Inquiry: a Sourcebook of New Paradigm Research.* London: John Wiley.

Roberts H (ed.) (1981). *Doing Feminist Research.* London: Routledge & Kegan Paul.

Rose D (2008). Service user produced knowledge. *Journal of Mental Health*, 17:447–51.

Rose D (2009). Is Collaborative Research Possible? In: Wallcraft J, Schrank B, Amering M (eds.) *Handbook of Service User Involvement in Mental Health Research.* West Sussex: Wiley-Blackwell.

Royle J et al. (2001). *Getting involved in research: a Guide for Consumers.* London: INVOLVE.

Russo J (2004). Forschung mit uns statt über uns [*Research with us instead of on us*]. *Rundbrief des Bundesverbands Psychiatrieerfahrener e.V [Magazine of the German Federal Organization of Mental Health Service Users]*, 4:5–9.

Russo J (2012). Survivor-controlled Research: a New Foundation for Thinking about Psychiatry and Mental Health. *Forum Qualitative Sozialforschung,* 13(1).

Russo J, Stastny P (2009). Beyond Involvement. Looking for a Common Perspective on Roles in Research. In: Wallcraft J, Schrank B, Amering M (eds.) *Handbook of Service User Involvement in Mental Health Research.* West Sussex: Wiley-Blackwell.

Simmons R, Powell M, Greener I (eds.) (2009). *The Consumer In Public Services: choice, values and difference.* Bristol: Policy Press.

Social Care Institute for Excellence (SCIE) (2013/2015). Co-production in social care: What it is and how to do it. SCIE Guide 51.

Staley K (2009). Exploring Impact: public involvement in NHS, public health and social care research. Available at: (http://www.invo.org.uk/wp-content/uploads/2011/11/Involve_Exploring_Impactfinal28.10.09.pdf (accessed 22 December 2016).

Staniszewska S, Denegri S (2013). Patient and public involvement in research: future challenges. *Evidence Based Nursing,* 16:69.

Sweeney A, Morgan L (2009). The Levels and Stages of Service User/Survivor Involvement in Research. In: Wallcraft J, Schrank B, Amering M (eds.) *Handbook of Service User Involvement in Mental Health Research.* West Sussex: Wiley-Blackwell.

ViBIS. Available at: https://danskepatienter.dk/about-danish-patients (accessed 21 February 2017).

Wadsworth Y (1998). What is Participatory Action Research? *Action research international, Paper 2.* Available at: http://www.aral.com.au/ari/p-ywadsworth98.html (accessed 27 June 2018).

Wilson P et al. (2015). ReseArch with Patient and Public invOlvement: a RealisT evaluation – the RAPPORT study. *Health Services and Delivery Research,* 3.

World Health Organization (1978). Declaration of Alma-Ata. International Conference on Primary Health Care, USSR.

World Health Organization (2006). Ninth futures forum on health systems governance and public participation. Copenhagen: World Health Organization Europe.

7 | *Listening to people: measuring views, experiences and perceptions*

ANGELA COULTER, GIUSEPPE PAPARELLA, ANDREW MCCULLOCH

Introduction

The universal challenge facing health policy-makers is how to ensure the delivery of high-quality health care to a given population with a defined level of resource. While there is often disagreement on how to achieve this goal, most agree that health care should aim to be clinically effective, safe, equitable, efficient and responsive to those it aims to serve. The concept of responsiveness is often equated with the notion of person-centredness. Person-centred care means ensuring that care delivery responds to people's physical, emotional, social and cultural needs, that interactions with staff are informative, empathetic and empowering, and that patients' values and preferences are taken into account. This is important, not just because people want it, but also because their health care experiences can influence the effectiveness of their treatment and ultimately their state of health.

The best way to check whether services are meeting these person-centred standards is to ask the users themselves. This chapter looks at why patients' perceptions on the quality of care are viewed as a key indicator and how people's views and experiences can be measured. In thinking about the scope of measurement we include all aspects of care that are important to patients and observable by them, either as a result of their direct experience or through their perceptions and beliefs about health systems.

Why patients' perspectives matter

Patients' experiences of health care are important for both intrinsic and extrinsic reasons. Numerous studies have looked at what people value when using health services and what they prefer to avoid. While there are demographic, cultural, socioeconomic and health status variations in people's values and priorities, there is a great deal of agreement on

173

what matters to us when we are patients. We all hope to be treated with dignity, kindness, compassion, courtesy, respect, understanding and honesty when using public services and we expect our rights to information and privacy to be respected. We want the security of knowing that appropriate health services will be readily accessible when we need them, that our physical and emotional needs will be carefully assessed by competent staff, that our rights to information and involvement will be acknowledged and acted upon, that we will be listened to and treated with empathy and understanding, and that our treatment and care will be well coordinated and speedily delivered.

Various conceptual frameworks have been developed to categorize these issues into distinct domains to enhance understanding and facilitate measurement. Starting with the Picker/Commonwealth Dimensions of Patient-Centred Care, the first of the international efforts to categorize and measure issues of importance to patients (Gerteis et al., 1993) and their incorporation into the Institute of Medicine's Six Aims for Improvement (Institute of Medicine, 2001), the field was later strengthened by the World Health Organization's work on system responsiveness (Murray, Kawabata & Valentine, 2001) and many subsequent academic and policy initiatives (*see* Chapter 2). These frameworks view patient experience, or responsiveness, as a unique dimension of health care quality, to be used alongside more traditional indicators of clinical effectiveness, equity and efficiency. Many countries have introduced systems for monitoring performance against these or similar frameworks. For example, in England the focus on measuring and improving patients' experience of care is underpinned by the publication of quality statements outlining specific criteria against which performance can be monitored and evaluated (National Institute for Health and Care Excellence, 2012).

Person-centred care incorporates functional aspects – access arrangements, organizational issues, physical environment and amenities – and interpersonal or relational aspects, especially communications between patients and professional staff. Both are very important but relational aspects, while more complex and difficult to change, probably have the greatest influence on the way patients evaluate the care they receive (Entwistle et al., 2012). The subjective features of care are important at a basic human level but also because there is evidence that those who report better experiences tend to have better health outcomes. Clinical care that is technically correct is crucial, but if this is delivered in a brusque manner without demonstrating empathy or respect for individual autonomy, then the results are likely to be less than optimal. For example, studies have found that more positive experiences are associated with better clinical indicators such as blood glucose levels, fewer complications or side-effects, better functional ability and quality of life, greater adherence to treatment recommendations, lower resource use, and less likelihood of premature death (Doyle, Lennox & Bell, 2013; Price et al., 2014).

The precise mechanisms underlying the positive associations between experience and health outcomes are not well understood. While it may appear intuitively obvious that patients who trust and respect their physicians are more likely to follow their advice, leading to improved adherence and better self-care, the connections are not always straightforward and may not be directly causal (Price et al., 2014). There is some evidence that hospitals with better work environments (as reported by nurses) and lower nurse-to-patient ratios are more highly rated by patients (Aiken et al., 2012). Perhaps those hospitals or departments that attract high ratings from patients are better resourced or better managed, or maybe clinicians in these facilities are more likely to follow evidence-based guidelines, leading to safer or higher quality care.

Critics have sometimes argued that patients' judgements are too subjective to be useful, but these objections miss the point. Measurement of patients' experience is not intended as a substitute for more objective clinical measures (Manary et al., 2013; Anhang Price et al., 2015). Instead it taps into an important dimension of health care not represented by more traditional indicators.

Purpose, methods and scope of measurement

The main reasons for adopting a systematic approach to the elicitation of patients' views are to inform quality improvement policy and practice and to hold providers to account for maintaining quality standards. Specific goals may include the following:

- to track public attitudes to the health system;
- to identify and monitor problems in care delivery;
- to facilitate performance assessment and benchmarking between services or organizations;
- to help professionals reflect on their own, their team's or their organization's performance;

- to inform service redesign and monitor the impact of any changes;
- to promote informed choice of provider by patients and/or clinicians; and
- to enable public accountability and transparency (Coulter, Fitzpatrick & Cornwell, 2009).

There are many ways to collect data for these purposes, including qualitative methods (such as focus groups or in-depth interviews) and analysis of administrative data or written complaints. Quantitative surveys using structured self-completion questionnaires are the most commonly used type of patient-based measure. Structured surveys are popular because they can be analysed statistically and used to compare results for whole populations or sub-groups. Data can be collected by mail, telephone or electronic means, as well as by more expensive face-to-face surveys. Questionnaires that are well designed, tested with patients to ensure salience and comprehensibility, checked for validity and reliability using appropriate psychometric methods, and rigorously implemented to achieve adequate response rates and minimize bias can yield useful information (Beattie et al., 2015).

Surveys do have important limitations, however. Questions are usually 'closed', offering a specific set of pre-coded response options. This necessarily imposes restrictions, so awareness of the design process is crucial for interpreting the findings and identifying potential sources of bias. Response rates are sometimes low, raising the risk of systematic error if certain groups in the population are less likely to respond. For example, it is known that responses to postal surveys tend to be lower among males, younger adults, the very old, people in poorer health, and those in socioeconomically deprived groups (Zaslavsky, Zaborski & Cleary, 2002). Systematic biases can also affect surveys with high response rates; for example, 'acquiescence bias' when respondents tend to answer 'yes' to questions instead of other response options, or 'social desirability bias' when respondents choose options that they think are socially desirable but may not be accurate indications of their behaviour or beliefs. The likelihood of responding positively to questions about health experiences tends to vary by health status too (Hewitson et al., 2014; Paddison et al., 2015). These issues can be handled statistically through adjustment if enough is known about the factors influencing specific responses, but users of survey data should always interpret the results cautiously (Raleigh et al., 2015).

Qualitative, unstructured feedback methods also have an important part to play. These may include in-depth face-to-face interviews, focus groups, patient stories, web-based free-text comments, suggestion boxes, video boxes, direct observations and shadowing, or mystery shopping (Ziebland et al., 2013). These methods usually yield a deeper understanding of the meanings that people attribute to their health care experiences, but they are generally unsuitable for use as performance indicators.

Routine health data can be used to assess certain elements of patients' experience, for example waiting times, lengths of stay, place of death, etc. There is also scope for more systematic use of complaints, looking for patterns and trends instead of just treating each complaint as an isolated event. No single method is ideal for every purpose and each of the approaches has strengths and weaknesses (Coulter, Fitzpatrick & Cornwell, 2009). It is often a good idea to use multiple sources to gain the fullest picture. For example, qualitative data from interviews, focus groups or observations can be used to inform the scope and wording of structured surveys; conversely, survey results may be used to identify issues requiring more in-depth investigation using qualitative methods.

Patient experience and satisfaction

Quantitative patient or public surveys are used to inform health policy in three main ways: monitoring patients', service users' or carers' experience of, and satisfaction with, care; measuring health outcomes from the patients' point of view; and assessing public attitudes, health beliefs and behaviours. Selected examples of how this is being tackled in various European countries are illustrated below.

Most people working in health care are familiar with the notion of patient satisfaction, but there is often confusion between this and the related notion of patient experience. Satisfaction is a broad and often ill-defined concept that has been measured in many different ways. Derived from marketing theory, it looks at the extent to which health care fulfils people's expectations (Batbaatar et al., 2015). Satisfaction surveys ask patients to evaluate the quality of care they have received, often using pre-defined response categories. A typical question might be: 'Please rate the care you received at this hospital' – 'excellent/very good/good/fair/poor.'

Patient satisfaction is sometimes treated as an outcome measure (satisfaction with health status following treatment) and sometimes as a process measure (satisfaction with the way in which care is delivered). It is generally recognized as multi-dimensional in nature, and there is no consensus on what domains should be included, nor which are most important. The best questionnaires are developed with patient involvement, covering topics that are known to be important to patients. Very general questions are often less informative than more specific, detailed ones. While it can be useful to know how satisfied people are with the process and outcomes of care, satisfaction ratings can be hard to interpret because they may be influenced by individual expectations and preferences, health status, personal characteristics or cultural norms, as well as the actual quality and outcomes of care received. Nevertheless, there is continuing interest in gauging people's satisfaction with services, and newer methods include inviting unstructured feedback via websites and brief 'exit' surveys designed to produce rapid results.

Many researchers now believe that the complexities of modern health care and the diversity of patients' expectations and experiences cannot be reliably evaluated by asking general satisfaction-style rating questions such as 'How satisfied were you with your care in hospital x?' or, as is sometimes the case, by focusing solely on food and amenities while ignoring people's concerns about their clinical care or the way staff dealt with them. More recently, therefore, the focus has shifted to asking people to give factual reports on what actually happened to them during an episode of care, instead of evaluative ratings. This style of questionnaire is known as a patient experience survey, sometimes referred to as Patient Reported Experience Measures (PREMs).

PREMs questionnaires are designed to elicit responses to specific questions about people's experiences of a particular service, hospital episode, general practice or clinician, or in other words to provide factual information instead of evaluations. Experience surveys are often quite lengthy, posing detailed questions about a specific episode or time period. For example, a typical experience question about a recent hospital episode might be: 'When you had important questions to ask a doctor, did you get answers you could understand?' – 'Yes always/ yes sometimes/no.' This type of question tends to be easier to interpret and respond to than responses to more general questions about levels of satisfaction, and hence it is more actionable. Patient experience questionnaires form the basis of the national patient survey programme in England and several other countries (Box 7.1).

Box 7.1 Measurement of patients' experience in England

The promotion of person-centred care has been a key policy goal for the British NHS for more than twenty years since the publication of the original Patients' Charter in 1991, later reconstituted as the NHS Constitution (Department of Health, 2015). To monitor this policy national patient experience surveys have been conducted in England since 2002 under the auspices of the Care Quality Commission.

The national patient experience surveys, which are mostly carried out on an annual basis, are specially designed for each of the following services: inpatient, outpatient, emergency hospital care, maternity, and community mental health services (http://www.cqc.org.uk/content/surveys). Questionnaires and sampling strategies are designed and tested by a national survey coordination centre run by Picker Institute Europe, but individual health care facilities are responsible for implementation, with most employing external survey companies to carry them out. Results are fed back to staff and made available to the public via a national website (www.nhs.uk).

A large survey of general practice patients is also carried out on behalf of NHS England (https://gp-patient.co.uk/), together with a cancer patient experience survey (https://www.quality-health.co.uk/surveys/national-cancer-patient-experience-survey) and a national staff survey (http://www.nhsstaffsurveys.com/).

Other countries collecting patient experience data at a national level include France, the Netherlands, Norway, Sweden, Switzerland and the United States (Rechel et al., 2016). Elsewhere a combination of approaches is used, including satisfaction surveys and household health surveys. For example, in Poland a set of standardized questionnaires on patient satisfaction, called PASAT, was developed by the Centre for Quality Monitoring in Health Care, a World Health Organization Collaborating Centre. Separate questionnaires were distributed to hospital patients (PASAT HOSPIT), parents of treated children (PASAT PEDIATRIA) and users of primary health care (PASAT PHC). In addition, a household health survey conducted by the Chief Statistical Office was recently expanded to include a set of questions on health care quality (Boulhol et al., 2012).

In countries with devolved responsibility for health care, Germany (Box 7.2), Italy (Box 7.3) and Spain for example, data collection tends to be coordinated at regional level.

Box 7.2 Measurement of patients' experience in Germany

Responsibility for the health care system in Germany is shared between the 16 Länder (states), the federal government and civil society organizations, while health insurance is provided by competing, not-for-profit, non-governmental 'sickness' funds and private agencies. This devolved system of care has led to multiple initiatives for gathering data on patients' experiences rather than a single national approach, and quality assurance is the responsibility of a number of agencies.

Germany does not currently run a systematic national survey of patients' experience, but this situation has changed following the establishment of a new federal institute. The Institute for Quality Assurance and Transparency in Health Care (IQTIG) was established in 2016 to monitor quality across the German health care system, with a particular focus on hospitals (IHS Markit, 2015). It is charged with developing quality indicators and measurement instruments, including patient surveys.

Patient satisfaction surveys in ambulatory and hospital care are also undertaken by sickness funds in cooperation with the Bertelsmann Foundation twice a year, and by professional stakeholders, such as the National Association of Statutory Health Insurance Physicians.

Box 7.3 Measurement of patients' experience in Italy

Since 1980 ISTAT (the Italian National Institute of Statistics) has conducted a five-yearly Health Conditions and Use of Medical Services Survey which includes some aspects of patients' experience, in particular questions about access to care. The questionnaire is comprised of more than 70 pages, with the most recent publication in 2013 (ILO, 2013).

Box 7.3 (cont.)

National legislation requires the Ministry of Health, in collaboration with patients' and citizens' associations, to establish a set of indicators to systematically measure the quality of health services from the patient's point of view. The indicators cover four areas: personalizing and humanizing care, citizens' information rights, quality of hospital accommodation services, and disease prevention policies. A Ministerial Decree published on 15 October 1996 identified 79 patient satisfaction indicators in these areas. Topics under 'personalized and humanized care' include the ability to book appointments by telephone and the percentage of general practitioners who set up out-of-hours services. The implementation of this national framework on patients' rights and empowerment has not been uniform: regions such as Emilia-Romagna, Tuscany and Veneto have given systematic attention to this issue, while others have not. Since each region has adopted distinctive and different solutions to seeking patients' views, there is a lack of comparability across the country about this aspect of person-centred care (Paparella, 2016).

At regional level data on Italian citizens' satisfaction compiled by ISTAT show that satisfaction varies across the north–south divide, with the northern and central regions consistently obtaining above average results, whereas all southern regions score below average.

The turnaround time between data collection and publication of results of patient experience surveys can sometimes be lengthy due to the number of health care organizations involved, the need to check sampling and mailing procedures (an initial mailing plus up to two reminders is usually required to secure a good response), the quantity of data obtained, analytical complexities and other bureaucratic reasons. Frustration with this lack of timeliness has led to a search for briefer, easy-to-implement measures.

The introduction of a new type of national patient survey for England, the Friends and Family Test (FFT), was an attempt to deal with this problem. Based on the Net Promoter Score (www.netpromotersystem.com), a marketing concept used extensively by retail companies, the FFT is an on-site or exit survey that asks people to evaluate their experiences using a single question: 'How likely are you to recommend our [hospital/ward/maternity service/GP practice] to friends and family if they needed similar care or treatment?', followed by an invitation to provide free text comments. It was hoped that use of this simple form of 'real-time' feedback would provide relevant and timely data to inform quality improvement efforts. This approach has certainly succeeded in amassing a great deal of data, some of which has been used to stimulate quality improvements, but problems of interpretation due to unsystematic approaches to data collection hamper its reliability as a performance measure (Coulter, 2016; Sizmur, Graham & Walsh, 2015).

Social media is an important source of data on people's experiences of health care and independent websites gathering unstructured feedback are becoming popular. Examples include Patient Opinion in the UK (https://www.careopinion.org.uk/), iWantGreatCare (https://www .iwantgreatcare.org/), and PatientsLikeMe (https://www.patientslikeme .com/). Their primary purpose is to collect feedback on people's experiences to improve quality, but people's accounts of their care are also used to inform other patients and to stimulate research.

There is considerable interest in using patient experience indicators to compare performance between countries. This is the purpose of the US-based Commonwealth Fund's international health policy surveys (www.commonwealthfund.org) (Box 7.4).

Box 7.4 Commonwealth Fund international surveys

The Commonwealth Fund's international surveys have been conducted on a regular basis since 2000. Now (2018) covering eleven countries (Australia, Canada, France, Germany, the Netherlands, New Zealand, Norway, Sweden, Switzerland, the UK and the USA), these telephone surveys include questions both about recent experience of using health care and about people's opinions of their local systems. The surveys target nationally representative random samples using common questionnaires that are translated and adjusted for country-specific wording. The published comparisons,

Box 7.4 (cont.)

which are weighted to reflect the demographic characteristics of the adult population in each country, tend to attract considerable interest among governments and the media in the various countries.

Inter-country comparisons face considerable methodological problems, especially if there is a lack of consistency in what is being measured and how the measurement is carried out. The Organisation for Economic Cooperation and Development's (OECD) Health Care Quality Indicators project is an attempt to encourage greater international coordination of patient experience surveys to facilitate inter-country comparisons (Fujisawa & Klazinga, 2016) (Box 7.5).

Box 7.5 OECD Health Care Quality Indicators

The OECD Health Care Quality Indicators project (HCQI), working in conjunction with the Directorate General for Health and Consumers of the European Commission, has been striving since 2006 to develop better methods for comparing the quality of health service provision in different countries on a routine basis, including measurement of patients' experiences (Fujisawa & Klazinga, 2016).

As part of this programme a number of countries have agreed to field OECD-proposed questions in their national surveys to stimulate cross-national learning, including Belgium, Estonia, Italy, Poland and Spain. The agreed list of indicator questions about patients' experience of ambulatory care covers the following topics:

- costs to the patient of medical consultations;
- costs to the patient of medical tests, treatment or follow-up;
- costs to the patient of prescribed medicines;
- waiting times to get an appointment with a specialist;
- doctor spending enough time with patient during the consultation;
- doctor providing easy-to-understand explanations;
- doctor giving opportunity to ask questions or raise concerns; and
- doctor involving patient in decisions about care and treatment.

Patient-reported outcomes

While patient experience surveys ask respondents to report on the process of care, patient-reported outcome measures (referred to as PROs or PROMs) ask them to report on their health state following a clinical intervention, the outcome of care. PROMs are standardized questionnaires that are designed to elicit subjective reports of the personal impact (outcomes) of illness and treatment, focusing on physical functioning (ability to maintain daily activities) and emotional well-being, often referred to more generally as health-related quality of life. The aim is to obtain important information that is not reflected in traditional clinical measures. This is done by asking respondents to describe their current state, by means of a structured interview or self-completion questionnaire, either paper-based or electronic. The resulting reports can then be compared to previous measurements from the same individual or group (to measure change over time) or to those from a reference group or sub-groups (to compare against an external norm or standard).

PROMs must be carefully developed and tested to conform to accepted statistical and psychometric standards, including evidence of validity, reliability and sensitivity to change. The best PROMs are developed with extensive input from patients, ensuring that they cover topics that are salient and meaningful from the patient's perspective. While they are intended primarily for use at two or more time points to measure health gain (or loss), for example before and after treatment, or at various time points during a period of illness or recovery, they can also be used to obtain a single snapshot of the prevalence of quality of life problems.

PROMs fall into three distinct types (Table 7.1). Some measure general health status regardless of the clinical diagnosis (generic PROMs), while others ask about health perceptions in relation to specific conditions (condition-specific PROMs). A third type is patient-generated measures, where respondents are asked to define their own outcome goals and achievement of these is then assessed after a period of time.

Most PROMs cover a number of quality of life dimensions or domains. For example, the widely used EuroQol measure (EQ-5D) (EuroQol Group, 1990) includes five domains (mobility, self-care, usual

Table 7.1 *Types of PROM*

Type	Examples
Generic	Medical Outcomes Study: SF-36 (Ware & Sherbourne, 1992); EuroQol: EQ-5D (EuroQol Group, 1990)
Condition-specific	Osteoarthritis of the hip: Oxford Hip Score (Dawson et al., 1996); Depression: PHQ-9 (Kroenke, Spitzer & Williams, 2001)
Patient-generated	Measure Yourself Medical Outcome Profile: MYMOP (Paterson, 1996); Schedule for Evaluation of Individual Quality of Life: SEIQol (Joyce et al., 2003)

activities, pain/discomfort, anxiety/depression) and an overall rating of the respondent's health state. The results can be scored separately for each domain or summarized in a single index score to monitor variations and time trends or for ranking providers. The EQ-5D has been adopted by the Department of Health in England for inclusion in its national PROMs programme (Box 7.6) and is also included in NHS England's large general practice patient survey mentioned earlier, giving population data that can be used as a 'normal population' reference for comparison purposes.

Condition-specific PROMs ask about issues relating to the specific problem (for example, 'Have you had trouble washing or drying yourself because of your knee?'). Like EQ-5D, the results can be used descriptively or summed to produce a single score. Condition-specific measures tend to be more responsive to change than generic measures, but both types can be used to describe pre- and post-treatment health status and health gain.

Patient-generated measures are intuitively appealing, but they are not often used for large-scale data collection because it is harder to score and summarize the results. Their primary use is for facilitating the exchange of information in clinical consultations and in care planning for long-term conditions.

PROMs are currently being collected on a routine basis in Denmark, England, Estonia, the Netherlands and Sweden, as well as in numerous individual studies of treatment effects.

Box 7.6 National PROMs programme in England

Since 2009 the Department of Health in England has funded a programme of work to measure patient-reported outcomes of elective surgery. The aim of the national PROMs programme is to measure and describe outcomes in a meaningful way in the hope that patients, GPs and health care commissioners would use the data to seek out those hospitals and clinicians that achieve the best outcomes, thereby driving up standards. Alongside this experiment in routine data collection from elective surgery patients, a research programme was launched to pilot the use of PROMs for patients with other conditions, including long-term conditions, mental health, coronary revascularization and cancer care.

The national surgical PROMs programme, also launched in 2009, monitors outcomes of care for patients undergoing hip replacement, knee replacement, hernia repair and varicose veins surgery. Everyone undergoing these procedures (i.e. a census, not a sample) is invited to complete a questionnaire before their operation. Those who complete the pre-surgery questionnaire are then sent a postal questionnaire three to six months after their operation to measure changes in their health status. A single generic standardized PROM (EQ-5D) is included in all questionnaires, together with condition-specific PROMs for three of the four diagnostic groups. Results from this continuous survey are collated, linked with data from the Hospital Episode Statistics, case-mix adjusted, and published at regular intervals by the NHS.

Response rates to individual surveys have been good to date – during 2016–2017, response rates were 86% for the pre-operative hip questionnaires and 76% for the post-operative ones – but the final response rate is subject to some attrition when before-surgery and after-surgery surveys are matched up. Not surprisingly, the results show that most patients experience improvements in their health-related quality of life, especially those undergoing hip or knee surgery where more than 80% of patients report better health six months after undergoing the procedure. Factors external to the health system, such as socioeconomic and environmental influences, do seem to make a difference to how quickly people are treated and how well they recover (Soljak et al., 2009; Neuburger

---

Box 7.6 (cont.)

et al., 2013), but somewhat surprisingly these and other studies (Varagunam, Hutchings & Black, 2014; Varagunam et al., 2014; Black, Varagunam & Hutchings, 2014; Appleby et al., 2013) suggest that there is in fact a great deal of uniformity across England in quality of life outcomes after these surgical procedures. Instead of the expected variations in quality of care, all providers appear to be performing at similar levels of competence, producing similar results.

It is important to consider carefully how the outputs will be used before planning PROMs data collection. Decisions about where and in what way the information will be gathered, when and from whom, are likely to vary according to its intended purpose. In theory, PROMs can be used for a variety of purposes, the most common of which is as an outcome measure in clinical trials to evaluate medical interventions and technologies. They can also be used to monitor performance across specialties, organizations, departments or whole systems, and in clinical care to inform diagnosis, treatment and provider choice (Devlin & Appleby, 2010) (Table 7.2).

Table 7.2 *Potential uses of PROMs*

Level of aggregation	Purpose	Relevance
Health system	System-wide performance assessment	To monitor variations in health outcomes between population sub-groups and provider organizations
	Determining value for money	To determine the extent to which the current pattern of service provision is delivering good value for money
Commissioners/ payers	Procurement/ contracting	To encourage providers to monitor health outcomes and to incentivize better care
	Monitoring quality	To use as a key performance indicator to monitor health outcomes and value for money

Table **7.2** *(cont.)*

Level of aggregation	Purpose	Relevance
Provider organization/ specialty	Clinical audit	To better understand patients' needs and assess how well these are being met by the organization
	Quality improvement	To help plan innovations, monitor progress and incentivize staff
Clinical trials	Trial recruitment	To screen for eligibility for participation in trials and for use as a baseline measure
	Trial outcomes	To measure outcomes in intervention and control groups
Clinical care	Screening and diagnosis	To help make a diagnosis, including co-morbidities and impact on quality of life
	Health needs assessment and monitoring	To improve communication, identify needs for self-management support and monitor how the patient is getting on
	Choosing providers	To select 'the best' provider for an individual patient
	Choosing treatments and self-management support	To inform patients to facilitate shared decision-making and personalized care planning

Population surveys

People's views on the general functioning of a health system and their opinions on the efficiency of its administration are of considerable interest to policy-makers, so a number of countries have invested in regular opinion surveys. These usually target general population samples instead of just health service users. For example, the British Social Attitudes survey regularly includes the following question: 'All in all, how satisfied or dissatisfied would you say you are with the way in which the National Health Service runs nowadays?' (Appleby & Robertson, 2016). Such questions enable comparison of attitudes and perceptions between different population groups and, if repeated at regular intervals, can throw light on trends over time.

Estonia has been monitoring public views on its health care system since the late 1990s (Lai et al., 2013). Annual population surveys measure public perceptions of health care quality, access to, and satisfaction with, family doctors, specialists, dentists and hospitals. Since 2003 there has been a steady improvement in perceptions of care quality and in 2012, 79% of the Estonian population expressed their satisfaction with the quality of care.

In Poland research on public attitudes to the health care system is regularly carried out by the Public Opinion Research Centre (Centrum Badania Opinii Społecznej – CBOS). While access to primary care doctors and availability of health information received positive reports, in the most recent survey conducted in July 2014, two-thirds (68%) of respondents were dissatisfied with waiting times and the overall efficiency of the system (CBOS Public Opinion Research Centre, 2014).

Comparison across countries can also be informative, so national efforts have been complemented by the European Commission's Eurobarometer surveys, some of which have focused on attitudes to health care across countries (Box 7.7).

Box 7.7 Eurobarometer surveys

The European Commission's series of Eurobarometer surveys has provided a useful source of comparison of public attitudes to health systems in all 28 Member States. The surveys elicit responses from people aged 15 years and over, resident in each of the countries, and the results are weighted to be representative of the local populations. Interviews are conducted face-to-face in people's homes in the appropriate local language.

The most recent health survey, which focused on people's perceptions of the safety and quality of health care in their country, was carried out in 2013 and repeated questions first used in 2009 (European Commission, 2014).

A majority of EU citizens (71%) felt that the overall quality of health care in their country was good, but there were considerable differences between countries. Respondents in western and northern areas tended to give more positive responses than those in the south and east of Europe. People's main priorities were well-trained staff and effective treatment. Awareness of patient safety issues was fairly high, at over 50%, but this varied between countries from 82% of respondents in Cyprus to 21% of those in Austria.

Interpretation of the results of opinion surveys must take account of the local context. People's attitudes are influenced by many factors, including personal experiences and those of family and friends, media reports, commercial and lobby groups, and political affiliations. For example, the question about satisfaction with the NHS tends to produce more positive responses from people with recent experience of health care than from those who have not used it recently, and from supporters of the government in power than from supporters of opposition parties (Appleby & Robertson, 2016). People's expectations are also likely to influence their experiences. For example, those who believe their local health system is deteriorating may be pleasantly surprised if they receive acceptable care, whereas those who expect a prompt service at all times may be disappointed if they have to wait. For these reasons, such surveys should not be seen as definitive measures of performance.

Population surveys are also used to gather epidemiological data and explore health needs. For example, the Spanish Institute of Statistics organizes a national health survey at periodic intervals to gather data on the population's state of health and social determinants, broken down by autonomous region (Instituto Nacional de Estadistica, 2013). In Germany the Robert Koch Institute, an agency subordinate to the Federal Ministry of Health and responsible for the control of infectious diseases and health reporting, conducts the German Health Interview and Examination Survey for Adults every two or three years (Robert Koch Institute, 2013). While primarily a face-to-face epidemiological survey, this also includes some questions about patients' experience and subjective health status. Similarly, the Health Survey for England, a regularly conducted face-to-face household survey, includes questions about people's needs for health and social care and the support needs of family carers. Health needs surveys may also include questions about health behaviours and attitudes to lifestyle change, for example smoking cessation or dietary modification. These are used to monitor the impact of public health programmes and to identify sub-groups where more precise targeting of health education may be required.

Using the data

Capturing public and patients' perspectives on health care is becoming increasingly important as systems strive to be more responsive to the needs of those using their services. As outlined above, many European countries now have programmes of work that include national or regional surveys undertaken at regular intervals, either as a component of household-based epidemiological health surveys or as patient experience or outcome surveys focused on health care facilities. Countries where these are in place include Austria, Belgium, the Czech Republic, Denmark, Estonia, Finland, France, Germany, Iceland, Ireland, Italy, Luxembourg, the Netherlands, Norway, Poland, Portugal, Spain, Sweden and the UK (Fujisawa & Klazinga, 2016).

Publication of PREMs and PROMs is seen as an important mechanism for holding providers to account for the quality of care ('voice') and for empowering patients to act as discerning consumers ('choice') (Coulter, 2010). Policy-makers hope that giving people (providers, patients and public) access to comparative information on performance will stimulate improvements. There is evidence that some providers do take note of published survey results leading to improvements (Hafner et al., 2011), but change is often hard to discern at a national level and public disclosure does not seem to have made much impact on the behaviour of patients as yet (Ketelaar et al., 2014). While better performing organizations will often act on the results of patient surveys, those at the lower end of the rankings probably need stronger stimuli to provoke action, for example financial incentives (Raleigh et al., 2012). Patients do make choices about their care, but their choice of provider is often based on informal information from family and friends rather than statistical information (Coulter, 2010).

It is self-defeating, and arguably unethical, to ask patients to take time to report on their health care experiences if the results are not used to make improvements. It is therefore discouraging to note that after more than ten years of gathering patient experience data in England, only a minority of hospital providers had taken effective action leading to demonstrable change (DeCourcy, West & Barron, 2012). Similar disappointing results have been reported in other countries, despite the presence of incentives such as public disclosure, pay-for-performance and encouragement to patients to exercise choice of provider. While many policy-makers are convinced of the usefulness of patient and public survey data, clinicians are often more sceptical. Lack of clinical engagement is a significant barrier to improvement (Asprey et al., 2013; Rozenblum et al., 2013).

Identifying the reasons for the failure to act is not straightforward. Lack of understanding of the issues is unlikely to be sufficient explanation – a considerable amount is known about which aspects of care matter to patients (Robert & Cornwell, 2011). A recent systematic review identified several barriers to improvement, including lack of time or resources to collect, analyse and act on the data; competing priorities, including workload and financial pressures; survey results that were insufficiently timely or too general to be relevant at the provider level; and a lack of effective leadership (Gleeson et al., 2016).

The good news is that change is possible, as evidenced by many successful local initiatives (Haugum et al., 2014). The challenge is to mainstream this learning across whole health systems. This requires committed leadership, clear goals, active engagement of patients and families, human resources policies that embed quality improvement skills in training and staff development, adequate resourcing and effective institutional support, and effective dissemination of the results (Coulter et al., 2014). There is considerable scope for cross-country learning in this field. The OECD initiative to develop a common set of principles and indicators is of major importance, offering a real opportunity to raise standards and ensure that patients' views really count in health policy development (Fujisawa & Klazinga, 2016). A similar effort may be needed to share best practice in using the data to improve the quality of patient care.

Future developments

This field is likely to develop in various directions over the next few years, leading to greater diversity of methods for obtaining feedback from patients and the public. Electronic data collection is becoming more prevalent and the days of paper-based surveys must be numbered. Online surveys that can provide automated data collection, instant analysis and feedback in a well-presented comprehensible format could provide a much more efficient and effective means of generating valuable information.

As the focus of policy interest turns increasingly towards integrated care, methods that focus on single episodes, institutions, services or conditions may become less relevant. The development of survey tools or sets of indicators that adequately reflect people's experiences across clinical pathways and service boundaries will be challenging, but work is currently under way to develop such measures (Strandberg-Larsen & Krasnik, 2009; Graham et al., 2013). There is great interest in the development of more broad-based indicators that better reflect service users' goals and outcome preferences (Hunter et al., 2015; Peters et al., 2016). Better measures are needed of concepts such as empowerment, autonomy, care coordination and self-management capabilities.

Public use of web-based ratings and social media to share information about health experiences is growing apace (Rozenblum & Bates, 2013). Historically, use of unstructured comments has been restricted to local quality initiatives, but new methods of data analysis offer the potential to gain generalizable insights from these types of data. There may be scope to collate this information electronically to supplement or even replace traditional surveys (Greaves et al., 2012; Bardach et al., 2013). Techniques such as 'sentiment analysis' could be used to produce overviews of patients' experiences as expressed on social media, for example (Greaves et al., 2013). Patient narratives are often more interesting to staff than statistics, and the availability of collections of video interviews of patients talking about their experiences may prove to be a useful adjunct to statistical reports of survey data. These videos are already being used in quality improvement initiatives such as experience-based co-design (Locock et al., 2014).

More work is needed to develop efficient means of combining patient narratives and PROMs data into user-friendly decision aids to support shared decision-making (Coulter et al., 2013). These tools can help patients understand treatment choices and participate in decisions about their care, but they are time-consuming to produce, and dissemination and uptake have proved challenging (Stiggelbout et al., 2012).

Use of electronic data collection to incorporate patient feedback directly into clinical record systems is attracting considerable interest at present (Kotronoulas et al., 2014; Etkind et al., 2014). Many experts are convinced that incorporation of PROMs into regular patient care is the way forward, recognizing that a number of challenges will need to be overcome (Gilbert et al., 2015). For example, the use of e-PROMs in routine primary care to monitor the impact of long-term conditions and multi-morbidities on people's physical and emotional health over time could transform the management of these conditions. Personalized care planning, in which patients and clinicians work together to agree goals and develop proactive action plans, reviewing these at regular intervals, could be facilitated by the use of these instruments, enabling clinicians and patients to better understand symptom fluctuations and identify effective self-management strategies.

The establishment of 'virtual' clinics using e-PROMs has also been mooted, enabling remote monitoring to avoid unnecessary post-treatment appointments (Gilbert et al., 2015). Patients could be called up only when their PROMs scores indicate unmet needs for specialist help, potentially leading to more efficient use of resources and a reduction in the 'treatment burden' for patients. Trials are under way to evaluate this type of system for use by cancer patients, but it may have the potential for wider application (Absolom et al., 2017).

Maintaining clarity of purpose will be essential if patients' perspectives are to be usefully incorporated into efforts to improve equitable and responsive delivery of health care. Governments, health authorities or health care organizations may be primarily concerned to gauge public views on the adequacy of arrangements made for health care delivery, the quality of care processes or the effectiveness of treatments. Each of these goals requires a thoughtful and well-designed approach to measurement. The seven principles for establishing national systems of patient experience measurement proposed by an OECD expert group should be given serious consideration:

1. Patient measurement should be patient-based, using survey instruments formulated with patient input.
2. The goal of patient measurement should be clear, whether for external reasons such as provision of information for consumer choice, public accountability or pay-for-performance, or for internal use by providers as part of quality improvement schemes.
3. Patient measurement tools should undergo cognitive testing by patients and their psychometric properties should be known.
4. The actual measurement and analyses of patient experiences should be standardized and reproducible.
5. Reporting methods should be carefully designed and tested.
6. International comparability should be enhanced with the development of agreed indicator questions.
7. National systems for the measurement of patient experiences should be sustainable, supported by appropriate infrastructure (OECD, 2010).

We would propose the addition of one further principle – that countries should work together to develop and test methods for ensuring that the results of these types of surveys are taken seriously and incorporated into quality improvement initiatives, leading to real, measurable improvements in the quality of health care. This will require the establishment of appropriate structures and mechanisms to facilitate sharing and learning.

Ultimately, the success or failure of the initiatives described in this chapter will rest on the extent to which the information generated stimulates real improvements in our health systems.

Note

We are most grateful to Niek Klazinga for allowing us to see a pre-publication copy of the recent OECD report on measuring patient experiences (Fujisawa & Klazinga, 2016).

References

Absolom K et al. (2017). Electronic patient self-Reporting of Adverse-events: Patient Information and aDvice (eRAPID): a randomised controlled trial in systemic cancer treatment. *BMC Cancer*, 17:318.

Aiken LH et al. (2012). Patient safety, satisfaction, and quality of hospital care: cross sectional surveys of nurses and patients in 12 countries in Europe and the United States. *BMJ*, 344:e1717.

Anhang Price R et al. (2015). Should health care providers be accountable for patients' care experiences? *Journal of General Internal Medicine*, 30:253–6.

Appleby J, Robertson R (2016). Public satisfaction with the NHS in 2015: Results and trends from the British Social Attitudes survey. Available at: http://www.kingsfund.org.uk/sites/files/kf/BSA-public-satisfaction-NHS-Kings-Fund-2015.pdf (accessed 19 August 2016).

Appleby J et al. (2013). Using patient-reported outcome measures to estimate cost-effectiveness of hip replacements in English hospitals. *Journal of the Royal Society of Medicine*, 106:323–31.

Asprey A et al. (2013). Challenges to the credibility of patient feedback in primary healthcare settings: a qualitative study. *British Journal of General Practice*, 63:e200–8.

Bardach NS et al. (2013). The relationship between commercial website ratings and traditional hospital performance measures in the USA. *BMJ Quality & Safety*, 22:194–202.

Batbaatar E et al. (2015). Conceptualisation of patient satisfaction: a systematic narrative literature review. *Perspectives in Public Health*, 135:243–50.

Beattie M et al. (2015). Instruments to measure patient experience of healthcare quality in hospitals: a systematic review. *Systematic Reviews*, 4:97.

Black N, Varagunam M, Hutchings A (2014). Influence of surgical rate on patients' reported clinical need and outcomes in English NHS. *Journal of Public Health (Oxford)*, 36:497–503.

Boulhol H et al. (2012). Improving the health-care system in Poland. Available at: http://www.oecd.org/officialdocuments/publicdisplay-documentpdf/?cote=ECO/WKP%282012%2934&docLanguage=En (accessed 24 August 2016).

CBOS Public Opinion Research Centre (2014). Polish Public Opinion: Functioning of the Healthcare System Available at: http://www.cbos.pl/PL/publikacje/public_opinion/2014/07_2014.pdf (accessed 24 August 2016).

Coulter A (2010). Do patients want a choice and does it work? *BMJ*, 341:c4989.

Coulter A (2016). Patient feedback for quality improvement in general practice. *BMJ*, 352, i913.

Coulter A, Fitzpatrick R, Cornwell J (2009). Measures of patients' experience in hospital: purpose, methods and uses. Available at: https://www.kingsfund.org.uk/sites/default/files/kf/Point-of-Care-Measures-of-patients-experience-in-hospital-Kings-Fund-July-2009_0.pdf (accessed 11 December 2019).

Coulter A et al. (2013). A systematic development process for patient decision aids. *BMC Medical Informatics and Decision Making*, 13 Suppl 2:S2.

Coulter A et al. (2014). Collecting data on patient experience is not enough: they must be used to improve care. *BMJ*, 348:g2225.

Dawson J et al. (1996). Questionnaire on the perceptions of patients about total hip replacement. *Journal of Bone and Joint Surgery (British)*, 78:185–90.

DeCourcy A, West E, Barron D (2012). The National Adult Inpatient Survey conducted in the English National Health Service from 2002 to 2009: how have the data been used and what do we know as a result? *BMC Health Services Research*, 12:71.

Department of Health (2015). The NHS Constitution. Available at: https://www.gov.uk/government/uploads/system/uploads/attachment_data/file/480482/NHS_Constitution_WEB.pdf (accessed 24 August 2016).

Devlin NJ, Appleby J (2010). *Getting the most out of PROMs*. London: King's Fund.

Doyle C, Lennox L, Bell D (2013). A systematic review of evidence on the links between patient experience and clinical safety and effectiveness. *BMJ Open*, 3.

Entwistle V et al. (2012). Which experiences of health care delivery matter to service users and why? A critical interpretive synthesis and conceptual map. *Journal of Health Services Research & Policy*, 17:70–8.

Etkind SN et al. (2014). Capture, Transfer, and Feedback of Patient-Centered Outcomes Data in Palliative Care Populations: Does It Make a Difference? A Systematic Review. *Journal of Pain and Symptom Management*, 49(3):611–24.

European Commission (2014). Patient Safety and Quality of Care. Available at: http://ec.europa.eu/public_opinion/archives/ebs/ebs_411_sum_en.pdf (accessed 24 August 2016).

EuroQol Group (1990). EuroQol – a new facility for the measurement of health related quality of life. *Health Policy*, 16:199–208.

Fujisawa R, Klazinga N (2016). *Measuring patient experiences (PREMS): progress made by the OECD and its member countries between 2006 and 2015*. Paris: OECD.

Gerteis M et al. (1993). *Through the patient's eyes: understanding and promoting patient-centred care*. San Francisco: Jossey Bass.

Gilbert A et al. (2015). Use of patient-reported outcomes to measure symptoms and health related quality of life in the clinic. *Gynecologic Oncology*, 136, 429-39.

Gleeson H et al. (2016). Systematic review of approaches to using patient experience data for quality improvement in healthcare settings. *BMJ Open*, 6:e011907.

Graham C et al. (2013). Options appraisal on the measurement of people's experience of integrated care. Available at: http://www.pickereurope.org/wp-content/uploads/2014/10/Options-appraisal-on...-integrated-care.pdf (accessed 24 August 2016).

Greaves F et al. (2012). Associations between Internet-based patient ratings and conventional surveys of patient experience in the English NHS: an observational study. *BMJ Quality & Safety*, 21:600–5.

Greaves F et al. (2013). Harnessing the cloud of patient experience: using social media to detect poor quality healthcare. *BMJ Quality & Safety*, 22:251–5.

Hafner JM et al. (2011). The perceived impact of public reporting hospital performance data: interviews with hospital staff. *International Journal for Quality in Health Care*, 23:697–704.

Haugum M et al. (2014). The use of data from national and other large-scale user experience surveys in local quality work: a systematic review. *International Journal for Quality in Health Care*, 26:592–605.

Hewitson P et al. (2014). People with limiting long-term conditions report poorer experiences and more problems with hospital care. *BMC Health Services Research*, 14:33.

Hunter C et al. (2015). Perspectives from health, social care and policy stakeholders on the value of a single self-report outcome measure across long-term conditions: a qualitative study. *BMJ Open*, 5:e006986.

IHS Markit (2015). IQTiG established in Germany to evaluate quality in medical care. Available at: https://www.ihs.com/country-industry-forecasting.html?ID=1065997751 (accessed 24 August 2016).

ILO (2013). Health interview survey. Available at: http://www.ilo.org/surveydata/index.php/catalog/923/related_materials (accessed 24 August 2016).

Institute of Medicine (2001). *Crossing the quality chasm: a new health system for the 21st century*. Washington: National Academy Press.

Instituto Nacional de Estadistica (2013). National Health Survey (ENSE). Available at: http://www.ine.es/dyngs/INEbase/en/operacion.htm?c=Estadistica_C&cid=1254736176783&menu=resultados&idp=1254735573175 (accessed 24 August 2016).

Joyce CR et al. (2003). A theory-based method for the evaluation of individual quality of life: the SEIQoL. *Quality of Life Research*, 12:275–80.

Ketelaar NA et al. (2014). Exploring consumer values of comparative performance information for hospital choice. *Quality in Primary Care*, 22:81–9.

Kotronoulas G et al. (2014). What is the value of the routine use of patient-reported outcome measures toward improvement of patient outcomes, processes of care, and health service outcomes in cancer care? A systematic review of controlled trials. *Journal of Clinical Oncology*, 32:1480–501.

Kroenke K, Spitzer RL, Williams JB (2001). The PHQ-9: validity of a brief depression severity measure. *Journal of General Internal Medicine*, 16:606–13.

Lai T et al. (2013). Estonia: health system review. *Health Systems in Transition* [Online], 6. Available at: https://www.sm.ee/sites/default/files/content-editors/Ministeerium_kontaktid/Uuringu_ja_analuusid/Tervisevaldkond/hit-estonia.pdf (accessed 24 August 2016).

Locock L et al. (2014). Testing accelerated experience-based co-design: a qualitative study of using a national archive of patient experience narrative interviews to promote rapid patient-centred service improvement. *Health Services and Delivery Research*, 2.

Manary MP et al. (2013). The patient experience and health outcomes. *New England Journal of Medicine*, 368:201–3.

Murray CJ, Kawabata K, Valentine N (2001). People's experience versus people's expectations. *Health Affairs (Millwood)*, 20:21–4.

National Institute for Health and Care Excellence (NICE) (2012). Patient experience in adult NHS services. Available at: https://www.nice.org.uk/guidance/QS15/chapter/quality-statement-1-respect-for-the-patient#quality-statement-1-respect-for-the-patient (accessed 24 August 2016).

Neuburger J et al. (2013). Socioeconomic differences in patient-reported outcomes after a hip or knee replacement in the English National Health Service. *Journal of Public Health (Oxford)*, 35:115–24.

OECD (2010). Improving value in health care: measuring quality. *OECD Health Policy Studies*.

Paddison CA et al. (2015). Why do patients with multimorbidity in England report worse experiences in primary care? Evidence from the General Practice Patient Survey. *BMJ Open*, 5:e006172.

Paparella G (2016). Person-centred care in Europe: a cross-country comparison of health system performance, strategies and structures. Available at: http://www.pickereurope.org/wp-content/uploads/2016/02/12-02-16-Policy-briefing-on-patient-centred-care-in-Europe.pdf (accessed 24 August 2016).

Paterson C (1996). Measuring outcomes in primary care: a patient generated measure, MYMOP, compared with the SF-36 health survey. *BMJ*, 312:1016–20.

Peters M et al. (2016). The Long-Term Conditions Questionnaire: conceptual framework and item development. *Patient Related Outcome Measures*, 7:109–25.

Price RA et al. (2014). Examining the role of patient experience surveys in measuring health care quality. *Medical Care Research and Review*, 71:522–54.

Raleigh V et al. (2012). Do some trusts deliver a consistently better experience for patients? An analysis of patient experience across acute care surveys in English NHS trusts. *BMJ Quality & Safety*, 21:381–90.

Raleigh V et al. (2015). Impact of case-mix on comparisons of patient-reported experience in NHS acute hospital trusts in England. *Journal of Health Services Research & Policy*, 20:92–9.

Rechel B et al. (2016). Public reporting on quality, waiting times and patient experience in 11 high-income countries. *Health Policy*, 120:377–83.

Robert G, Cornwell J (2011). *What matters to patients? Developing the evidence base for measuring and improving patient experience*. Warwick: NHS Institute for Innovation and Improvement.

Robert Koch Institute (2013). Positive signals and warning signs – 34 articles with results of the "German Health Interview and Examination Survey for Adults" published (press release). Available at: http://www.rki.de/EN/Content/Service/Press/PressReleases/2013/05_2013.html (accessed 24 August 2016).

Rozenblum R, Bates DW (2013). Patient-centred healthcare, social media and the internet: the perfect storm? *BMJ Quality & Safety*, 22:183–6.

Rozenblum R et al. (2013). The patient satisfaction chasm: the gap between hospital management and frontline clinicians. *BMJ Quality & Safety*, 22:242–50.

Sizmur S, Graham C, Walsh J (2015). Influence of patients' age and sex and the mode of administration on results from the NHS Friends and Family Test of patient experience. *Journal of Health Services Research & Policy*, 20:5–10.

Soljak M et al. (2009). Is there an association between deprivation and pre-operative disease severity? A cross-sectional study of patient-reported health status. *International Journal for Quality in Health Care*, 21:311–15.

Stiggelbout AM et al. (2012). Shared decision making: really putting patients at the centre of healthcare. *BMJ*, 344:e256.

Strandberg-Larsen M, Krasnik A (2009). Measurement of integrated healthcare delivery: a systematic review of methods and future research directions. *International Journal of Integrated Care*, 9:e01.

Varagunam M, Hutchings A, Black N (2014). Do patient-reported outcomes offer a more sensitive method for comparing the outcomes of consultants than mortality? A multilevel analysis of routine data. *BMJ Quality & Safety*, 24(3):195–202.

Varagunam M et al. (2014). Impact on hospital performance of introducing routine patient reported outcome measures in surgery. *Journal of Health Services Research & Policy*, 19:77–84.

Ware JE Jr, Sherbourne CD (1992). The MOS 36-item short-form health survey (SF-36). I. Conceptual framework and item selection. *Medical Care*, 30:473–83.

Zaslavsky AM, Zaborski LB, Cleary PD (2002). Factors affecting response rates to the Consumer Assessment of Health Plans Study survey. *Medical Care*, 40:485–99.

Ziebland S et al. (eds.) (2013). *Understanding and Using Health Experiences.* Oxford: Oxford University Press.

8 | *Choosing providers*

MARIANNA FOTAKI

Introduction

Choice of health care provider has become an increasingly important feature of health care policy in many countries (Thomson & Dixon, 2006; Bevan & Helderman, 2010; Or et al., 2010), particularly in countries where choice had been previously unavailable. It was introduced as a means to generate competition among providers, thereby improving quality, efficiency and responsiveness, while in some cases choice was also meant to improve equity of access (Reid, 2003; Ringard et al., 2013). Moreover, giving patients and users choice of who, when and what forms of care will be available to them is in keeping with the political declarations and policy commitments towards more person-centred health services (Cacace & Nolte, 2011). Increasingly, individual patients and users are being thought of as consumers and expected to play a key role in their own care, while helping to shape the health system that serves them. Yet the market-type patient choice has not worked as intended, producing little benefit under specific conditions, which limits its usefulness as a policy tool in public health systems.

The types of choice introduced in European health systems reflect their structural and institutional requirements and the wider policy environment in which they operate. Understanding what motivates the adoption of certain policies can help to predict and evaluate the effects of choice on the intended objectives (e.g. efficiency, quality, responsiveness, equity and personalization). This chapter seeks to systematically explore the different types of choice of provider in primary and specialist care implemented in selected European health systems. It considers policy drivers behind expanding (or in some cases restricting) provider choice in an attempt to better understand the potential benefits and limitations. In examining the rationale for introducing patient and user choice, it critically appraises evidence of how choosing primary and specialist care providers works in a small number of single-payer health systems, where such options were previously limited. It does not consider insurance-based systems, where choice and competition among insurers operate simultaneously, although these could increase or limit patient choice of provider; this is discussed in greater detail in Chapter 9 on choice of health insurer.

The chapter draws on the theories of choice and empirical evidence to analyse the impact by considering the following:

- To what values, besides 'choice', does the theory explicitly or implicitly appeal? In other words, is choice a means to achieve other goals such as equity or efficiency or is it a value of its own?
- At what point do conflicts arise (i.e. 'tensions', 'trade-offs', 'contradictions', 'inconsistency') between choice and these other values?
- What practical constraints on the exercise of choice are implied (e.g. limits on the amount of complex technical knowledge patients can be expected to process, financial and structural constraints, or asymmetries of power and unwillingness of professionals to enable choice)?

It reviews the evidence of the impact of choice on care outcomes, efficiency, equity and patient empowerment and it puts forward proposals for empirical evaluation of choice in different settings and for models of choice that are closer to the reality of patient care. The institutional conditions necessary to realize effective patient choice are also discussed. The final section argues for recognizing the value and importance of the variety of aspects involved in patient choice, to propose a more balanced framework of choice taking account of users' diverse needs and the resources they can realistically draw on when making their care-related decisions. The chapter concludes by assessing whether choice in its present forms has contributed to person-centred health systems or can support this objective in the future.

The concept of choice: origin, logic and rationale

The literature on choice is wide-ranging and closely associated with the concepts of freedom, autonomy and democracy (Fotaki, 2006). Normative theories assert that people would exercise choice if they chose 'rationally'. Policy-makers often rely on these theories to identify the possible outcomes resulting from policies promoting patient choice, the mechanisms which would produce such outcomes, and the required conditions for these mechanisms to work effectively (Fotaki et al., 2006). Additionally, descriptive theories have been used to explain how people actually exercise choice.

Larkin & Mitchell (2016) have argued that choice supported by competition in care services can be seen to be intrinsically a 'good thing'. It can help in achieving desirable policy goals such as improving efficiency and quality of care by allowing patients and users of services to decide which services best meet their needs, and it provides the means for individuals to acquire a greater sense of control (Iyengar & DeVoe, 2003) and intrinsic motivation. Research from the adjacent fields of social care and elderly care points to the potential positive psychological effects that choice has on increasing one's sense of personal independence (Arksey & Glendinning, 2007; Sandman & Munthe, 2010), as well as individual physical and mental well-being (Morris, 2006; Rabiee & Glendinning, 2010), which are also relevant in the context of health and long-term care. Moreover, choice is frequently associated with principles of citizenship (Markus & Schwartz, 2010). In short, choice has intrinsic value to patients; it feels good to be able to choose as it enables each person to pursue precisely those objectives and activities that best satisfy their own preferences within the limits of their resources (Saltman, 1994). Choice of provider in primary care settings could promote continuity of care while fostering a trusting relationship between doctor and patient, and contribute to positive health outcomes (Starfield, 1994; Goold, 1999). However, choice can also lead to anxiety, stress and regret (Loomes & Sugden, 1982; Daly, 2012; Baxter & Glendinning, 2013). Patients and service users may avoid exercising choice due to fears of potential or anticipated negative consequences (Ryan, 1994; Goold, 1999; Fotaki, 2014). This raises the issue of the patient's right to refuse treatment from providers that they did not choose, the option of a second opinion, and the option not to choose.

Choice in the policy context: motivation, drivers and expectations

In health policy, choice was influenced by the neoclassic economics and neoliberal ideology developed throughout the 1970s, now permeating all aspects of society (Chang, 2014). At the same time, choice can also be seen as a response to long-standing demands by patient and user groups for autonomy and for greater control over the health care resources available to them (Barnes, 1999; Fotaki, 2011), enabling them to better manage their own conditions.

The following sections provide a brief overview of choice policies in selected European countries. The focus here is on countries where patient choice of provider was introduced from the 1990s and include Denmark, England, Norway and Sweden.

Denmark

In 2007 Denmark embarked on the most radical reform of the political administrative system since the first democratic constitution in 1849 with the thirteen counties merging into five regions and the 271 municipalities being amalgamated into 98 (Andersen & Jensen, 2010). Denmark has a decentralized system with regions having relative freedom to choose the volume of hospital activity allocated to different specialisms but central government is responsible for legislating these regional initiatives and their financing (Vrangbæk et al., 2012).This semi-decentralized model of health care was expected to stimulate active participation by local people in their own health care and to ensure the responsiveness of the system to the specific needs in each local area (Stubbs, 2015).

In a move to improve the efficiency of the health care system, in 1993 the government in Denmark introduced user choice of hospital. In 2002 the government introduced a waiting time guarantee ('extended free choice') of two months from referral, subsequently reduced to one month (Larsen & Stone, 2015). The 2007 reform also gave patients the option of choosing a specialist provider from outside their region if they were unhappy with the treatment offered or if waiting times were too long. However, primary care doctors continue to be responsible for referrals, acting as gatekeepers to the system; for example, in 2011 GPs chose the hospital on behalf of 76% of their patients (Pedersen, Bech & Vrangbæk, 2011). At the same time, introducing patient choice of hospital has led to each region in Denmark offering hospital services according to demand (Vrangbæk et al., 2007). Early evaluations of choice reforms in Denmark (as well as in Sweden and Norway) found limited use of choice by patients due to their lack of knowledge regarding reforms, insufficient support from GPs and limited information, although there was an upward trend in the uptake of choice (Vrangbæk et al., 2007).

England

In England a series of legislative changes have introduced increased levels of choice in all aspects of patient care in the National Health Service (NHS) over the last decades. The first attempts to introduce elements of choice date to experiments with quasi-market reforms aiming to introduce competitive mechanisms in health care services in the early 1990s, the so-called internal market (Le Grand, 2003). The policy sought to make services more responsive to users' needs by giving health authorities a budget to contract services from hospitals, which had to compete for contracts. At the same time, general practitioners' practices were encouraged to take up a portion of the budget to purchase some services for patients on their own lists, again requiring providers to compete (GP Fundholding). This enabled the referral of patients to a hospital of their own or their GP's choice. However, in practice this kind of choice was not vigorously pursued, resulting in half-hearted and isolated responses rather than a choice revolution (Tuohy, 1999). If anything, choice of provider is likely to have diminished during this time, because the internal market set up contracts with specific hospitals, so that GPs and patients could only choose from among these options (Robinson & Le Grand, 1994; Fotaki, 1999).

In 2003, under the New Labour government, patients in England (Scotland, Wales and Northern Ireland have followed different non-market approaches since devolution) were offered a choice of five providers for elective treatments, such as hip or cataract surgery; this was expanded to about 150 approved providers from public, private or not-for-profit sectors in 2006 and took the form of an 'extended choice network' in 2008. Although there was no evidence of strong public demand for choice of hospital as such, there was considerable public concern about waiting times, and the newly introduced choice options particularly benefited patients in areas where existing services were poor and had long waiting times (Coulter, Le Maistre & Henderson, 2005; Dawson et al., 2004). In addition to improving quality and efficiency, the policy of offering choice to all was intended to extend the opportunity to choose different providers beyond the articulate and those who could afford to access private health care (Department of Health, 2003). This second attempt at creating a market within a single payer system was justified on the basis of having to keep up with the presumed demands of patients who were increasingly thought of as consumers and who were expected to 'reveal their preferences' through choice (Le Grand, 2007). There was, however, little evidence of whether market-based choice could work in publicly funded health services.

The 2012 Health and Social Care Act further expanded the commitment to provider choice. From 2015 patients may choose to register with a GP practice outside the GP-practice's catchment area, although this scheme is voluntary for GP practices. In addition, patients, along with their GPs, have been given the possibility to choose the best services for their needs from an NHS, third sector or independent private sector provider as long as these are approved by the commissioners.

Norway

In Norway the structural reform of 2001 divided the responsibility for health care between the state, the four regions and the 428 municipalities (Lian, 2003). The reform also introduced choice of GP to improve accessibility, continuity and quality of primary health care (Ringard et al., 2013), especially for older people and those with chronic health problems, while addressing the problem of low recruitment of GPs (Holte et al., 2015). It introduced free registration with any physician licensed by municipalities, including those in private practice, to work in primary care (capacity permitting) as it was expected that this would strengthen the physician's personal responsibility for continuity of care and availability (Grasdal & Monstad, 2011). In parallel with the reform, the capacity of primary care doctors increased by about 10% (Iversen & Lurås, 2011). Evaluations found that the reform has been popular among doctors and that the population has become more satisfied with access to care. There are also indications of improved equity in access to specialist services (Grasdal & Monstad, 2011). However, while mostly beneficial for improving equity of access, continuity of care and patient satisfaction, it is difficult to disentangle these outcomes from the increases in capacity in primary care. Also, challenges remain regarding the integration between independent private primary care doctors' services, in particular for those working mostly in small practices, and other primary and specialist care activities. Finally, there is recognition of a need for more patient orientation, and more decentralized services close to where patients live to reduce costs (Rørtveit, 2015).

Sweden

The Swedish health system is similar to those in other Nordic countries in that it shares the same commitment to universal access and equality, and it is characterized by a decentralized structure. It differs, however, with regard to primary care, with an overall lower investment and fewer providers; also, GPs do not act as gatekeepers (Anell, 2015). Choice of health care provider has been introduced gradually since the 1990s (Fotaki & Boyd, 2005). The 1994 national family physician reform introduced an element of choice in primary care but this was discontinued the following year when the government changed from conservative to social-democrat over a dispute about extending choice to private providers in primary care.

Beginning in January 2010 the government made it compulsory for county councils to provide patients with a choice of primary care provider and freedom of establishment for those private units that did accept requirements and payment principles determined by county councils (Anell, 2015). Patients had to be given the option of a public or private provider, with county council funding allocated according to the individual patient's choice. In keeping with the decentralized model of the Swedish health system, ten out of the 21 counties already had some arrangements in place at that time (Anell, 2011). In 2015 the government introduced unrestricted choice of provider in primary care and outpatient specialist care. These latest reforms led to the establishment of over 270 new private primary care practices operating for profit throughout the country, with some researchers foreseeing potentially negative impact on equity (Burström, 2002), which will be discussed below.

In specialist care, most county councils have adopted some form of public competition since the mid-1990s, particularly in Stockholm and other urban areas (Winblad, 2008), offering increased choice of hospital. However, only a minority of patients (who in many cases could self-refer themselves) and physicians exercised their right to choose a hospital at this point. Research has found that referrals are mostly based on medical grounds while the patient's wish to choose a specific provider is considered less important (Burström et al., 2017). The 2015 health reform supports choice in outpatient specialist services and choice related to second opinion for treatment of life-threatening diseases nationally; there is no national policy related to choice of inpatient care in general.

However, choice in primary care remains a controversial issue in the Swedish debate, although much of the criticism does not revolve around choice as such but rather concerns the free establishment of private providers, which has found increasing support over time.

In summary, policies introducing patient choice of provider in various countries differed in content and context, and reform agendas have changed over time. For instance, in Norway and Sweden the emphasis was on improving access to primary care, while choice policies in Denmark and England were driven, at least initially, by policy concerns about waiting times, although in England the focus progressively shifted towards introducing competition in specialist services. A common feature for all systems described was the growing importance of individualized market-based forms of choice, although this may now be changing with the shift towards person-centred care as will be discussed in the concluding section of this chapter.

Implementation and the evidence of impact: how far has provider choice delivered on its promises?

Do patients want choice and feel empowered by it?

Choice has been used not only as a policy instrument for achieving the policy goals of efficiency, quality and equity, but also to promote service user empowerment and autonomy (Fotaki, 2011). The development of the active, critical consumer is considered an important end in itself, even if people cannot always act as a perfectly informed agent.

A 2012 survey of patients' involvement in health across the EU found that some expressed a desire for a more balanced relationship with their doctors, which would allow patients to participate more actively in their care. This finding was particularly strong for younger and well-educated people, those with chronic conditions, and those living in western Europe (Eurobarometer, 2012). However, these observations do not necessarily imply a demand for more choice. At the same time, a review of how people use choice in public services in England found that 'having choice' was seen to be important by the vast majority of respondents (Boyle, 2013). Those with lower education were more likely than those with at least a degree to respond positively to having this opportunity, although people from disadvantaged backgrounds may be less able to exercise choice and are therefore less likely to benefit from it.

The individual characteristics and circumstances of patients and users of health services are likely not only to influence their choices, but also to determine whether they exercise choice at all. For example, an evaluation of the London Patient Choice Project, which was established to offer NHS patients in England more choice over where and when they receive treatment, found that old age, low educational attainment, family commitments or low income all had an impact on patients' choice of a non-local hospital, meaning that they were less likely to travel to a non-local hospital if they were offered the choice (Burge et al., 2004). Distance remains an issue for many people and a lack of public transport can make choice difficult for people who are unable to afford a car (Dixon et al., 2010).

The London Patient Choice Project also found that differential access to information for people with low educational attainment and those for whom English is not their first language could lead to variations in uptake of choice (Dixon et al., 2010). A related empirical study concluded that patients in England who are not highly numerate and health-literate were less able to use the available information to make complex decisions about hospital choice without some expert support (Boyce et al., 2010). Comprehending the options and making trade-offs between quality, safety, patient experience and location posed difficulties, and the way information was presented made a difference to how patients used it. Similar difficulties were observed in other health systems such as in Sweden regarding accessibility (Anell, 2015; Victoor et al., 2012) and the role of information when choosing hospitals in Denmark (Birk & Henriksen, 2012; Pedersen, Bech & Vrangbæk, 2011). This highlights the need for adequate support structures to be put in place if choice is meant to work for all. Evidence from shared decision-making suggests that structured support may help reduce health inequalities when the intervention is adapted to disadvantaged groups' needs (Durand et al., 2014) (*see also* Chapter 11).

The type and degree of choice patients want and value is not self-evident either. Research by the UK-based consumers' association *Which?* in 2005 found that choice was seen to be of relatively low priority for many people compared with other aspects of service delivery in the NHS. The majority of respondents were more concerned with having safe, good quality services provided locally, and not so much about having diverse providers to choose from (*Which?*, 2005). Patients tend to favour a provider they know and trust and opt for choice only when no such provider is available (Taylor-Gooby & Wallace, 2009). The evidence from across Europe further suggests that in addition to satisfaction with the health system (Eurobarometer, 2012), perceptions of choice are influenced by an individual's personal health situation, age and gender. For instance, early studies from Sweden found that older patients appeared to be both interested in choice of primary care doctor and happy about the amount of choice offered, while highly educated young people, and women in particular, were found to both exercise and favour choice more when compared to other population groups (Rosén, Anell & Hjortsberg, 2001; Anell, Rosén & Hjortsberg, 1997). These age and gender factors were also confirmed for England. Overall, evidence suggests that patients appear to be more interested in choosing treatments especially when they are chronically ill and have knowledge about their disease (Coulter, 2010). The willingness to engage in treatment decisions is, however, often influenced by the severity of the medical condition and the complexity of the procedure involved: the more life-threatening the disease and technologically advanced the treatment, the lower tends to be the patient's desire for choice (Fotaki et al., 2008). Patients' preference for choice might also be different in primary care as opposed to specialist services but there is little comparative research on these issues.

It is important to note that, for example, in England retaining the public and universal aspects of the health system has tended to be of greater concern than demands for choice, and the marketization of public services has been considered as a threat to universal and free provision of health services provided by the NHS. When ranked on a scale of one to five in a 2010 MORI survey, fairness in public services came first, while choice and the personalization of services was last for the majority (63%) of the British population (2020 Public Services Trust, 2010). Similar public concerns about the impact of recent privatization have been noted for Sweden, with evidence suggesting that while the public may be in favour of provider choice, they were sceptical about profit incentives in tax-funded markets and about the payment of dividends by health care providers to their owners (Anell, 2015).

In summary, patients' willingness to exercise, and demand for, choice differs by age, gender, social characteristics and personal circumstances. Although service users might be attracted to the idea of having a choice in general, research shows that not all populations are equally able to exercise choice, as will be discussed next.

What are the impacts of choice on equity?

As noted earlier, one aim of individual patient choice of provider is to improve equity by removing barriers to access, although there are other important equity considerations such as improving health outcomes for those in greater need (Fotaki, 2010). Thus, the introduction of choice of primary care provider in Norway and Sweden was, at least initially, intended to improve access to primary care, while elsewhere relevant policies served to provide greater choice of specialist care, such as in Denmark and England. In England the introduction of choice of elective treatment in 2003 described earlier was specifically intended to enhance equity of access by permitting those unable to afford private health care a choice of provider already enjoyed by those who could afford to pay for it (Reid, 2003).

In Sweden some population groups in urban areas enjoyed improved access to primary care because of the increased number of private providers entering the market following the choice reforms (Anell, 2015; Dietrichson, Ellegård & Kjellson, 2016). However, the higher number of new primary care providers in densely populated urban areas might have negatively affected equality of access for patients outside urban areas (Burström et al., 2017). Also, evidence from some county councils from the 1990s suggested that relatively healthy people benefited more following the choice reforms than did others in terms of access to primary care (Saltman, 1994). This risk of inequality might be higher for specialist services (Devaux, 2015) as they generally tend to favour the better off while primary care is more pro-poor (Grasdal & Monstad, 2011). However, in the case of Norway, introducing choice and contracting of a higher number of primary care doctors operating in the private sector improved patient access to specialist services as well as decreasing the marginal effect of income on utilization (Grasdal & Monstad, 2011).

Evaluations of pilots introducing choice of hospital in various regions in England in 2002–2003 found that age, class, income and family obligations affected patients' ability to travel to a non-local provider, and therefore their choices (Burge et al., 2004). Other studies reported no evidence of inequalities of access for patients participating in the same projects but these studies did not consider patients who were not offered choice (Coulter, Le Maistre & Henderson, 2005; Dawson et al., 2004). In many cases choice was only offered to a minority of patients, for example excluding older and sicker patients (Appleby, Harrison & Devlin, 2005).

Empirical research on the effects of reforms introduced into the English NHS during the 1990s suggest that socioeconomic differences that lead to variations in health care utilization are deeply ingrained, and that in the context of universal and comprehensive health systems small doses of 'quasi market' competition (with a few providers competing) modifies providers' behaviour while having little or no effect on socioeconomic inequalities in health care (Cookson et al., 2010). Nevertheless, there is a risk of creating new inequalities over and above those that already exist and this might differ by the type of service and setting (primary or specialist care). This is because some patients receive preferential access and treatment under certain schemes, as was the case with the patients of GP fundholders in the UK (Manion, 2005).

There is also evidence that physicians are likely to change their behaviour to fit the market, which could benefit some patients more than others. For example, following the introduction of competition and choice in Sweden, GPs and specialists reported that these changes had enhanced their autonomy, income and employment prospects, while at the same time they could reduce their commitment to the normative foundation of the system, that is ensuring equal access according to clinical need (Bergmark, 2008). Thus, although choice and privatization might have improved access to primary care in Sweden in general, the reforms have also raised serious questions regarding their impact on equity, leading to calls for future regulation of providers (Anell, 2016). The full impact of choice on equity cannot be assessed without suitable data on quality or outcomes of care, which is currently lacking in the Swedish context. A study from the Netherlands found that surgeons felt they had to 'sell themselves' by advertising or marketing their performance when patients had the option to choose between them (Dwarswaard, Hilhorst & Trappenburg, 2011). It was noted that better performance would be easier to demonstrate for relatively minor routine conditions, such as varicose veins and hernia, which represented a significant source of income for hospitals; therefore, surgeons began to pay more attention to patients with such conditions, following patients' preferences rather than medical need. Recent work by Visser et al. (2018), also in the Netherlands, noted that the introduction of consumerist communication technology in health care would assume a 'universal individual', creating tensions for health care professionals who aim for equal treatment of all patients, and which has paradoxically led to new inequalities among patients with differential abilities to access technology.

In summary, countries differed in their objectives by which introducing choice of provider should improve equity. There is evidence of choice leading to improved access to certain services, for some populations, and in some settings. Yet there might also be different and potentially negative consequences for equity where there is little additional support offered to those who are less able to exercise the option of choice. Indeed, patient choice of provider might exacerbate inequities in access due to pre-existing inequalities in income, class and individual circumstances, with the additional risk of individual choice leading to new inequalities.

Does choice improve the quality of care?

Quality is an intrinsically difficult concept to define, with definitions including a wide range of dimensions and indicators of process, such as waiting times, as well as the outcome of care, such as patient experience (Berwick, 2002). The economic assumptions driving choice policies in public systems where prices are fixed, such as the National Health Service in the UK, is that providers will strive to attract patients by improving quality if the market contains a sufficient number of competitors: hospitals in these instances will compete in terms of quality and not price (Gaynor, Morreno-Serra & Propper, 2012). Empirical studies measuring the relationship between competition and quality of care suggest that there are positive as well as negative consequences, and sometimes neither. For example, in the Netherlands there were reports of perceived decreases in quality of care after the introduction of regulated competition (Dwarswaard, Hilhorst & Trappenburg, 2011; Victoor et al., 2012; *see also* Chapter 9). The estimated impact of competition on quality of care has been considered to be small in other health systems such as in England (Dixon et al., 2010) and Sweden (Anell, 2015).

For example, empirical evidence from England found an association between the introduction of choice policies and improvements in the quality of care. For example, Cooper et al. (2011) demonstrated that death rates from acute myocardial infarction were slightly lower in geographical areas where there was greater potential competition between hospitals facing fixed prices. These competitive pressures were attributed to the effects of patient choice initiatives, although patients exercised choice mainly in relation to elective treatment, which was not the subject of the evaluation in this specific study (Pollock et al., 2011). Conversely, an evaluation of the impact of the internal market in England in the 1990s using negotiable prices found that greater competition was associated with higher mortality among patients with acute myocardial infarction (Propper & Burgess, 2004). However, as many other factors besides competition influence the quality of hospital services, including price structure, payment methods, internal organization and pre-existing culture, in addition to quality regulation systems and protocols, it remains difficult to clearly attribute observed outcomes to choice policies per se (Sutton et al., 2012; Ferlie et al., 2004).

There is also evidence from market-based systems such as that in the USA of providers tending to compete on quality by introducing expensive technology (particularly when they do not face hard budget constraints) that can lead to higher costs and squeeze out cost-effective care (Pauly, 2005). This appeals mainly to doctors but it also aims to attract patients by offering novel and usually more expensive treatments and diagnostic procedures.

Overall, most research on the impact of choice and competition in relation to quality is conducted in the context of specialist care. The available evidence of the impact of choice in terms of improved outcomes remains inconclusive. Alongside methodological weaknesses, reported improvements tend to be small or were derived from a very narrowly defined set of clinical indicators. Moreover, studies are often conducted under specific conditions that may not be universally applicable.

There is a lack of comparable studies in primary care, along with a lack of suitable data on quality of care besides patient satisfaction surveys. There is some, albeit limited, evidence for Sweden, and studies have failed to find a substantial impact on the quality of care following the introduction of patient choice in primary care (Dietrichson, Ellegård & Kjellsson, 2016; Fogelberg, 2014) and few patients compare providers before making their choice (Glenngård, Anell & Beckman, 2011; Swedish Agency for Health and Care Services Analysis, 2013; Wahlstedt & Ekman, 2016). There is some indication of improved patient satisfaction (in areas with alternative providers) but there is no general trend suggesting that satisfaction or quality of care has improved overall and as a consequence of the choice reforms alone (Gaynor, Morreno-Sella & Propper, 2013; Gaynor, Propper & Seiler, 2016; Gravelle et al., 2014; Moscelli, Gravelle & Siciliani, 2016) as these will often depend on precise institutional arrangements (Cellini, Pignataro & Rizzo, 2000). Population surveys show that trust in primary care has increased between 2009 and 2012 (Anell, Glenngård & Merkur, 2012) but this trend reversed after 2013. In Norway there have been improvements in patient satisfaction in most aspects since the 2001 reform, but it is not clear to what extent this can be explained by the parallel capacity increase in the number of primary care doctors (Iversen & Lurås, 2011).

On the whole, there is little robust empirical evidence that choice of provider leads to substantial quality improvements. Studies on increased patient choice of hospitals have shown mixed effects on health outcomes.

Does choice improve the efficiency of health care?

We noted in the introduction to this chapter that competition between health care providers has been considered central to improving the efficiency of publicly funded health systems. Efficiency in this context can be defined as the optimal allocation of scarce resources and providing the best value for money (Palmer, 1999). It is seen by some as a solution to rising costs and demand (Le Grand, 2007). Choice, then, can – at least in theory – enhance efficiency by favouring providers who offer better services at lower cost (Bartlett, Roberts & Le Grand, 1998). However, the principles of the commercial sector do not readily apply in health care. This is because service users often have to base their choices on insufficient information (Arrow, 1963) or they may be induced to make choices that suit providers, especially when there is a financial incentive to do so (Rice, 2002).

The evidence of whether patient choice of provider does positively impact efficiency remains mixed. For instance, one review of the impact of choice in England concluded that any increases in efficiency that were observed after the introduction of related policies (as measured by, for example, an increase in the number of elective surgery patients treated as day cases, a decrease in the length of inpatient stays, or reductions in avoidable admissions) could not be attributed to patient choice alone as there were also other policies and trends which could have encouraged such results (Civitas Institute, 2010). There is limited evidence from Sweden suggesting that implementing provider choice may be associated with an increase in costs (Bergmark, 2008).

In the context of specialist services, when these involve fee-for-service payments, providers may classify treatments as being more risky and expensive in order to generate additional revenues in these instances, a practice which can be found in the market-type based health systems (Kuttner, 2008). This gaming of the system, combined with an increased supply of specialist services that followed the introduction of competition, choice and per case payment in the 1990s in Sweden, made strategic priority setting and resource allocation by county councils more difficult, creating new threats to efficiency (Bergmark, 2008). Another form of gaming was observed under the internal market in the NHS in the 1990s where hospitals competing with each other became intentionally less productive shortly before obtaining trust status, so as to look more efficient under the new arrangements when compared with those that did not (Söderlund et al., 1997).

In summary, the evidence that patient choice of provider leads to greater efficiency is not persuasive because it is difficult to single out a specific policy initiative as the 'cause' of a specific 'effect'. Any measured efficiency gain may also be achieved by gaming the system and compromising quality. Furthermore, introducing competition and choice between providers to improve efficiency relies on an implicit belief that existing public providers with restricted choice are intrinsically inefficient (and private providers with extended choice for patients are intrinsically efficient), which has little basis in evidence, although non-market systems may create their own inefficiencies due to the suboptimal allocation of resources.

The limitations of provider choice: policy lessons

The key implication that policy-makers need to consider concerns the usefulness of provider choice for promoting the goals of public health systems and for supporting person-centred care. The introduction of provider choice in single-payer systems such as Denmark, England, Norway and Sweden were shown to produce some benefits for some population groups in some settings, in particular those who are most likely to benefit from a higher supply of providers and those who are willing and able to use the information available. At the same time, there are a number of undesirable effects, especially in specialist and/ or hospital services. Evaluations of choice policies in health care find that they rarely lead to more social efficiency or increases in welfare (Schwartz & Cheek, 2017) at a population level. This is because of the complexity of the choices involved and patients' unequal ability to navigate these. Choice policies in health care may also negatively impact on equity, and may fail to meet patients' interest in improving the quality of services provided locally (which patients prefer), once policy assumes their willingness to travel afar to find the best provider since patients with caring commitments (Burge et al., 2004) and those who do not own a car are less likely to travel any distance (Dixon et al., 2010).

The theory of market imperfections in health care considers how choices are actually made, and demonstrates the problems of replicating simplistic economic choice models in health care. People's ability and willingness to make choices is influenced by their beliefs, cultural values and expectations as well as by their life circumstances, personal characteristics and experiences of health care services (Fotaki et al., 2006; Visser et al., 2018). People are seldom rational choosers, least of all in relation to health or care services, a reality that psychologists and economists both acknowledge (Kahneman & Tversky, 1979; Thaler & Sunstein, 2008; Hansen et al., 2015).

Although these limitations may apply more to some types of care than others, choice is often impaired in health care and cannot on its own promote person-centred care for all. Patients often lack the information needed to make meaningful choices about providers and their care, and there is therefore a need to better understand the information needs of people to help their choices or indeed, where people are unwilling to exercise choice, to provide appropriate support. At the same time, as it was noted earlier, there are population subgroups that are more motivated and better able to make informed choices about their own care, such as people with long-term conditions. This can be turned into a strong argument for choice in primary care, where the role of the service is to support them in their choice but with a default option available for those who do not want, or who are unable, to choose.

Although it is possible to treat people who seek support from the health service as customers, this may not be compatible with ways of thinking and acting that are crucial to good quality health care. Good care grows out of collaborative and continuing attempts to attune professional knowledge and technologies to diseased bodies and complex lives (Mol, 2008). When making complex health decisions, patients often rely on their intuition and emotions, which also involves the avoidance of regret (Ryan, 1994; Loomes & Sugden, 1982) as well as trusted networks (Pescosolido, 1992), rather than the impersonal data.

Framing the issue of choice in the context of market competition roots it in assumptions originating in neoclassical economics about humans as disembodied and socially disembedded individuals pursuing their self-interest. This leads to a significant narrowing of the concept of choice, and of the users of health services as rational 'choosers' exercising their preferences. Choice and independence are indeed powerful concepts, but interdependency is an essential part of social life and never more so than in relationships involving care (Fotaki, 2015).

Innovations and future developments: implications for person-centred care

The desire of service users for more autonomy and greater control over the health care they receive should not be discarded along with the consumerist market model but rather should be seriously addressed on its own terms (Beresford, 2008). In many ways patients are obliged and increasingly willing to make health-related decisions as co-producers of their health together with health care professionals, and as citizens and community members they participate in co-designing health services. Often these choices are governed by social values and the need for cooperation and recognition, not by mere self-interest (Taylor-Gooby, 1999); patients' involvement is most effective when used as part of a broader ethos of care (Health Foundation, 2012).

Various practical ways of strengthening elements of 'voice' in the system should be considered. Enabling people to use voice, beyond the option to exit and choose a different provider, would allow patients and service users to assume responsibility for their health in ways that are different from the individualistic personalization agenda. The example of co-production of public services, with the users of services as active asset-holders of resources rather than passive consumers, demonstrates the benefits of promoting collaborative rather than paternalistic relation-ships between staff and service users, where the focus is on the delivery of outcomes rather than the services (Needham & Carr, 2009). The degree to which patients and professionals each hold agency for these co-produced outcomes varies widely, but the concept has profound implications for improving health care quality, safety and value.

Overall, the expansion of choice can empower patients, if it is appropriately linked to their direct participation in decision-making processes. This can occur, for instance, by involving them (individually or collectively) in managing their health resources as in existing co-production schemes (Batalden et al., 2016; Baker, 2010; Needham & Carr, 2009) and by assisting them in deciding what is best for them (Barry & Edgman-Levitan, 2012). Supporting patients in the process of choosing can help overcome the information disadvantage and some of the socioeconomic barriers associated with market-based choice. In all cases, patients and service users should be clear about what is involved in their choices, and the potential consequences, not just for their immediate care but for the future provision of care for them and their families and community.

Choice is also a key value embedded in contemporary approaches to framing the delivery of health care services as can be seen in the emphasis placed upon it and its integration in the movement towards person-centred care. The idea of person-centredness implies that an individual's decisions and preferences are at the heart of all their interactions with health care practitioners, who are expected to support these despite the degree of confusion over what is meant by 'person-centredness' and the types of changes that are needed to promote it (*see* Chapter 2).

Conclusions

Promoting market-based individual patient choice, first introduced in the planned health systems in the UK and Sweden in the 1990s, has become a standard health policy objective in health and social care in many other countries. Two rationales typically make the case for consumer choice in health systems. First, it is as a method to stimulate providers to improve the quality of services offered; and second, as a benefit in its own right that is valued and desired by patients. Moreover, in many western societies choice is increasingly seen as an expression of an individual's unique identity (Schwartz & Cheek, 2017).

However, the idea of offering patients choice and making them act as consumers in a market-place has serious limitations when applied to health and social care. Overall, policies based on these assumptions have been found wanting, for both theoretical and empirical reasons. People have various needs, which are further augmented in times of dislocation, vulnerability and stress, and many cannot or do not want to make such complex choices themselves. Choice works best in instances where it is supported by trusted people and with the help of decision aids.

Furthermore, any impact on quality and costs will depend on the precise institutional setting in which choice of provider is implemented. Reliance on competition to promote choice in health carries the risk of reproducing existing inequalities while simultaneously introducing new ones related to health literacy and access to information linked to users' educational status and ability to pay.

Choice is more likely to work if policy design reconsiders what it means and what types of choice are important to patients. Policy design should be informed by the social and psychological factors affecting individuals' health-related decisions, such as their previous experience and social bonds as family and community members. To achieve this, policy-makers might consider interdisciplinary frameworks and alternatives to market mechanisms which could offer a more balanced view of how choice works and what choices matter to patients if they are to promote person-centred care.

Note

I would like to thank Professor Colin Leys, Dr Sally Ruane and David Roland for commenting on an earlier version of the policy report on this topic produced for the Centre for Health and the Public Interest. I would also like to thank Professor Anders Anell for his valuable comments and insights offered, in particular on Sweden and Norway. Any errors are mine alone.

References

2020 Public Services Trust (2010). What People Want, Need and Expect from Public Services. London: 2020 Public Services Trust at RSA prepared by Ipsos MORI.

Andersen PT, Jensen JJ (2010). Health Care Reform Denmark. *Scandinavian Journal of Public Health*, 38(3):246–52.

Anell A (2011). Choice and privatization in Swedish primary care. *Health Economics, Policy and Law*, 6(4):549–69.

Anell A (2015). The public–private pendulum – Patient choice and equity in Sweden. *New England Journal of Medicine*, 371(1):1–4.

Anell A (2016). Striving for a harmonized approach – a macro perspective. Presentation given to the International Forum for Quality and Safety in Healthcare, Goteborg, April 2016.

Anell A, Glenngård AH, Merkur S (2012). Sweden: Health system review. *Health Systems in Transition*, 14(5):1–159. Copenhagen: World Health Organization.

Anell A, Rosén P, Hjortsberg C (1997). Choice and participation in the health services: a survey of preferences among Swedish residents. *Health Policy*, 40(2):157–68.

Appleby J, Harrison A, Devlin N (2003). *What is the real cost of more patient choice?* London: King's Fund.

Arksey H, Glendinning C (2007). Choice in the context of informal caregiving. *Health and Social Care in the Community*, 15(2):165–75.

Arrow K (1963). Uncertainty and welfare economics in health care. *American Economic Review*, 53(6):941–73.

Baker J (2010). *Co-production of local services*. London: Local Government and Research Councils.

Barnes M (1999). Users as citizens: Collective action and the local governance of welfare. *Social Policy and Administration*, 33(1):73–90.

Barry MJ, Edgman-Levitan S (2012). Shared decision making — the pinnacle of patient-centered care. *Journal of General and Internal Medicine*, 366:780–1.

Bartlett W, Roberts J, Le Grand J (eds.) (1998). *A revolution in social policy: Lessons from developments of quasi-markets in the 1990s*. Bristol: Policy Press.

Batalden M et al. (2016). The co-production of health services. *BMJ Quality and Safety*, 25:509–17.

Baxter K, Glendinning C (2013). The role of emotions in the process of making choices about welfare services: the experiences of disabled people in England. *Social Policy and Society*, 12(3):439–50.

Beresford P (2008). Time to get real about personalisation. *Journal of Integrated Care*, 16(2):2–4.

Bergmark Å (2008). Market reforms in Swedish health care: normative reorientation and welfare state sustainability. *Journal of Medicine and Philosophy*, 33:241–61.

Berwick D (2002). A user's manual for the IOM's 'Quality Chasm' report. *Health Affairs*, 12(3):80–90.

Bevan G, Helderman J-K (2010). Changing choices in health care: implications for equity, efficiency and cost. *Health Economics, Policy and Law*, 5(3):251–67.

Birk HO, Henriksen LO (2012). Which factors decided general practitioners' choice of hospital on behalf of their patients in an area with free choice of public hospital? A questionnaire study. *BMC Health Service Research*, 12:126.

Boyce T et al. (2010). *Choosing a high quality hospital. The role of nudges, scorecard design and information*. London: King's Fund.

Boyle D (2013). *The barriers to choice review. How are people using choice in public services?* London: Cabinet Office.

Burge P et al. (2004). Do patients always prefer quicker treatment? A discrete choice analysis of patients' stated preferences in the London Patient Choice Project. *Applied Health Economics and Health Policy*, 3(4):183–94.

Burström B (2002). Increasing inequalities in health care utilization across income groups in Sweden during the 1990s. *Health Policy*, 62(2):117–29.

Burström B et al. (2017). Equity aspects of the primary health care choice reform in Sweden – a scoping review. *International Journal for Equity in Health*, 16:29.

Cacace M, Nolte E (2011). *Healthcare services: strategy, direction and delivery.* In: Walshe K, Smith J (eds.) *Healthcare Management*. Maidenhead: Open University Press, 145–68.

Cellini R, Pignataro G, Rizzo I (2000). Competition and efficiency in health care: an analysis of the Italian case. *International Tax and Public Finance*, 7:503–19.

Chang H-J (2014). *Economics: The User's Guide. A Pelican Introduction.* London: Penguin Books Limited.

Civitas Institute (2010). *The impact of the NHS market. An overview of the literature.* London: Civitas Institute for the Study of Civil Society.

Cookson R et al. (2010). Competition and inequality: evidence from the English National Health Service 1991–2001. *Journal of Public Administration Research and Theory*, 20:1181–1205.

Cooper Z et al. (2011). Does hospital competition save lives? Evidence from the English NHS patient choice reforms. *Economic Journal*, 121:228–60.

Coulter A (2010). Do patients want choice and does it work? *BMJ*, 341:972–5.

Coulter A, Le Maistre N, Henderson L (2005). *Patients' experience of choosing where to undergo surgical treatment. Evaluation of the London Patient Choice Scheme.* Oxford: Picker Institute.

Daly G (2012). Citizenship, choice and care: an examination of the promotion of choice in the provision of adult social care. *Research, Policy and Planning*, 29(3):179–89.

Dawson D et al. (2004). *Evaluation of the London Choice Project: System wide impacts. Final report. A report to the London Patient Choice Project.* York: Centre for Health Economics, University of York.

Department of Health (2003). *Fair for all, personal to you: a consultation on choice, responsiveness and equity.* London: Department of Health.

Devaux M (2015). Income-related inequalities and inequities in health care services utilization in 18 selected OECD countries. *European Journal of Health Economics*, 16:21–33.

Dietrichson J, Ellegård LM, Kjellsson G (2016). Effects of increased competition on quality of primary care in Sweden. Working Paper 2106:36. Lund: Department of Economics, School of Economics and Management, University of Lund.

Dixon A et al. (2010). *Patient choice. How patients choose and providers respond?* London: King's Fund.

Durand A-M et al. (2014). Do interventions designed to support shared decision-making reduce health inequalities? A systematic review and meta-analysis. *PLoS ONE*, 9(4):e94670.

Dwarswaard J, Hilhorst M, Trappenburg M (2011). The doctor and the market: about the influence of market reforms on the professional medical ethics of surgeons and general practitioners in the Netherlands. *Health Care Analysis*, 19:388–402.

Eurobarometer (2012). *Eurobarometer qualitative study. Patient involvement. Aggregate report.* Conducted for European Commission by TNS Qual+.

Ferlie E et al. (2004). *NHS London Choice Project evaluation. Organisational process strand. Final report. Findings and key learning points.* London: Centre for Public Services Organisations, Royal Holloway College, University of London.

Fogelberg S (2014). Effects of competition between healthcare providers on prescription of antibiotics. Mimeo: Stockholm University.

Fotaki M (1999). The impact of the market oriented reforms on information and choice. Case study cataract surgery in Outer London and County Council of Stockholm. *Social Science & Medicine*, 48(10):1415–32.

Fotaki M (2006). Choice is yours. A psychodynamic exploration of health policymaking and its consequences for the English National Health Service. *Human Relations*, 59(12):1711–44.

Fotaki M (2010). Patient choice and equity in the British National Health Service: towards developing an alternative framework. *Sociology of Health & Illness*, 32(6):898–913.

Fotaki M (2011). Towards developing new partnerships in public services: users as consumers, citizens and/or co-producers driving improvements in health and social care in the UK and Sweden. *Public Administration*, 89(3):933–95.

Fotaki M (2014). Can consumer choice replace trust in the National Health Service in England? Towards developing an affective psychosocial conception of trust in health care. *Sociology of Health & Illness*, 36(8):1276–94.

Fotaki M (2015). Why and how is compassion necessary to provide good quality healthcare? *International Journal of Health Care Policy Management*, 4(1):1–3.

Fotaki M, Boyd A (2005). From plan to market: a comparison of health and old age care policies in the UK and Sweden. *Public Money & Management*, 25(4):237–43.

Fotaki M et al. (2006). *Patient Choice and the Organization and Delivery of Health Services: Scoping Review. A Report to the National Institute for Health Research*. London: SDO/NIHR.

Fotaki M et al. (2008). What benefits will choice bring to patients? Literature review and assessment of implications. *Journal of Health Services Research and Policy*, 13:178–84.

Gaynor M, Morreno-Serra R, Propper C (2012). Can competition improve outcomes in UK health care? Lessons from the past two decades. *Journal of Health Services Research & Policy*, 17(1):49–54.

Gaynor M, Morreno-Serra R, Propper C (2013). Death by market power: reform, competition and patient outcomes in the British National Health Service. *American Economic Journal: Economic Policy*, 5(4):134–66.

Gaynor M, Propper C, Seiler S (2016). Free to choose? Reform, choice, and consideration sets in the English National Health Service. *American Economic Review*, 106(11):3521–57.

Glenngård A, Anell A, Beckman A (2011). Choice of primary care provider: Results from a population survey in three Swedish counties. *Health Policy*, 103:31–7.

Goold SD (1999). The doctor–patient relationship. Challenges, opportunities, and strategies. *Journal of General and Internal Medicine*, 14(Suppl 1):S26–S33.

Grasdal AL, Monstad K (2011). Inequity in the use of physician services in Norway before and after introducing patient lists in primary care. *International Journal for Equity in Health*, 10:25.

Gravelle H et al. (2014). *Patient choice and the effects of hospital market structure on mortality for AMI, hip fracture and stroke patients*. CHE Research Paper 106.

Hansen P et al. (2015). The future of health economics: the potential of behavioral and experimental economics. *Nordic Journal of Health Economics*, 3(1):68–86.

Health Foundation (2012). Evidence: Helping people share decision making. A review of evidence considering whether shared decision making is worthwhile. London: Health Foundation. Available at: http://www.health.org.uk/sites/health/files/HelpingPeopleShareDecisionMaking.pdf (accessed 6 August 2017).

Holte JH et al. (2015). General practitioners' altered preferences for private practice vs. salaried positions: a consequence of proposed policy regulations? *BMC Health Services Research*, 15:119.

Iversen T, Lurås H (2011). Patient switching in general practice. *Journal of Health Economics*, 30(5):894–903.

Iyengar SS, DeVoe SE (2003). Rethinking the value of choice: Considering cultural mediators of intrinsic motivation. In: Murphy-Berman V, Berman John J (eds.) *Cross-Cultural Differences in Perspectives on the Self*, vol. 49:129–74, of the Nebraska Symposium on Motivation. Lincoln, Neb./London: University of Nebraska Press.

Kahneman D, Tversky A (1979). Prospect theory: an analysis of decision under risk. *Econometrica*, 47:263–91.

Kuttner R (2008). Market-based failure – a second opinion on U.S. health care costs. *New England Journal of Medicine*, 358(6):449–501.

Larkin M, Mitchell W (2016). Carers, choice and personalisation: what do we know? *Social Policy and Society*, 15(2):189–205.

Larsen LT, Stone D (2015). Governing Health Care through Free Choice: Neoliberal Reforms in Denmark and the United States. *Journal of Health Politics, Policy and Law*, 40(5):941–70.

Le Grand J (2003). *Motivation, agency and public policy*. Oxford: Oxford University Press.

Le Grand J (2007). *The other invisible hand*. Princeton University Press.

Lian OS (2003). Convergence or divergence? Reforming primary care in Norway and Britain. *Milbank Quarterly*, 81(2):305–30.

Loomes G, Sugden R (1982). Regret theory: an alternative theory of rational choice under uncertainty. *Economic Journal*, 92:805–24.

Mannion R (2005). *Practice-based budgeting: Lessons from the past; prospects for the future*. Report to the Department of Health. York: Centre for Health Economics, University of York.

Markus HR, Schwartz B (2010). Does choice mean freedom and well-being? *Journal of Consumer Research*, 37(2):344–55.

Mol A (2008). *Choice. The logic of care*. London: Routledge.

Morris J (2006). Independent living: the role of the disability movement in the development of government policy. In Glendinning C, Kemp P (eds.) *Cash and care: policy changes in the welfare state*. Bristol: Policy Press, 235–48.

Moscelli G, Gravelle H, Siciliani L (2016). Market structure, patient choice and hospital quality for elective patients. CHE Research Paper 139.

Needham C, Carr S (2009). *Co-production: An Emerging Evidence Base for Adult Social Care Transformation.* London: Social Care Institute for Excellence.

Or Z et al. (2010). Are health problems systemic? Politics of access and choice under Beveridge and Bismarck systems. *Health Economics, Policy and Law*, 5(3):269–93.

Palmer S (1999). Definitions of efficiency. *BMJ*, 318:1136.

Pauly MV (2005). Competition and new technology. *Health Affairs*, 24(6):1523–35.

Pedersen KM, Bech M, Vrangbaek K (2011). *The Danish health care system: an analysis of strengths, weaknesses, opportunities and threats. The Consensus Report.* Copenhagen: Copenhagen Consensus Center.

Pescosolido BA (1992). Beyond rational choice – the social dynamics of how people seek help. *American Journal of Sociology*, 97(4):1096–138.

Pollock A et al. (2011). No evidence that patient choice in the NHS saves lives. *Lancet*, 378(9809):2057–60.

Propper C, Burgess C (2004). Does competition between hospitals improve the quality of care? Hospital death rates and the NHS internal market. *Journal of Public Economics*, 88(7–8):1247–72.

Rabiee P, Glendinning C (2010). Choice: what, when and why? Exploring the importance of choice to disabled people. *Disability and Society*, 25(7):827–39.

Reid J (2003). *Choice for all, not the few.* Speech on 16 July 2003. Press Release 2003/0267. London: Department of Health.

Rice T (2002). *The economics of health reconsidered.* 2nd edition. Chicago: Health Administration Press.

Ringard Å et al. (2013). Norway. Health Systems Review. *Health Systems in Transition*, 15(8):1–162. Copenhagen: World Health Organization.

Rørtveit G (2015). Future primary care in Norway: valid goals without clear strategies. *Scandinavian Journal of Primary Health Care*, 33(4):221–2.

Robinson R, Le Grand J (1994). *Evaluating the NHS reforms.* Berkshire: King's Fund Institute.

Rosén P, Anell A, Hjortsberg C (2001). Patients' views on choice and participation in primary health care. *Health Policy*, 55(2):121–8.

Ryan M (1994). Agency in health care: lessons for economists from sociologists. *American Journal of Economics and Sociology*, 53:207–17.

Saltman RB (1994). A conceptual overview of recent health care reforms. *European Journal of Public Health*, 4(4):287–93.

Sandman L, Munthe C (2010). Shared decision making, paternalism and patient choice. *Health Care Analysis*, 18(1):60–84.

Schwartz B, Cheek NN (2017). Choice, freedom and well-being: considerations for public policy. *Behavioural Public Policy*, 1(1):106–21.

Söderlund N et al. (1997). Impact of the NHS reforms on English hospital productivity: an analysis of the first three years. *BMJ*, 315:1126–9.

Starfield B (1994). Is primary care essential? *Lancet*, 344(8930):1129–33.

Stubbs E (2015). *Devolved healthcare in Denmark*. London: Civitas.

Sutton M et al. (2012). Reduced mortality with hospital pay for performance in England. *New England Journal of Medicine*, 367(19):1821–8.

Swedish Agency for Health and Care Services Analysis (2013). *Vad vill patienten veta för att välja? Vårdanalys utvärdering av vårdvalsinformation*. Stockholm: Swedish Agency for Health and Care Services Analysis.

Taylor-Gooby P (1999). Markets and motives trust and egoism in welfare markets. *Journal of Social Policy*, 28(1):97–114.

Taylor-Gooby P, Wallace A (2009). Public values and public trust: Responses to welfare state reform in the UK. *Journal of Social Policy*, 38(3):401–19.

Thaler RH, Sunstein CR (2008). *Nudge: Improving decisions about health, wealth, and happiness*. New Haven, CT: Yale University Press.

Thomson S, Dixon A (2006). Choices in health care: the European experience. *Journal of Health Service Research and Policy*, 11(3):167–71.

Tuohy C (1999). Dynamics of a changing health sphere: the United States, Britain, and Canada. *Health Affairs*, 18(3):114–34.

Victoor A et al. (2012). Determinants of patient choice of healthcare providers: a scoping review. *BMC Health Services Research*, 12:272.

Visser LM et al. (2018). Unequal consumers: Consumerist healthcare technologies and their creation of new inequalities. *Organization Studies*, OnlineFirst.

Vrangbæk K et al. (2007). Patient reactions to hospital choice in Norway, Denmark, and Sweden. *Health Economics, Policy and Law*, 2(2):125–52.

Vrangbæk K et al. (2012). Choice policies in Northern European health systems. *Health Economics, Policy and Law*, 7(1):47–71.

Wahlstedt E, Ekman B (2016). Patient choice, Internet based information sources, and perceptions of health care: Evidence from Sweden using survey data from 2010 and 2013. *BMC Health Services Research*, 16:325.

Which? (2005). Which choice? Health. London: *Which?* Available at: https://www.which.co.uk/ (accessed 6 August 2017).

Winblad U (2008). Do physicians care about patients' choice? *Social Science & Medicine*, 67(10):1502–11.

9 | Choosing payers: can insurance competition strengthen person-centred care?

EWOUT VAN GINNEKEN, RUTH WAITZBERG, ANDREW
BARNES, WILM QUENTIN, MARTIN SMATANA,
THOMAS RICE

Introduction

Individual choice of insurance is used in several health systems as a means to empower citizens. This is based on the assumption that the insurers will act strategically on behalf of their clients to meet their needs and preferences and ensure access to high quality services, or else risk losing them to a competing insurer. Competition among insurance funds is expected to lead to improved health system efficiency, higher satisfaction with insurer services for clients (such as timely provision of information, easy administration, low waiting times, waiting list mediation, etc.). There is also an expectation that insurance competition will lead to improved care quality and could stimulate the development of more person-centred services.

The degree of choice and competition between insurers varies between health systems that have introduced this approach, as do the expectations that policy-makers in individual settings associate with choice and competition. Related policies range from those that only allow choice of insurance fund or company (with the ability to switch between insurers within defined periods) to those that expect (and incentivize) insurers to compete on quality and cost of their purchased care. Insurers may be given additional instruments to do so, including the possibility to offer different insurance premiums (while ensuring the same benefits) to attract more customers; others involve selective contracting, that is, insurers only contract with providers that are expected to deliver better value services in terms of cost and quality.

A number of countries have introduced (various degrees of) insurance choice and competition. In Europe, these are Belgium, the Czech Republic, Germany, the Netherlands, Slovakia and Switzerland. Other examples include Israel and the United States of America (USA). These countries have systems or subsystems in place that allow people to choose among a (varying) number of health insurance funds and they may switch between funds on a periodic basis. Such schemes are typically highly regulated to ensure that they are affordable, minimize risk selection and do not undermine health care coverage.

This chapter discusses insurance choice and competition models in six countries: Germany, Israel, the Netherlands, Slovakia, Switzerland and the USA. We selected these countries because they represent varying degrees of insurance choice and competition. More importantly perhaps, these countries have explicitly pursued choice and competition in health care more broadly (Smatana et al., 2016; Kroneman et al., 2016; Rosen, Waitzberg & Merkur, 2015; Rice et al., 2013), compared to, for example, Belgium and the Czech Republic (Alexa et al., 2014; Gerkens & Merkur, 2010). We begin by briefly discussing the theoretical framework underpinning insurance choice and competition. We then describe the systems of insurance choice in place in the six countries, along with the types of choice available to the population and the tools to support choice. Subsequent sections explore the evidence about the degree to which people exercise choice of insurance and their use of available support tools; the underlying motivations for exercising choices; the nature of the choices made (that is, whether people make choices that are in their best interest); and the frequency with which people change insurers. We then explore the impact of choice policies on care quality and satisfaction, and on the development of more person-centred care arrangements. We conclude by providing lessons for countries that may be contemplating introducing insurance choice into their system.

Insurance choice and competition: theoretical considerations

The conceptual basis for introducing competition between insurance companies is often attributed to the American economist Alain Enthoven (1978; 1993). Originally Enthoven referred to consumer-choice health plans, emphasizing the role of consumer choice in driving efficiency, but subsequently described the concept as 'managed competition'. This underlines the key role ascribed to a regulatory framework to ensure that insurer competition achieves socially desirable outcomes, namely improved quality and economic efficiency and minimizes 'cream skimming', that is, selection of low-cost customers. Regulation is also necessary to help ensure that the system provides equitable access to coverage and care. This is usually achieved through risk adjustment (*see* below), the explicit definition of an essential basket of benefits, and, where necessary, subsidies for customers to purchase insurance who would otherwise not be able to do so because of, for example, low income.

Insurance competition relies on the interplay between three sets of stakeholders: consumers, providers, and insurers (Van Ginneken & Swartz, 2012). Insurers are assumed to compete for customers based on the quality of the care (arrangements) they purchase and the customer services they provide, as well as the premiums they charge. In such a market, providers in turn are assumed to compete with other providers for contracts with insurers by offering quality services at reasonable cost. People are expected to choose insurers and providers based on the quality and convenience of the services offered. They may also select an insurer based on the quality of their purchased care. As noted above, a risk adjustment mechanism would define compensation payments for different 'insurance risks' so that insurers that have a high proportion of high-cost customers are not disadvantaged, reducing incentives for insurers to enrol low-cost customers only (Van de Ven, van Kleef & van Vliet, 2015). Each of these elements forms a critical part of the theory, but in practice countries that are considering a system of competing health insurers may choose not to use some of these elements. For example, a country might introduce a system of competing insurers, but competition would be permitted on the basis of quality only (and not price) or they may not be allowed to selectively contract with particular providers.

In this chapter, we focus on the relationship between customers and insurers. This relationship is a strong driver for insurance competition because, in theory, competing insurers would be expected to lose customers if they do not ensure good quality care and services at acceptable cost. This theory then assumes that customers are informed about differences in quality and costs and that they are willing to act (switch insurer) based on this information. The following sections illustrate the degree to which these assumptions are realized, or indeed are realizable, in practice by looking at the experiences in six multiple-insurer systems that introduced choice and competition.

Insurer choice and competition in Europe, Israel and the USA

Germany, Israel, the Netherlands, Slovakia and Switzerland, all countries with multiple insurers, have to varying degrees introduced choice and competition among insurers in their health systems from the 1990s onwards. This has also included providing insurers with more tools to purchase care (Table 9.1). It was hoped this move would stimulate improved efficiency in health care and better respond to people's preferences. The USA has seen a somewhat different trajectory in that choice and competition formed the central tenets of the private health insurance market, which is characterized by less regulation than that in other countries, and which covered 49% of the population in 2016 (Kaiser Family Foundation, 2018). However, similar to the European settings reviewed here, choice and competition were also successively introduced into public schemes such as Medicaid and Medicare from the 1990s onwards.

In Germany, choice of insurer (statutory health insurance (SHI) fund) was introduced by the 1993 health reform. From 1996 people who were previously assigned an SHI fund based on their profession or region of residence were able to freely choose an SHI fund of their choice. At the time there were considerable differences in contribution rates between different SHI funds, ranging between 9% and 18% of gross monthly salary (Busse et al., 2017). Therefore, a risk-equalization mechanism (RSA scheme) was introduced simultaneously to ensure that SHI funds that covered a larger share of older people were not disadvantaged because of the higher costs of their customer base. The RSA scheme was further refined in 2009 to also incorporate morbidity into the reallocation formula. All SHI funds are required to offer a minimum benefits package, and the insured population has, in principle, free choice of hospitals and office-based physicians in ambulatory care. The number of SHI funds has fallen considerably since the mid-1990s, from some 960 funds in 1995 to 113 in 2017, because of mergers, mostly within groups of SHI funds (e.g. regional funds). In 2016 the five largest funds insured almost 50% of the population (Statista, 2017a). Prices of most services are determined by nationally agreed fee schedules, but insurers can negotiate lower prices for pharmaceuticals, and larger funds have greater leverage in these negotiations. Provisions for selective contracting were introduced in the early 2000s and were initially restricted to integrated care programmes,

Table 9.1 *Overview of insurance choice in Germany, Israel, the Netherlands, Slovakia, Switzerland and the USA (2017)*

	Funding source	Number of insurers	Market concentration	Selective contracting allowed?	Insurers negotiate prices
Germany*	Income-dependent contributions	113 statutory health insurance (SHI) funds	Five largest SHI funds hold 50% of statutory insurance market	Yes (for integrated care programmes)	Only pharmaceuticals
Israel	Taxes and income-dependent contributions	Four health plans	Largest insurer holds about 54% of the market	Yes	Yes
Netherlands	Income-dependent contributions (employers), community rated premiums (citizens)	26 health insurers	Four health insurers hold about 90% of the market	Yes	Most hospital care
Slovakia	Income-dependent contributions	Three health insurers	Largest insurer holds about 63% of the market	Yes	Yes
Switzerland	Community rated premiums	58 health insurers	Four insurers hold about 56% of the market	Yes (for managed care plans)	Yes (managed care insurance plans)
USA**	Premiums/ contributions	1300 health insurance companies	Varies according to type of insurance (e.g. Medicare, private)	Yes	Yes

Note: * only statutory insurance schemes, **total market for private insurance

Sources: Busse et al., 2017; De Pietro et al., 2015; Kroneman et al., 2016; Rice et al., 2013; Rosen, Waitzberg & Merkur, 2015; Smatana et al., 2016

although this stipulation was broadened with the 2015 health reform which introduced other forms of selective contracting to strengthen care coordination in the system.

In Israel, the health insurance system emerged from originally four non-profit health insurers (Health Plans, HPs) that were established between 1920 and 1940 by political parties or trade unions and that insured their members and provided medical services. The planning, regulation and supervision of the HPs was subsequently (1948) taken on by the Ministry of Health, which also began to provide selected health services and operate hospitals. Although health insurance was still voluntary, by 1995 almost all citizens (96%) had insurance, with the insurer Clalit holding a 62% share of the market. At that time HPs could define the range of benefits offered, as well as premiums; they were also able to select applicants (Brammli-Greenberg, Waitzberg & Gross, forthcoming). This changed with the 1995 national health insurance (NHI) law, which provided for universal coverage and sought to combine progressive financing (through taxes) and competition in an equitable and sustainable manner. The NHI law established health (and health insurance) as a right for all citizens and permanent residents and guaranteed full freedom of choice among the four HPs (Rosen, Waitzberg & Merkur, 2015). Since then, the four competing HPs are responsible for providing and managing a broad benefits package specified by government. Within the public system, HPs provide care (as listed in the NHI benefits package) in the community and they may purchase selectively inpatient and outpatient care from hospitals. Residents are not able to opt out of the NHI system. HPs do not compete on the level of price but on the basis of quality of care and service quality, as well as on a co-payments rate (which must be approved by the Ministry of Health) and voluntary health insurance (VHI) packages.

The Netherlands moved in 2006 from a social health insurance system that covered about two-thirds of the population, and in which people with incomes above a certain threshold purchased private health insurance, to one of managed competition. This move aimed to reduce the emphasis on government regulation of health care supply, increase efficiency through strategic purchasing and, ultimately, offer more affordable and more patient-driven health care (Thomson et al., 2013). Health insurance covers a comprehensive set of benefits for acute care. All residents are required to purchase statutory health insurance from private insurers, and insurers must enrol all applicants. Insurers compete on price for insurance policies, which cover a comprehensive set of benefits for acute care. Insurers can offer lower premiums for basic health insurance in exchange for charging higher voluntary deductibles; the level of these deductibles is set by government and they are in addition to the mandatory deductible all adults have to pay. The 2006 health reform also considerably increased the possibilities for health insurers to selectively contract with health care providers and so offer restricted or preferred provider insurance packages at a lower cost. The role of this type of policy is increasing but it remains small in terms of uptake. Some insurers waive the cost of the mandatory deductible if preferred providers are chosen. Furthermore, those with lower incomes are eligible to receive tax subsidies. The introduction of insurer competition led to a wave of mergers and acquisitions of insurance funds and by 2016 just four insurers held about 90% of the market (Vektis Zorgthermometer, 2016).

In Slovakia, insurance competition was gradually introduced between 2002 and 2006. A controversial reform, it established private insurers as purchasers of health care services and made them responsible for ensuring health care to their insured population. The reform aimed at more effective utilization of resources, to improve fairness and financial sustainability, as well as transfer responsibility for the health system from the state to the individual, health insurers and providers (Smatana et al., 2016). Ownership regulation allowed both the state and the private sector to be shareholders of health insurance companies. Changes in the insurance market led to increased consolidation through mergers, from seven health insurance companies to three in 2017: the state-owned Všeobecná ZP (General health insurance company), and two privately owned insurers (Dôvera and Union). Insurers do not compete on price and, as the benefits basket is quite comprehensive, there is also limited scope for insurers to compete for patients through, for example, offering additional benefits. Purchasing is based on selective contracting and health insurers can develop their own payment methods and set up their own pricing policy towards contracted providers (Smatana et al., 2016).

In Switzerland, the 1996 health reform sought to enhance equity of access to health insurance, to strengthen solidarity and to create incentives for organizational innovation and expenditure control (Thomson et al., 2013). The 1996 reform stipulated that all Swiss residents must purchase basic health insurance, which covers a comprehensive basket of goods and services defined at the federal level. The insurance market is not as concentrated as it is in the Netherlands as noted above, and in 2016 four insurers held 56.3% of the market (Statista, 2017b). Insurers can offer several 'basic' policies with standardized benefits; premiums are lower for insurance policies with higher deductibles and those that only cover managed care. All insurers are private; they must be non-profit-making (although they can make profits from selling complimentary and supplementary policies) and they must accept all applicants for membership during specified open-enrolment periods. The cantons (states) provide income-dependent tax subsidies to compensate those on low incomes (De Pietro et al., 2015; OECD/WHO, 2011; Van Ginneken, Swartz & Van der Wees, 2013). Similar to Germany, collective contracting remains the dominant approach to purchasing care, and competition between providers for contracts with insurers is limited. However, there is a possibility for selective contracting within managed care arrangements, the number of which is increasing rapidly. Thus, in 2014 about 24% of the insured population were enrolled in some form of managed care plan, involving some 75 physician networks or health maintenance organizations (HMOs), up from about 8% in 2008 (Ärztenetzerhebung, 2014). There are also network health insurance plans in which insurers determine a list of physicians that patients can consult, while Telmed models require patients to have a telephone consultation with a medical call centre first before they may arrange an appointment with a medical doctor in ambulatory care. In total, these 'alternative' forms of contracts accounted for 63% of all contracts in 2014 (BAG, 2016c).

In the USA, the largely unregulated private insurance market for employer-based insurance mainly includes three categories of private insurer, namely health maintenance organizations, preferred provider organizations, and high-deductible health insurance plans (Rice et al., 2014). As noted, in 2016 some 49% of the population were covered through their employer by a private health insurance. In addition, Medicare, the public insurance programme for people aged 65 years and older and for disabled persons, covered 14% of the population, while Medicaid, which covers those under a certain income threshold, covered 19% (Kaiser Family Foundation, 2018). The 2010 Affordable Care Act (ACA) introduced major insurance coverage expansions from 2014, and this has increased the share of the population with insurance. Provisions included the requirement that most Americans purchase health insurance (subsequently repealed, effective as of January 2019); the introduction of health insurance market-places, or exchanges, which offer premium subsidies to people with lower and middle incomes; and the expansion of Medicaid in many states, which involved raising the income threshold for eligibility to increase coverage for low-income adults. The state-based exchanges can be seen as a first attempt to establish managed competition in the individual insurance market in that all health plans sold through this marketplace must meet minimum standards ('essential health benefits'). Their structure and supporting regulation resemble the Dutch and Swiss regulated insurance models (Van Ginneken & Swartz, 2012; Rice et al., 2014). The Medicaid expansion and the exchanges (along with other provisions) together are colloquially referred to as Obamacare. Insurers negotiate prices with provider groups for services provided by in-network providers. There is a large number of insurers in the USA who offer an even larger number of insurance policies. Generally, there is an open enrolment period once a year, and people can switch insurer during that period. With a few notable exceptions (i.e. state-based health insurance exchanges), private health insurance policies are rarely standardized.

Type of choice and tools to support choice

Table 9.2 provides an overview of the types of choice offered in the reviewed countries. Slovakia offers the least choice, such that people can choose the insurer only. The Netherlands and Switzerland offer a greater level of choice, in that people may choose the insurer, the premium level and predefined levels of deductibles (and so pay a lower premium overall). Insurers in these countries also offer various (risk-rated) VHI policies, which they can use, in theory, to attract people to (or deter them from choosing) the basic insurance package they have to offer. Furthermore, as noted above, both countries allow limited network (preferred provider-type) health insurance policies, which offer restricted provider choice for a lower premium. In Germany, people have somewhat greater choice among SHI funds, with insurers permitted to charge a supplementary (income-dependent) premium above the legally set contribution rate (14.6% of gross monthly salary from 2015, shared equally between employers and employees), although in reality the differences in rates are comparatively small, ranging from 14.9% to 16.3% in 2018 (Krankenkassen Deutschland, 2018). SHI funds may also offer benefits in addition to the statutory benefits package. Furthermore, people can choose optional insurance policies, for example covering disease management programmes, optional deductibles

Table 9.2 *Type of choice in basic insurance in Germany, Israel, the Netherlands, Slovakia, Switzerland and the USA*

	Insurer	Insurance premium/ contribution level	Fixed or minimum benefit package	Cost-sharing requirements	Basic insurance providers also offer VHI	Limited network (preferred provider) policies available
Germany	Yes	Yes	Minimum	Bonus plans (e.g. deductible in exchange for bonus)	Yes	No
Israel	Yes	Not applicable	Minimum	Co-payment rates	Yes	No
Netherlands	Yes	Yes	Fixed	Deductible level (in exchange for lower premium)	Yes	Yes (budget policies)
Slovakia	Yes	No	Fixed	No	No	No
Switzerland	Yes	Yes	Fixed*	Deductible level (in exchange for lower premium)	Yes	Yes (managed care insurance plans)
USA	Yes	Yes	Varies	Varies	Yes*	Yes

Note: *Mainly Medicare (Medigap)

in exchange for a bonus, or no-claims policies. In 2016 about 25% of people with statutory insurance had opted for one of these optional policies (GBE, 2017).

In Israel, residents have a choice of insurer, additional benefits, cost-sharing levels and (community rated) VHI policies. For example, health plans may offer services or cover drugs that go above and beyond the legally mandated benefits package that all health plans have to offer, although individuals may not be aware about the differences between the 'voluntary' benefits offered by insurers. Individuals can also choose among different co-payment rates offered by health plans. There are slight differences among insurers, but here too individuals may not be very aware of them.

Among the countries reviewed here insurance choice is greatest in the USA. With a few notable exceptions, insurance benefits covered by private insurance policies vary considerably and people are therefore required to trade-off price (premium level), cost-sharing requirements (deductibles, co-payments, co-insurance), benefits and prescription drugs covered, as well as breadth and quality of provider networks covered by the individual plan. The public insurance scheme Medicaid is a jointly administered state–federal programme and insurance choice options (if any) may vary from state to state, with some but not all offering Medicaid beneficiaries a choice of insurer as part of managed care plans that restrict choice of providers within their networks. In the public Medicare programme, beneficiaries may choose between private sector Medicare (Medicare Advantage) or traditional Medicare (federal government-administered). Medicare beneficiaries also have the option to purchase supplementary VHI policies (known as Medigap plans) to cover costs not covered under the regular (original) Medicare, and these offer varying benefits, co-payments and deductibles (Rice et al., 2013).

The reviewed countries have introduced a range of tools both to support consumers in making informed choices and to avoid market failures due to information asymmetries. For example, in 2014 the Israel Ministry of Health launched a website, Call-Habriut, which provides independent, open and up-to-date information about insurance options, including VHI (benefits, eligibility conditions, co-payments set by HPs and VHI, etc.). There are plans to also include information about for-profit VHI, and to offer this information in additional languages such as Arabic and Russian. The launch of the website was accompanied by an advertising campaign for the public. The aim is to enhance people's knowledge of and awareness about their rights and eligibility to benefits, and so enable them to demand these from insurers; if refused, they can refer the case to the Ministry of Health.

In Germany, the Netherlands and Switzerland, webportals operated by private non-profit or for-profit organizations are the most important sources for comparative information about health insurers. They provide tailored information on insurance options, including benefits covered, contribution rates and VHI options. In the Netherlands, the government-operated portal KiesBeter.nl ('Choose better'), set up in 2005 to assist service users to choose between different health care providers, previously also provided independent information on health insurance policies but this was discontinued from 2013, based on the argument that there was a sufficient number of alternative, independent webportals available providing these data. This move was followed by some debate, with newspaper reports on widely differing recommendations for health insurance policies by different webportals using the same service user profile, highlighting that people may not be able to judge the degree to which these portals are indeed independent (Van Ginneken, 2016). In Switzerland, the government's online portal also provides general information on health insurance, but a more widely used source is comparis. ch, a leading commercial Swiss online portal providing comparative information on a range of services, including health insurance. Comparative information is freely accessible; health insurers pay a commission in the range of CHF 40–50 (€37–46) for every request for a quote through the comparis portal (Comparis, 2017). In Germany, there are various webportals hosted by different organizations, including those providing general service comparisons (e.g. check24 and verivox), as well as portals providing comparative information on health insurance specifically (e.g. krankenkassen.de and krankenkassenvergleich.de).

In the USA, there is a range of webportals providing comparative information on employer-based insurance policies (especially for large employers) and Medicare; these portals also provide some data on patient satisfaction. Employers often act as agents for their employees by providing information about provider quality on a webportal and they may coordinate with insurers to encourage employees to utilize recommended preventive care. Many of the aforementioned state-based health insurance exchanges that were established under the ACA also provide webportals and tools to support consumer choice. The quality of navigation tools, particularly those offered by employers, varies greatly. Both Medicare and the health insurance exchanges provide extensive tools to compare both the cost and the quality of insurance options. For example, the Medicare Part D Plan Finder, used by beneficiaries to choose prescription drug coverage, arrays plan choices from lowest to highest total estimated annual costs, and provides quality measures through a star rating system based on a number of measures grouped into five categories: staying healthy through screening tests and vaccines, managing chronic conditions, member experience with the health plan, member complaints and customer service (US Department of Health and Human Services, 2016). The insurance exchanges, which target a more vulnerable population, use so-called navigators to help consumers as well as small businesses and their employees in their search for health insurance policies. They also assist in completing eligibility and enrolment forms; the information and support tools are required to be unbiased and free to consumers.

Slovakia is the only country among those reviewed where a dedicated website to help people choose health insurance has not been established. This is perhaps due to the limited scope of choice. The Health Care Surveillance Authority, which among other things is responsible for supervising public health insurance in Slovakia, publishes data on waiting times for all specialties and individual insurers that people may use to make their decision.

Do people use available tools to support choice and do they exercise choice?

Much of the literature on how people exercise choice of health insurer originates from the USA, but there is also increasing evidence from the Netherlands and Switzerland. An important consideration is understanding whether people know how to exercise choice in the first place and how to move (switch) between insurers in practice. This requires knowing where to find relevant information, which, given that webportals are the prime source for information as noted above, may be especially challenging for people who do not have access to the internet or who are not able to use it (Sinaiko, Eastman & Rosenthal, 2012). Evidence further suggests that webportals should offer simple options, because too many options may be overwhelming and lead to confusion and inertia (staying with the same insurer), as has, for example, been documented for Switzerland (Frank & Lamiraud 2009) and the USA (Hanoch et al., 2011; Barnes et al., 2012; Zhou & Zhang, 2012; Abaluck & Gruber, 2013).

Indeed, in Switzerland in 2013 there were 58 insurers offering about 287 000 different insurance policies, with options varying by region (canton), the type of policy (e.g. managed care or combined accident insurance), and price, including the level of the (voluntary) deductible or whether it offers a no-claims bonus (BAG, 2016a; BAG, 2016b). In the Netherlands, the 26 health insurers (2014) offer 71 policies, which increases to 5940 insurance combinations when also considering VHI policies and deductible options (NZA, 2016). The Medicare Advantage programme in the USA varies by geographic area, averaging 19 insurers in 2016 (Kaiser Family Foundation, 2018) but as benefits are not standardized above a legally defined minimum benefits basket it is difficult to compare the relative value of the resultant variable insurance policies on offer. The state-based insurance exchanges offer various choices, ranging from a single insurer in five states to 15 insurers in Wisconsin in 2015 (with typically 67 insurance policies from which people can choose) (US Department of Health and Human Services, 2016). Conversely, in Slovakia and Israel people can only choose between three and four insurers, respectively.

Information on whether people exercise choice of insurer can be inferred from the rate of switching between insurers. Generally, the evidence suggests that switching rates range between a low of under 2% of the insured population in Israel (Ministry of Health, 2016b) to about 5–10% in Switzerland (FOPH, 2014). Switching rates tend to be high directly following the introduction of choice policies creating a (temporarily) volatile market, such as observed in Israel during 1995–97 subsequent to the 1995 NHI law and in the Netherlands after the 2006 health reform. However, usually switching rates fluctuate only within a limited range. For example, in the Netherlands from 2011 switching rates varied between 5.5% and 8.2% (Vektis Zorgthermometer, 2016), although it should be noted that the majority of people in the Netherlands switch as part of a collective group, that is, not as a result of their individual choice but rather that of their employer. Thus, at individual level rates have fluctuated between only 1.6% and 2.6% during the same period. In Slovakia, switching rates have been below 5% since 2007 (Smatana et al., 2016), while in the USA, switching between Medicare Advantage insurers appears to be within a similar range as those seen in Switzerland (Rice et al., 2014). In Germany, official data on switching between SHI funds are not available. A survey of just over 2000 insured people in 2015 found that only 3.2% had switched their SHI fund in the preceding year, with another 3% seriously considering doing so (Zok, 2016). However, it is important to note that some 40% of respondents reported to have switched their SHI fund in the past.

Interpreting switching rates remains challenging. Low rates could be taken to mean that insurance competition is not effective in achieving the goal of improved quality and cost of care. At the same time, high rates could imply increased transaction costs and prices, and, more importantly perhaps, they might discourage investment by insurers in health promotion and prevention, or the development of care programmes. Yet from the insurers' perspective, the prospect of even a small proportion of people switching to another insurer could trigger action to counteract people leaving. It is therefore important to understand which factors matter to people when they decide to switch insurer and whether switching rates impact on care quality and cost.

Who switches insurance policy and what are their motivations for doing so?

Empirical evidence from Germany, the Netherlands, Switzerland and the USA shows that people who switch insurers are mostly likely to be young, male, healthy and well-educated (Boonen, Laske-Aldershof & Schut, 2016; Thomson et al., 2013; Rooijen, de Joong & Rijken, 2011; Lako, Rosenau & Daw, 2011), although there are exceptions as the experience from Israel demonstrates (Box 9.1).

Box 9.1 Observed health insurance switching patterns in Israel

In Israel, data from the Ministry of Health show that unlike in other countries, switching between insurers is relatively more common among lower-income individuals (Figure 9.1). This was first observed by Shmueli, Bendelac & Achdut (2007) who found that in 2005–06 young people were more likely to switch insurer, as well as people on lower incomes, and those receiving income maintenance or unemployment benefits (controlling for age and gender). Switching rates were also found to be higher for persons who had a greater number of children under the age of 18 years. The authors explained these observations by implicit risk-selection strategies inherent in the risk-adjustment system, in which children represent a "predictable profit" under the formula which overcompensates for this age group.

Box 9.1 (cont.)

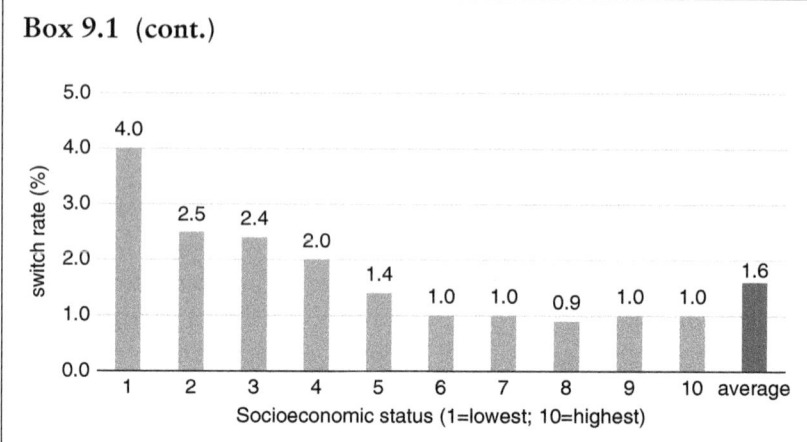

Figure 9.1 Switch rates in Israel by socioeconomic status (SES) of place of residence, 2015 (1 = lowest SES, 10 = highest SES)

Source: Ministry of Health, 2016

Available evidence suggests that where people do exercise choice by switching between insurers, this appears to be rarely motivated on the basis of quality of contracted care (providers). Table 9.3 summarizes the findings of a range of studies carried out in Israel, Germany and the Netherlands that have sought to understand the reasons for switching insurers among the eligible population. Thus, the main reasons included dissatisfaction with the services provided by the current insurer, the range of benefits covered, and price. Data from 2016 from Israel also provide insights into reasons for staying with the current insurer. Some 13% of respondents to a national survey (aged 22 years and over) indicated that they had considered switching insurers in the preceding year but ultimately remained in the health plan. The main reasons for not switching included: administration (switching procedure and loss of rights) (52%); thought that all health plans are the same (11%); wanting to remain with their physician (9%); proximity to health plan's clinic (7%); satisfaction with staff and services (6%); wanting to remain in the same health plan as their family (5%); waiting times for specialists (5%); uncertainty about the continuity of benefits/eligibility and the price of supplemental VHI offered by other health plans (4%);

Table 9.3 Reasons for switching insurer

Country	Reasons for switching (% of respondents, where applicable)
Israel (2016)[a]	• dissatisfaction with staff and service (20%) • wanted a specific physician not contracted by their current insurer (19%) • wanted to belong to the same health plan as their family (18%) • wanted to visit a closer clinic that was not contracted by their current insurer (12%) • financial considerations (9%) • wanted better quality of care and professional standards (9%) • wanted broader scope of services and providers (7%) • shorter waiting times and less bureaucracy (6%)
Germany (2015)[b]	• price (34%) • offered benefits (26%) • service of the sickness fund (17%)
Netherlands (various years)[c]	• a collective offer (e.g. from the employer) • dissatisfaction with the premium of the package offered • dissatisfaction with the coverage of the complementary insurance • dissatisfaction with the coverage of the package offered • dissatisfaction with the service of the insurer • dissatisfaction with the premium of the collective offer

Sources: [a] Brammli-Greenberg, Medina-Artom & Yaari, 2017; [b] Zok, 2016; [c] Boonen, Laske-Aldershof & Schut, 2016; Lako, Rosenau & Daw, 2011; Rooijen, de Jong & Rijken, 2011

and about the value of switching (2%) (Brammli-Greenberg, Medina-Artom & Yaarj, 2017).

There is only limited evidence from Slovakia, with some suggestion that waiting times for selected procedures can potentially influence choice. However, many people choose the state-owned General health insurance company as it is perceived to be the least likely to 'skimp' on the quality of reimbursed care (Smatana et al., 2016).

In the USA, a small number of studies examined the role of quality information included in health care report cards on choice of insurer and of provider. They found that report cards most commonly impact on the quality of services provided by health insurers but not necessarily on the quality of care delivered by contracted providers. Impacts are not large, however, and any effects will be limited to those who make use of the information presented in report cards (Rice & Unruh, 2015).

As indicated by the data from Israel reported above, one important consideration for the decision to switch insurer involves arrangements for (supplementary) VHI on offer, an issue of concern for people in the Netherlands and Switzerland also. In Israel, although VHI policies are community rated, individuals may refrain from switching insurers to avoid losing access to covered services, because this generally involves a waiting period of up to 12 months after purchasing VHI. The latter has recently been rectified in that insurers allow for enrolment in VHI without restricting access to benefits by means of a waiting period. In the Netherlands and Switzerland people with VHI may be reluctant to switch insurer out of concerns that they will not be able to access similar VHI benefits from another insurer of a comparable price and comprehensiveness (Dormant, Geoffard & Lamiraud, 2009; Duijmelinck & van de Ven, 2014).

Do people make 'good' choices?

Several studies have examined the degree to which people make choices of insurer that serve their own interest with regard to price and care quality. However, as noted earlier, in most settings exercising informed choice requires a good understanding of a myriad of insurance terms such as deductibles, co-payments, out-of-pocket maximum, and managed care, along with the range of benefits covered (health insurance 'literacy').

Studies set in the USA showed only low to moderate levels of health insurance literacy among the adult population (Loewenstein et al., 2013; McCormack et al., 2009). For example, a survey of adults aged 25–64 years found that only 11% of respondents could correctly answer an open-ended question about out-of-pocket liability from a hypothetical four-day hospital stay; respondents were provided with an overview table of benefits and the authors deemed the question to be "relatively simple" compared to other questions (Loewenstein et al., 2013). In Israel, a national cross-sectional survey of a random sample of the Jewish and Arab population found that knowledge about supplementary VHI contents and terms was generally low (Green et al., 2017).

As noted above, quality of contracted care seems to play a minor role when individuals make insurance choices and studies investigating whether people that use care quality information make insurance choices to their advantage are lacking. Although cost appears to play a greater role, the literature suggests that people do not always appear to make optimal choices on the basis of price, and they may choose a more expensive insurance policy than needed. Moreover, people tend to pay more attention to the level of insurance premiums instead of trading this against cost-sharing requirements. While it may be the case that some people knowingly choose to pay higher premiums at the price of a lower deductible, it is likely that most do not act in their best interest (Bhargava, Loewenstein & Sydnor, 2015; Gaynor, Ho & Town, 2015; Zhou & Zhang, 2012). For example, Van Winssen, van Kleef & van de Ven (2015) estimated that nearly half of the Dutch population would be financially better off if they had chosen a voluntary deductible (on top of the mandatory deductible), but in 2014 only 11% had done so. Cost considerations and trade-offs will be of less concern in Israel and Slovakia, where insurance policy options do not involve large financial incentives.

Has insurance choice led to novel person-centred care arrangements (and for which group of people)?

The question about whether insurance choice has encouraged insurers to invest in more person-centred services can be answered at two levels: first, whether insurers have tailored their customer services and health insurance policies to (certain) population groups and in what way, and second, whether insurers have organized and purchased new care arrangements for (defined) population groups.

In response to the first point, available evidence shows that in all reviewed countries, insurers have sought to tailor their services and (additional) benefits to attract certain groups of people, through, for example, offering special membership rates for diabetes patient groups. Risk-adjustment schemes play a key role in making certain population groups more attractive to insurers and thus increasing the likelihood of a tailored policy and care arrangements. For example, the risk-adjustment scheme in place in Israel only considers age, gender and place of residence and, as we have noted earlier, the capitation formula overcompensates people with a greater number of children and older men, and undercompensates older women (Brammli-Greenberg, Waitzberg & Glazer, 2017). As a consequence, insurers in Israel compete for children and men, and they have developed and enhanced their offers of specific services for children, such as developmental tests and treatments, and mental health services. Moreover, insurers advertise to attract large young families in particular (Shmueli, 2015). Conversely, the risk-adjustment systems disincentivizes attracting older women while possibly incentivizing 'skimping behaviour', meaning that they reimburse fewer services, although until now there is no hard evidence that such behaviour is realized in practice.

In the Netherlands, where a more sophisticated risk adjustment system has been implemented (Van de Ven et al., 2013), several strategies are being used to attract certain population groups. For example, while previously insurers could negotiate collective group contracts with employers only, the 2006 health reform introduced the possibility to also negotiate collective contracts with any group of individuals directly (following successful lobbying by the Dutch Patients Federation). By the end of 2007, two years after the implementation of the health reform, patient groups had negotiated around 40 collective contracts (Van Ginneken, Busse & Gericke, 2008), and this number had risen to 155 in 2015 (NZA, 2016). However, some (often smaller) chronic disease patient groups did not manage to secure a collective contract. This means that the risk adjustment scheme only inadequately compensates for these groups of patients to make them sufficiently attractive for insurers. It has been estimated that in 2014 insurers were undercompensated by an average of €331 per person per year for the 31% of the population who reported at least one chronic condition (Van de Ven, van Kleef & van Vliet, 2015).

In Slovakia, the two privately owned insurers also focus their marketing efforts on the young and healthy (Smatana et al., 2016). They have also introduced policies covering prevention and maternity care in an attempt to attract women specifically and to encourage them to register their newborn babies with them. These initiatives are, however, quite limited and not rolled out nationally.

Evidence in support of the question of whether insurance choice has led to the organization and purchasing of more person-centred care arrangements is difficult to assess. In Switzerland, the emergence and strong growth of managed care insurance policies (including HMOs and physician networks) could be seen as the result of insurance choice. Yet it is equally plausible that the risk-adjustment system in place does not sufficiently take account of the risk of ill health in the Swiss population since insurers are able to offer cheaper managed care type insurance policies to the young and healthy, while people at higher risk of ill health tend to remain covered by traditional health insurance policies (Beck et al., 2010). In the Netherlands, an evaluation found that insurers are reluctant to invest in more appropriate care models for high-cost (mostly chronic) patients (KPMG, 2015), yet it is this group that is most likely to benefit from more integrated care arrangements. In general, lack of investment in appropriate care models for high-cost patient groups is difficult to prove as it is unknown whether insurers would act differently if the incentive system was structured in favour of 'high risks' (Van de Ven, van Kleef & van Vliet, 2015).

In Slovakia, the private insurer Dovera implemented the MediPartner project that virtually integrated general practitioners (GPs) with the rest of the network of providers, and gave GPs a virtual budget to manage patients along the care pathway. The project was piloted in certain regions in the eastern part of Slovakia and although it achieved significant cost savings, these were often allegedly associated with under-provision of care; for example, GPs received a bonus if they did not refer patients upwards.

Most reviewed countries are increasingly experimenting with disease management programmes, managed care arrangements and integrated care initiatives more broadly, with the goal of providing more person-centred care, but these experiments are not necessarily linked to, nor indeed emerged as a result of, insurance choice. For example, in Germany the introduction of disease management programmes in 2002 was mandated by law as a means to improve the quality of care for people with chronic disease, in particular the prevention of long-term consequences and complications, and to ultimately reduce the costs of care (Nolte, Knai & Saltman, 2014). Elsewhere, relevant approaches also typically had improvement of quality of care at their core, while frequently also aiming to enhance efficiency and, in some instances, reduce utilization and costs. The USA has seen an increase in accountable care organizations, encouraged by provisions in the 2010 Affordable Care Act. Accountable care organizations are consortia of providers who agree to work together to coordinate care for patients across health systems and settings. While initially implemented in the context of Medicare, they are becoming increasingly common in the private insurance sector as well (Barnes et al., 2014).

Does insurer choice or competition lead to improved patient satisfaction or better care quality?

It has been suggested that countries with social health insurance systems are more responsive to people's expectations and show higher satisfaction levels when compared to countries with tax-funded systems (Busse et al., 2012). Clearly, this is not seen to be the result of the funding mechanisms or levels per se, but is based on the assumption that countries with social health insurance place more emphasis on consumer orientation, which includes choice of provider and purchaser, clearly defined entitlements and patient rights (Busse et al., 2012). It is not possible to say how much insurance choice contributes to this difference, and it may well be caused by other factors. These generalizations, therefore, should be made with great caution as considerable methodological issues remain with regard to the measurement and interpretation of satisfaction and lack of standardization of this term across countries, regions and even insurers.

The countries reviewed have a tradition of insurance choice and competition, which perhaps explains why no studies have looked at whether (increased) choice has led to improved patient satisfaction or care quality. Most insurers in most countries monitor satisfaction with their services, and satisfaction levels generally seem to be quite high (Busse et al., 2017; De Pietro et al., 2015; Kroneman et al., 2016; Rice et al., 2013; Rosen, Waitzberg & Merkur, 2015; Smatana et al., 2016). Earlier sections of this chapter have shown that where choice is exercised, this is often not based on considerations of quality, which can lead to opting for insurance policies that are not necessarily in people's best interest. Therefore, it is doubtful that the signals that are given by those switching will stimulate insurers to organize and purchase higher quality care. It could perhaps be argued that risk adjustment systems in place are more relevant in terms of ensuring that insurers contract for quality of care for certain groups than choice and competition. Indeed, systems could provide incentives for insurers to focus on specific population groups, although as a sole mechanism this is unlikely to automatically increase the quality of care.

Conclusions

Choice is valued by people and can contribute to ensuring that insurers offer better consumer services. But overall, there is little evidence that supports the notion that insurance choice has led to higher quality care or was a pivotal factor in the emergence of person-centred care arrangements in the six countries reviewed in this chapter. Available evidence points to the difficulty that people face in making informed insurance choices. Although switching rates are generally low, they should be sufficient to 'nudge' insurers in a certain direction if people exercise choice on the basis of the quality of the care covered by the insurance policy. This is not the case, however, given that the quality of contracted care as part of a given health insurance policy continues to play only a marginal role in the selection of insurer. This could change if more meaningful data on the quality of care became available and if they were presented in a transparent and easy-to-understand manner that would allow people to make better-informed choices. Even in terms of the cost of a given insurance policy, which is more often a factor in switching, evidence shows that people do not tend to select the highest value insurance plan. Indeed, the many insurance options and concepts in some countries require a level of health insurance literacy that may not be present. For these reasons, it is doubtful whether the signals given by the switchers are sufficient to motivate insurers to purchase better quality care.

At best, insurance choice may have led to increased satisfaction of patients with the services of their insurers and perhaps better-tailored health insurance policies in terms of benefits and services offered. It should be noted, however, that risk-adjustment plays a key role and the way the risk adjustment system compensates for certain population groups may be a more important factor in determining the range of policies offered by insurers, rather than insurance choice as such. Even in the Netherlands, which has one of the most sophisticated risk adjustment schemes (Van de Ven et al. 2013), there are identifiable population groups that remain less attractive for insurers because of the associated costs that are not sufficiently compensated for within the existing scheme. These are often people with (complex) chronic conditions who would benefit the most from more integrated care service arrangements. Therefore, risk selection still seems to be a much more profitable strategy than developing person-centred care arrangements for high-cost patients. Risk adjustment schemes that allow for improved risk sharing arrangements between insurer and regulators or involve overcompensating for certain risk combinations could potentially stimulate insurers investing in more advanced care arrangements for related population groups (Van Barneveld et al., 2001; Van Barneveld, van Vliet & van der Ven, 2001; Van de Ven, van Kleef & van Vliet, 2015; Van Kleef, van Vliet & van de Ven, 2016).

The question of whether countries should use insurance choice as a means to achieve more person-centred care has no easy answers. Countries would be well advised not to overestimate its impact on person-centredness or ultimately the quality of care. They also should not underestimate the wider implications of insurance choice and competition for health systems. These include the limited negotiation power of multiple insurers vis-à-vis providers (especially when compared to a single payer), increased administrative burden, incentives that may undervalue public health, and a possible further fragmentation of the system, which is likely to undermine rather than promote more person-centred care. There may be more effective ways to improve patient centredness in a given system. One is to better involve consumer and patient groups in the governance, design, operation, learning and purchasing decisions of insurers. Moreover, a range of regulation and accountability mechanisms exist that may be more effective in encouraging the development and adoption of person-centred care models. There is also a need to better understand the degree to which the population understands and values insurance choice, with regular debates in the Netherlands, Slovakia, Switzerland and the USA about the possibility of switching to a single national health insurance fund, a topic that was subject to a referendum in the case of Switzerland in 2014 (De Pietro et al., 2015).

That said, countries contemplating the introduction of (more) insurer choice and competition should take the following lessons to heart. First, periodic choice should be structured, simple and individualized and perhaps narrowed to a smaller number of options. Second, there should be regular monitoring and presentation of information on satisfaction with insurance services, on the quality of care provided under health insurance policies, and on the benefits covered and prices. Third, webportals that provide information to support people in making choices should be independent and transparent, an issue that will be especially important in the case of for-profit providers. Fourth, people should be given the opportunity to purchase mandatory insurance separately from additional VHI arrangements, and this should be enforced and monitored closely. Although this is the case in the reviewed countries, people are not always aware of these options. Fifth, there is a need for regularly improving and updating the risk adjustment system to minimize gaming and optimize incentives for insurers for contracting person-centred services. Finally, the use of navigators to assist consumers in making their choice and enrolling with insurers may help people to exercise more informed choices.

References

Abaluck J, Gruber J (2013). Evolving Choice. Inconsistencies in Choice of Prescription Drug Insurance. National Bureau of Economic Research, Working Paper 19163. Available at: http://www.nber.org/papers/w19163 (accessed 7 August 2017).

Alexa J et al. (2015). Czech Republic: health system review. Health Systems in Transition, 17(1):1–165.

Ärztenetzerhebung (2014). Available at: http://fmc.ch/fmc-impulse/archiv/artikel-detailseite/?tx_emagazine_article%5Barticle%5D=15&tx_emagazine_article%5Baction%5D=show&tx_emagazine_article%5Bcontroller%5D=Article&cHash=f02da79b31aee3e9281ef10e9d68cae1 (accessed 15 April 2017).

BAG (2016a). Statistik der obligatorischen Krankenversicherung 2015 (STAT KV 15). Available at: https://www.bag.admin.ch/bag/de/home/service/zahlen-fakten/statistiken-zur-krankenversicherung/statistik-der-obligatorischen-krankenversicherung.html (accessed 9 July 2018).

BAG (2016b). Die gesundheitspolitischen Prioritäten des Bundesrates (2013). Available at: https://www.bag.admin.ch/dam/bag/de/dokumente/nat-gesundheitsstrategien/gesundheit2020/g2020/bericht-gesundheit2020.pdf.download.pdf/bericht-gesundheit2020.pdf (accessed 7 July 2017).

BAG (2016c). Available at: https://www.bag.admin.ch/dam/bag/de/dokumente/kuv-aufsicht/stat/publications-aos/statistik-oblig-kv-2014-pdf-210seiten.pdf.download.pdf/statistik-oblig-kv-2014-pdf-210seiten.pdf (accessed 13 July 2017).

Barnes A et al. (2012). One Fish, Two Fish, Red Fish, Blue Fish: Effects of Price Frames, Brand Names, and Choice Set Size in Medicare Part D Insurance Plan Decisions. *Medical Care Research and Review*, 69(4):460–73.

Barnes AJ et al. (2014). Accountable care organizations in the USA: types, developments and challenges. *Health Policy*, 118(1):1–7.

Beck K et al. (2010). *Efficiency gains thanks to Managed Care? – evidence from Switzerland.* Lucerne: CSS Institute for Empirical Health Economics.

Bhargava S, Loewenstein G, Sydnor J (2015). Do individuals make sensible health insurance decisions? Evidence from a menu with dominated options. NBER Working Paper 21160.

Boonen LHHM, Laske-Aldershof T, Schut FT (2016). Switching health insurers: the role of price, quality and consumer information search. *European Journal of Health Economics*, 17:339–53.

Brammli-Greenberg S, Medina-Artom T, Yaari I (2017). Summary of Findings of Insuree Survey 2016 – Switching Health Plans. Jerusalem: Myers-JDC-Brookdale Institute. Available at: https://brookdale.jdc.org.il/en/switching-health-plans/ (accessed 28 August 2018).

Brammli-Greenberg S, Waitzberg R, Glazer K (2017). Payment mechanisms to mitigate incentive for (adverse) service selection among health plans in Israel. iHEA Boston 2017 Congress, Boston, USA, 8–11 July 2017.

Brammli-Greenberg S, Waitzberg R, Gross R (forthcoming). Integrating public and private insurance in the Israeli health system: an attempt to reconcile conflicting values. In: Thomson S, Sagan A, Mossialos E (eds.) *Paying for health care through private health insurance: history, politics, performance. An international perspective.* Cambridge: Cambridge University Press.

Busse R et al. (2012). Being responsive to citizens' expectations: the role of health services in responsiveness and satisfaction. In: Figueras J, McKee M (eds). *Health systems: health, wealth, society and well-being.* Maidenhead: Open University Press, 175–208.

Busse R et al. (2017). Statutory health insurance in Germany: a health system shaped by 135 years of solidarity, self-governance, and competition. *Lancet*, 390(10097):882–97.

Comparis (2017). Wir über uns. Available at: https://www.comparis.ch/comparis/info/wir (accessed 2 February 2017).

De Pietro C et al. (2015). Switzerland: Health system review. *Health Systems in Transition*, 17(4):1–288.

Dormont B, Geoffard P, Lamiraud K (2009). The influence of supplementary health insurance on switching behaviour: evidence from Swiss data. *Health Economics*, 18(11):1339–56.

Duijmelinck DMID, van de Ven WPMM (2013). Choice of insurer for basic health insurance restricted by supplementary Insurance. *European Journal of Health Economics*, 15(7):737–46.

Enthoven A (1978). Consumer-choice health plan – A national health-insurance proposal based on regulated competition in the private sector. *New England Journal of Medicine*, 298(13):709–20.

Enthoven AC (1993). The history and principles of managed competition. *Health Affairs* 12, Supplement: 24–48.

FOPH (2014). Statistiken zur Krankenversicherung – Statistik der obligatorischen Krankenversicherung 2013. Bern: Federal Office of Public Health. Available at: http://www.bag.admin. ch/themen/krankenversicherung/01156/index.html?lang=de&download=NHzLpZeg7t,ln p6I0NTU042l2Z6l n1acy4Zn4Z2qZpnO2Yuq2Z6gpJCMdHx_fWym162epYbg2c_JjKb NoKSn6A-- (accessed 23 October 2015).

Frank RG, Lamiraud K (2009). Choice, price competition, and complexity in markets for health insurance. *Journal of Economic Behavior and Organization*, 71:550–62.

Gaynor M, Ho K, Town RJ (2015). The industrial organization of health care markets. *Journal of Economic Literature*, 53(2):235–84.

GBE (2017). Gesetzliche Krankenversicherung: GKV Mitglieder/Versicherte. Gesundheitsberichterstattung des Bundes (GBE). Available at: http://www.gbe-bund.de/gbe10/trecherche.prc_them_rech?tk=700&tk2=2730&p_uid=gast&p_aid=30048177&p_sprache=D&cnt_ut=1&ut=2730 (accessed 18 June 2017).

Gerkens S, Merkur S (2010). Belgium: Health system review. *Health Systems in Transition*, 12(5):1–266, xxv.

Green MS et al. (2017). A national survey of ethnic differences in knowledge and understanding of supplementary health insurance. *Israel Journal of Health Policy Research*, 6(1):12. Available at: https://ijhpr.biomedcentral.com/track/pdf/10.1186/s13584-017-0137-4?site=ijhpr.biomedcentral.com (accessed 4 April 2017).

Hanoch Y et al. (2011). Choosing the Right Medicare Prescription Drug Plan: The Effect of Age, Strategy Selection and Choice Set Size. *Health Psychology*, 30(6):719–27.

Kaiser Family Foundation (2018). Health Insurance Coverage of the Total Population. Available at: https://www.kff.org/other/state-indicator/total-population/?currentTimeframe=0&sortModel=%7B%22colId%22:%22Location%22,%22sort%22:%22asc%22%7D (accessed 23 January 2017).

KPMG (2015). Evaluatie Zorgverzekeringswet [Evaluation of the Dutch Health Insurance Act], Eindrapportage, September 2014 [Internet]. Rotterdam: KPMG. Available at: https://zoek.officielebekendmakingen.nl/blg-384793 (accessed 8 July 2018).

Krankenkassen Deutschland (2018). Zusatzbeitrag der Krankenkassen. Available at: https://www.krankenkassen.de/gesetzliche-krankenkassen/krankenkasse-beitrag/kein-zusatzbeitrag/ (accessed 23 January 2017).

Kroneman M et al. (2016). Netherlands: Health System Review. Health Systems in Transition, 18(2):1–240.

Lako CJ, Rosenau P, Daw C (2011). Switching Health Insurance Plans: Results from a Health Survey. *Health Care Analysis*, 19(4):312–28.

Loewenstein G et al. (2013). Consumers' Misunderstanding of Health Insurance. *Journal of Health Economics*, 32:850–62.

McCormack L et al. (2009). Health Insurance Literacy of Older Adults. *Journal of Consumer Affairs*, 43(2):223–48.

Ministry of Health (2016). Switching between HMO – over who do HMO compete? Jerusalem: Ministry of Health. Available at: http://www.health .gov.il/publicationsfiles/switching_between_hmo2016.pdf (accessed 7 February 2017).

Nolte E, Knai C, Saltman R (eds.) (2014). *Assessing chronic disease management in European health systems. Concepts and approaches.* Copenhagen: World Health Organization, acting as the host organization for, and secretariat of, the European Observatory on Health Systems and Policies.

NZA (2016). Marktscan Zorgverzekeringsmarkt 2016. Utrect: NZA. Available at: https://puc.overheid.nl/nza/doc/PUC_3484_22/1/ (accessed 9 July 2018).

OECD/WHO (2011). OECD Reviews of Health Systems: Switzerland 2011 [Internet]. Paris: OECD.

Rice T, Unruh LY (2015). *The Economics of Health reconsidered.* Fourth edition. Chicago, IL: Health Administration Press/Arlington, VA: Association of University Programs in Health Administration.

Rice T et al. (2013). United States of America: health system review. *Health Systems in Transition*, 15(3):1–431.

Rice T et al. (2014). Challenges facing the United States of America in implementing universal coverage. *Bulletin of the World Health Organization*, 92(12):894–902.

Rooijen MR, de Jong JD, Rijken M (2011). Regulated competition in health care: switching and barriers to switching in the Dutch health insurance system. *BMC Health Services Research*, 11:95.

Rosen B, Waitzberg R, Merkur S (2015). Israel: Health System Review. *Health Systems in Transition*, 17(6):1–212.

Shmueli A (2015). On the calculation of the Israeli risk adjustment rates. *European Journal of Health Economics*, 16(3):271–7.

Shmueli A, Bendelac J, Achdut L (2007). Who switches sickness funds in Israel? *Health Economics, Policy and Law*, 2(3):251.

Sinaiko AD, Eastman D, Rosenthal MB (2012). How report cards on physicians, physician groups, and hospitals can have greater impact on consumer choice. *Health Affairs*, 31(3):602–11.

Smatana M et al. (2016). Slovakia: Health System Review. *Health Systems in Transition*, 18(6):1–210.

Statista (2017a). Größte gesetzliche Krankenkassen in Deutschland nach der Mitgliederanzahl in den Jahren 2014 bis 2017 (in Millionen). Available at: https://de.statista.com/statistik/daten/studie/218457/umfrage/groesstegesetzliche-krankenkassen-nach-anzahl-der-versicherten/ (accessed 18 June 2017).

Statista (2017b). Available at: https://de.statista.com/statistik/daten/studie/426582/umfrage/marktanteile-von-krankenversicherungen-in-der-schweiz/ (accessed 8 July 2018).

Thomson S et al. (2013). Statutory health insurance competition in Europe: a four-country comparison. *Health Policy*, 109(3):209–25.

US Department of Health and Human Services (2016). Website. Medicare.gov star ratings. Available at: https://www.medicare.gov/find-a-plan/staticpages/rating/planrating-help.aspx?termId=2018SS3 (accessed 8 July 2018).

Van Barneveld EM, van Vliet RC, van de Ven WP (2001). Risk sharing between competing health plans and sponsors. *Health Affairs*, 20(3):253–62. Available at: http://repub.eur.nl/pub/9767/11585175.pdf (accessed 9 July 2018).

Van Barneveld et al. (2001). Risk sharing as a supplement to imperfect capitation: a tradeoff between selection and efficiency. *Journal of Health Economics*, 20(2):147–68.

Van de Ven WP, van Kleef RC, van Vliet RC (2015). Risk Selection Threatens Quality Of Care For Certain Patients: Lessons From Europe's Health Insurance Exchanges. *Health Affairs (Millwood)*, 34(10):1713–20.

Van de Ven WP et al. (2013). Preconditions for efficiency and affordability in competitive healthcare markets: are they fulfilled in Belgium, Germany, Israel, the Netherlands and Switzerland? *Health Policy*, 109(3):226–45.

Van Ginneken E (2016). Governing competitive insurance market reform: cases studies from the Netherlands and Switzerland. In: Wismar M, Greer S, Figueras J (eds.) *Strengthening health system governance: better policies, stronger performance* Maidenhead: Open University Press, 129–42.

Van Ginneken E, Swartz K (2012). Implementing insurance exchanges – lessons from Europe. *New England Journal of Medicine*, 367(8):691–3.

Van Ginneken E, Busse R, Gericke CA (2008). Universal private health insurance in the Netherlands: the first year. *Journal of Management & Marketing in Healthcare*, 1(2):139–53.

Van Ginneken E, Swartz K, Van der Wees P (2013). Health insurance exchanges in Switzerland and the Netherlands offer five key lessons for the operations of US exchanges. *Health Affairs (Millwood)*, 32(4):744–52.

Van Kleef RC, van Vliet RC, van de Ven WP (2016). Overpaying morbidity adjusters in risk equalization models. *European Journal of Health Economics*, 17(7):885–95.

Van Winssen KP, van Kleef RC, van de Ven WP (2015). How profitable is a voluntary deductible in health insurance for the consumer? *Health Policy*, 119(5):688–95.

Vektis Zorgthermometer (2016). Verzekerden in Beeld 2016. Available at: https://www.vektis.nl/uploads/Publicaties/Zorgthermometer/ Verzekerden%20in%20beeld%202016.pdf (accessed 9 July 2018).

Zhou C, Zhang Y (2012). The Vast Majority of Medicare Part D Beneficiaries Still Don't Choose the Cheapest Plans that Meet Their Medication Needs. *Health Affairs*, 31:2259–64.

Zok (2016). Beitragssatzwahrnemung und Wechselbereitschaft in der GKV. WidoMonitor, 1. Available at: http://aok-bv.de/imperia/md/aokbv/presse/ pressemitteilungen/archiv/2016/wido-monitor_1_16_final.pdf (accessed 18 June 2017).

10 | *The service user as manager of care: the role of direct payments and personal budgets*

NICK VERHAEGHE

Introduction

Direct payments and personal budgets have gained prominence in a range of countries as a means to strengthen the role of people in their own care and support (Gadsby, 2013). The origin of personal budgets can be traced to the independent living and disability rights movements in western countries in the 1970s that argued for greater self-determination and the right of people with disabilities to make decisions about the services that affect their lives. Subsequently, the concept of 'user-directed care' (which includes personal budgets and direct payments) was widened to include other target populations such as older people and people with long-term care needs, and, more recently, to health care (Gadsby, 2013; Kodner, 2003; Tilly & Wiener, 2001). Most commonly, personal budget schemes were introduced as part of a move towards personalization of care promoting choice, independence and autonomy by giving individuals control of a budget to purchase services to tailor their care to meet their specific needs (Gadsby, 2013).

This chapter traces the evolution of personal budgets and similar schemes in health and social care, describes the different types of scheme that have been implemented in different countries, explores the approaches that have been used and the goals different schemes are pursuing, and assesses the evidence of the impact of personal budgets and similar schemes on outcomes and their role towards more person-centred health systems. The chapter concludes with a set of recommendations to inform further research and policy. The chapter will not address 'medical savings accounts' which have emerged in a different context in response to concerns around inefficiencies in the private health insurance market, such as escalating costs, moral hazard, adverse selection and gaps in coverage (Hsu, 2010).

Personal budgets: defining terms and concepts

The terminology of what can be broadly subsumed under the heading of personal budgets varies widely across countries and includes, in addition to 'personal budgets' (Germany, the Netherlands, England), and 'direct payments' (England), concepts such as 'cash and counseling' (United States of America), 'cash payments for care' (Germany), 'cash for care' (France), 'personal assistance budgets' (Belgium), 'cash payments' (Austria), 'home care service vouchers' (Finland), 'assistance allowances' (Sweden), 'individualized funding' (Canada) and 'consumer directed care' (Australia), among others (Forder et al., 2012; Kaambwa et al., 2015).

As the terminology varies, so do the nature, scope and target populations of the different schemes that have been implemented in different countries. This variation reflects, mainly, differences in contexts between countries in terms of structures, organization, and financing of health and social care systems, along with differences in societal values and cultures. At the same time, personal budgets and related schemes share some commonalities, in general seeking to promote choice, independence and autonomy, and the personalization of health and social care more broadly (Alakeson et al., 2016). For ease of flow, this chapter uses the term 'personal budgets' throughout as an overarching concept, which we define as 'an amount of money to be spent by individuals to purchase services to tailor care to meet specific needs'.

Independent from the type of model used, Gadsby et al. (2013) identified four 'primary' motivations for introducing personal budget schemes including: (1) giving individuals more choice; (2) expanding the options for care; (3) improving outcomes; and/or (4) reducing expenditures. Underlying these motivations is the assumption that more choice will lead to greater autonomy, which will in turn improve outcomes at lower costs. Other motivations may include efforts to reduce the fragmentation of services, to stimulate private sector provision, or to improve the family's capacity to take on caring responsibilities (European Platform for Rehabilitation, 2013).

As noted, by allowing individuals to decide on how to spend an allocated budget, they have – at least in theory – more choice, control and flexibility over the services they wish to use and that best meet their individual needs (Gadsby, 2013). In practice, however, the degree to which people have choice and control varies. In general, two models can be identified (Alakeson, 2010). At the one end there are 'open models'.

In such programmes, individuals are allocated cash payments that they can choose to spend how they wish, and there are few or no accounting mechanisms in place. The only condition is that the individual must obtain adequate care and this is monitored at regular points in time. Examples of such models can be found in Austria, Germany and Finland (Alakeson, 2010). At the other end are the 'planned or budgeted models'. These programmes provide for a more direct connection between an individual's needs and the goods or services purchased. There are a number of restrictions on how the money can be spent, in that individuals must account for purchases against an approved spending plan by regularly submitting a record of the purchases, or limitations may exist in the types of goods or services that can be purchased. Examples of this type of model can be found in Canada, England, the Netherlands and the USA. Personal budget schemes may also contain elements of both models, such as in Belgium or France (Alakeson, 2010).

There are different ways in which personal budgets can be managed. These are:

1. direct payment model (or direct payments): the individual as the budget holder receives a cash payment or vouchers to purchase services or support (Health Foundation, 2010);
2. third party payment model: the budget is held by a third party service (for example, a professional, care manager or broker) who will assist the individual to access funding; service provision is monitored according to an approved care plan (European Platform for Rehabilitation, 2013);
3. notional budget model: commissioners are responsible for purchasing services, but the individual is aware of the treatment or service options and the corresponding costs (Welch et al., 2016); and
4. combined model: this model combines one or more features of models 1–3.

Personal budgets in practice: an overview of country experiences

This section provides an overview of recent developments in personal budgets and related schemes in Australia, Belgium, England, the Netherlands, Scotland, Sweden and the USA. This selection of countries was informed by an earlier analysis of such schemes in England, Germany, the Netherlands and the USA by the Commonwealth Fund

(Alakeson, 2010), and broadened to also include countries for which information was available in English or Dutch. Germany was excluded as there was only little published information in English available. We excluded Canada from this analysis as disability policy and service provision are determined at the provincial level, with different solutions developed across provinces, making an overview of Canada difficult. We recognize that other countries have also introduced personal budgets or similar schemes – including Austria, Denmark, Finland, France, Italy and New Zealand – but we were unable to identify sufficiently robust information that would allow satisfactory presentation of these schemes.

The principal features of each scheme are summarized in Table 10.1. As highlighted earlier, countries differ in the nature and scope of personal budget models and in the drivers behind the introduction of such schemes. Overall, however, the main idea or driver is to place the individual, who receives a certain amount of funding, at the centre of the process of identifying needs and making choices over the services they expect to best meet their needs. Other drivers include, among others, cost savings (Australia), reducing care home admissions (Belgium), and strengthening the private sector and diversification in the care market in particular, so increasing service options (the Netherlands). Differences with regard to organizational boundaries, eligibility criteria, funding structure and target populations were also observed. For example, target populations differ in terms of age group ('older people' in Australia, 'youth' in the Netherlands), in terms of care needs and nature of 'disability' (e.g. 'long-term care needs' in Belgium, England and the USA; 'physical or mental disabilities' in Sweden, 'psychiatric problems' in the Netherlands). In all but one country (Australia), the budget can be managed in more than one way (e.g. direct payments and budgets held by third parties in England, the Netherlands, Scotland, Sweden and the USA). There is a tendency in the literature to use different terms as they relate to the person receiving the personal budget interchangeably, such as 'individuals', 'people', 'users', 'persons', 'participants', 'patients' (Gadsby et al., 2013; O'Shea & Bindman, 2016; Pike, O'Nolan & Farragher, 2016). Pragmatically, we use the term 'individual' throughout this chapter.

Australia

The origins of personal budgets in Australia can be traced to a 2011 report by the Productivity Commission, which highlighted that the disability support arrangements in place at that time provided fairly limited

Table 10.1 *Overview of the use of personal budgets in a number of countries*

Country	Scheme	Drivers	Target populations	Budget deployment	Financial reporting
Australia	self-directed care	choice and control; cost savings	people with disabilities; older people	provider holds the budget	depends on the type of support
Belgium	personal assistance budget; personal budget	choice; autonomy; reduce care home admissions	people with long-term care needs	notional budgets; direct payments	depends on the type of support
England	personal (health) budget; direct payment	choice; autonomy; personalization of health and social care	people with long-term needs	direct payments; budgets held by commissioners or third parties	detailed financial accounting
the Netherlands	personal budget	choice and control; address limitations in current system; stimulate private sector provision	people with long-term needs; disability; psychiatric problems; youth	direct payments; budgets held by third parties	financial accounting
Scotland	self-directed care; direct payments	choice and control; recovery; rehabilitation	people in need of social care	direct payments; budgets held by third parties	compulsory accounting, but varies according to locality
Sweden	assistance allowances	personalization; autonomy; choice	people with severe physical or mental disabilities	direct payments; budgets held by third parties	limited responsibilities for the patients
USA	cash & counselling; self-directed care	expand options for home- and community-based long-term care	older people; disabled people with long-term care needs	direct payments; budgets held by third parties	detailed financial accounting

choice to individuals with disabilities (Productivity Commission, 2011). This was followed, in 2013, by the National Disability Insurance Scheme Act, which aimed to give individuals 'true' choice and control over "care and support that is objectively assessed as being reasonable and necessary over the course of their lifetime", including the ability to manage their own funding (Pike, O'Nolan & Farragher, 2016). The driving force behind the legislation was a perceived need to halt the rising costs of the national disability system (Pike, O'Nolan & Farragher, 2016). More recent years saw the introduction, in 2015, of consumer-directed care, including publicly subsidized home care services that are designed to assist individuals aged 65 years and older to remain independent. The individualized budget is managed by an approved provider on behalf of the individual. A control and decision-making framework outlines how the individual should, in conjunction with their provider, manage their care plan and the services they receive (Kaambwa et al., 2015). The plan distinguishes between 'general' and 'reasonable and necessary' support. The former refers to coordination, strategic or referral service or activity over which the individual has a high degree of flexibility regarding provision and implementation. Reasonable and necessary support is more narrowly defined in that the funding and the way in which related services are to be provided are specified to help ensure that expected outcomes are attained. Funds can be used for services that are aimed at pursuing individuals' goals, maximizing their independence and their ability both to live independently and to be included in the community as fully participating citizens. Support services will not be provided or funded if they are likely to cause harm to the individual or pose a risk to others (Pike, O'Nolan & Farragher, 2016).

Belgium

The foundations for personal budgets in Belgium were set in 1997, with the introduction of a pilot programme for individuals with disabilities to enhance their autonomy in managing their own care. However, it was only in 2000 that the Flemish government developed a legal framework for the introduction of personal assistance budgets for disabled individuals (Breda et al., 2004; Flemish Government, 2015). From 2017 this scheme switched to a two-phase system consisting of a 'basic support budget' ('basis ondersteuningsbudget') and a 'personal budget' ('persoonsvolgende budget'). The major drivers behind this system can be seen to be situated within a shift towards more demand-driven care and support for the disabled. There was also an expectation that personal budgets would reduce the demand for care home places (Flemish Government, 2013). The 'basic support budget' consists of a fixed amount of funds aimed at individuals with a disability with limited care needs. The budget can be used for home-based support or transport services, and this does not need to be formally reported. The 'personal budget' is personalized and directed at disabled individuals with intensive or recurring care needs. It involves the agreement of a care plan between the individual and the Flemish Agency for People with a Disability which sets out the types of service that are required. The budget is determined based on a needs assessment tool, using parameters that correspond with nationally fixed budget levels. Funds can be obtained in cash, through a voucher, or a combination of both (Flemish Agency for People with a Disability, 2017).

England

Direct payments were first introduced by the 1997 Community Care (Direct Payments) Act. It was targeted at working age disabled individuals with long-term care needs. Eligibility was subsequently expanded to include older individuals (2000), parents of disabled children (2001), and those with mental health problems (2009) (Alakeson, 2010; European Platform for Rehabilitation, 2013). In 2007 personal budgets were further promoted as part of the new approach to adult social care to reduce public spending in social care (Government of the United Kingdom, 2007). This was followed, in 2009, by the piloting of personal budgets within the National Health Service (NHS), and the 2014 Care Act created a legal framework for the development of care and support for all adults with needs for care and support. The personal budget pilot provided for a spectrum of flexibility for individuals in managing their budget. Thus, eligible individuals could choose whether to manage the budget themselves (direct payments) or use a third party to do so on their behalf (Department of Health, 2014; Department of Health, 2015; NHS England, 2015). As some individuals included in the pilot also used funds to purchase health-related services, the government introduced a further pilot scheme for personal health budgets, which operated from 2009 to 2012 (Alakeson et al., 2016; European Platform for Rehabilitation, 2013).

Similar to personal budgets and direct payments in social care, eligible individuals could choose to receive the funds as a direct payment, or have the funds managed by the NHS or by a third party (Gadsby, 2013; NHS England, 2015). Following completion of the pilot phase, personal health budgets were introduced from 2013 for individuals with diabetes, chronic obstructive pulmonary disease, Parkinson's disease, and serious mental illness receiving long-term complex care (Forder et al., 2012; Gadsby, 2013). From October 2014 personal health budgets were to be rolled out to include all individuals eligible for continuing health care (Department of Health, 2012). Central to the scheme is a care plan which is planned and agreed between the individual (or their representative) and the local clinical commissioning group (the purchasers of most care in the English NHS). Individuals can choose to manage their personal health budgets in different ways depending on the level of financial responsibility they wish to take (Alakeson et al., 2016). Individuals have considerable freedom in the services they can purchase, ranging from home-based support services to psychological and physical therapies, as well as nursing services, transport services and leisure activities (O'Shea & Bindman, 2016). The budgets are typically determined by using 'indicative budgets' based on best estimates and/ or previous care packages. Local authorities are responsible for setting the level of funding to meet the individual's needs (Gadsby, 2013; Pike, O'Nolan & Farragher, 2016).

In April 2015 the Integrated Personal Commissioning Programme was launched as a partnership between NHS England and the Local Government Association. It is aimed at individuals with high health and social care needs. A key element of the programme consists of personalized commissioning and payment enabling a wider range of care and support options tailored to individual needs and preferences (Bennett, 2016).

The Netherlands

Active promotion and campaigning by the patients' rights and disability movements in the 1980s and 1990s paved the way for personal budgets in the Netherlands (Pike, O'Nolan & Farragher, 2016). In 1995 personal budgets were introduced for individuals with disability, chronic illness, mental health problems, or age-related impairments (European Platform for Rehabilitation, 2013) and regulated under the long-term care legislation (Pike, O'Nolan & Farragher, 2016). Individuals were required to complete a needs assessment to justify their choice of services (European Platform for Rehabilitation, 2013) and also submit a care agreement. In 2007, under the 'Social Support Act', municipalities were given responsibility for personal budgets to fund domestic care (Pike, O'Nolan & Farragher, 2016). A relaxation of the accounting requirements in the early 2000s led to a substantial growth in overall costs and since 2014 only those who would otherwise have had to move into care or a nursing home were able to keep their personal budget or apply for one. The new mechanisms allowed individuals to keep tailored services, but financial limits were defined by the authorities (Alakeson, 2010; European Platform for Rehabilitation, 2013). In 2015 the system was further reformed with personal budgets allowed under the following acts:

1. the 'Long-term Care Act', for people with severe long-term care needs including vulnerable old people and people with severe disabilities. The budget can be used for intensive care or close supervision, with care determined based on a needs assessment;
2. the 'Social Support Act', which aimed at enabling people to live independently and to participate in society. The municipalities determine how social support is delivered;
3. the 'Youth Act', which includes personal budgets for mental health care, parenting support and social support for children less than 18 years old. The municipalities are responsible for the budget; and
4. the 'Healthcare Insurance Act', which included additional benefits for a number of services such as nursing care, care related to sensory disabilities (low vision, blindness, deafness), and inpatient mental health care.

The Dutch government, the municipalities and the health insurers are jointly responsible for long-term care, including personal budgets. The vast majority of personal budget payments are made under the 2015 Social Support Act. Personal budgets for elements of long-term care and for nursing care are also covered under the Long-term Care Act and the Healthcare Insurance Act respectively (Government of the Netherlands, 2015; Pike, O'Nolan & Farragher, 2016). The personal budget schemes have been designed explicitly to stimulate private sector provision of care services (Pike, O'Nolan & Farragher, 2016).

Scotland

The 'Community Care and Health Act 2002' introduced direct payments for social care that aimed at providing greater independence for eligible individuals (Ridley et al., 2011). Following this, the 10-year strategy 'Self-directed care support: a national strategy for Scotland' was introduced in 2010 focusing on the delivery of care and support for all categories of individuals in need of social assistance, including people with disabilities, and also for caregivers. It was assumed that involving carers in the assessment process of required care for the individual can help identify and deliver support that is personalized, preventative, responsive and sustainable. This would then lead to greater satisfaction with the process and can contribute to improved outcomes for the individual, as well as for the carer (e.g. stress relief, improved quality of life). This strategy promoted choice and control and linked these concepts to the goals of recovery and rehabilitation (Scottish Government, 2010). In 2014 the 'Social Care (Self-directed Support) Scotland Act 2013' came into force, which provided for direct payments (Scottish Government, 2014). Local authorities determine the amount of money that individuals may receive as a direct payment and for which services they can be used. 'Eligible needs' are established according to national eligibility criteria that determine the level of these needs. Services can include care from a personal assistant or family member, nursing care, housing support services, equipment and adaptations (Pike, O'Nolan & Farragher, 2016).

Sweden

In 1993, following campaigns by the Swedish Independent Living Movement and as part of a broader disability policy reform, two acts were established: the 'Act concerning Support and Service to Persons with Certain Functional Impairments' and the 'Assistance Benefit Act'. The Acts' main objective was to provide support for people with severe physical or mental disabilities so they could live like others in the community. Personal assistance budgets, through direct payments (based on assistance hours), were established in 1994, subject to the personal assistance needs of the individual and without means-testing. Thus, payments are made without consideration of personal or family income. When applying for assistance individuals have to submit an assessment by a physician that describes their functional disabilities and the impact they have on their quality of life. Eligible patients can choose to receive direct payments, purchase services from their municipalities or private bodies, or privately employ personal assistants. The payment can be used for 'fundamental needs' and other activities, such as assistance with household tasks, work, childcare or leisure activities. There are few restrictions on how the money can be spent, but budget-holders are required to send a monthly report on the number of hours of work performed by the assistants (Gadsby, 2013; Independent Living Institute, 2010).

The United States of America

Many US states have financial and care assistance programmes, usually associated with Medicare, which provide the beneficiary with cash assistance and with the flexibility to self-direct the spending of the cash on care providers of their choosing. Formerly called 'Cash and Counseling', this model is now referred to as 'Consumer Direction', 'Participant Direction', 'Self-Directed Care' and a variety of other state-specific names.

The term 'Cash and Counseling' originated in the mid-1990s – with a pilot run in fifteen states – aiming to give Medicaid beneficiaries with disabilities the flexibility to self-direct the spending of the cash on care providers of their choice (American Elder Care Research Organization, 2017). The target population consisted of children, adults and older people with disabilities who were eligible for personal care or home-based and community-based services (Alakeson, 2010). The budget is managed by third-party financial management organizations to improve financial control and simplify the accounting process (Doty, Mahoney & Simon-Rusinowitz, 2007; O'Shea & Bindman, 2016). The budget is determined by an assessment of the number of care hours required and is then calculated using the number of care hours and cost of care for a geographic area. The budget can be increased or decreased as the individual's needs change. The budgets can be used for some health care services (e.g. nursing, rehabilitation) and for hiring and supervising of personal assistants for a specified number of hours per week aimed at reducing the demand for places in care homes (Kaambwa et al., 2015; O'Shea & Bindman, 2016). Since the success of the pilot, the model has been adopted in many states, as 'IndependentChoices' in Arkansas, 'In Home Supportive Services' in California and 'Choice Waiver' in Michigan.

Personal budgets: considerations

Personal budgets and similar schemes are about making the financial aspect of care more explicit at the individual level. By allowing the individual to determine how to spend the money, personal budgets can offer more choice and control to the budget-holder (Gadsby, 2013). However, there are a number of considerations that may impede the success of personal budgets, including: if increasing consumer choice leads to confusion; if people are unable to access the relevant information and support to make informed choices; and whether health professionals are comfortable in acknowledging patients' preferences, which may be different from their own (Gadsby et al., 2013).

Although personal budgets can increase an individual's sense of control and choice, and the money can be used in a more flexible way to respond to each individual's needs, allowing patients to determine which services they want to use poses the risk of them choosing services that increase rather than decrease their problems. For example, personal budgets can be spent in ways that do not conform to the current understanding of evidence-based medicine. There is yet a risk that the budget is spent on care that is ineffective or at worst even harmful and as a consequence is not meeting the needs of the patient. Moreover, increasing choice is accompanied by a number of responsibilities, constraints and consequences resulting in individuals losing a certain amount of security when third parties determine their needs, or even increased uncertainty (Spandler & Vick, 2006).

There are also concerns that complicated personal budget programmes may even reduce control and oversight for some service user groups (Ungerson, 2004). People without the ability or capacity to manage a personal budget themselves, or without the necessary support, risk being less able to benefit from, or being excluded from, access to such financial allowances (Galpin & Bates, 2009). So, a key element for the implementation of effective personal budget schemes is the availability of professional support (Welch et al., 2016). The need for support may, however, vary across different target populations. For example, older people and people with complex needs may need more extensive support to help them to manage their personal budgets effectively, particularly when direct payments are used (Health Foundation, 2010). In contrast, younger adults with physical disabilities have been found to be more capable in managing personal budgets themselves (Wise, 2016).

At present, there is only limited research examining the benefits of personal budgets for different demographic groups or people with different health conditions. There is only little comparative information available, suggesting that personal budget schemes are more effective for particular target groups (for example, Wise, 2016). Further, concerns remain for people who lack the capacity to manage their personal budget themselves. Family members or third parties may act as representatives, but they need to act in the best interest of the individual. Involvement of third parties is preferable if concerns exist about financial exploitation by family members (Alakeson et al., 2016; European Platform for Rehabilitation, 2013). However, in the Netherlands the involvement of third-party organizations, in the form of independent support brokerage agencies, was found to be problematic because they employed aggressive marketing tactics (Gadsby, 2013).

The availability of accurate information is crucial to make an informed choice; however, substantial differences in the availability of such information exist between countries. For example, in an evaluation of the use of personal budget schemes in 11 OECD countries, it was concluded that necessary information was not available in countries with more 'open models' because the provision of information was not incorporated into these programmes (Gadsby et al., 2013). Another consideration is the extent to which patients may want to make decisions about the services they want to use. For example, the findings of a review by Auerbach (2001) suggested that patients want information, but do not necessarily want to make decisions. This is congruent with the findings of a study that examined the experiences of receiving and using a budget by 58 English NHS patients with long-term conditions. An important factor that contributed to a sense of satisfaction with the budget was the feeling that 'somebody cared'. A number of respondents reported that they felt uncomfortable making choices about their health care and strongly argued for more professional support (Davidson et al., 2013). No evidence exists related to 'best practices' in terms of providing information, training or support to service users. Therefore, future research could examine the 'optimal support dose', which may vary across individuals, target populations and/or health conditions.

Other challenges persist which may prevent the successful implementation of personal budget schemes. The introduction of personal budgets often challenges the current way of working and it may take considerable time and effort to ensure successful implementation. Indeed, personal budget programmes may require substantial change across a number of existing service systems. Furthermore, the uptake by individuals is difficult to predict and may be slower than anticipated (Gadsby, 2013). Although some countries have endeavoured to expand personal budgets to include health care services (so-called 'personal health budgets'), concerns have been expressed that such an extension may pose the risk that governments will use such budgets to cap spending on health care and transfer the risk of unexpected health care needs to the individual (Alakeson, 2010). Flexible capacity is needed for personal health budgets because health systems need to be able to reallocate resources in favour of those services selected by patients in directing their own care. If this extra capacity is not available, then patients' choices will be limited (Appleby, Harrison & Devlin, 2003).

Personal budgets: what do we know about their effectiveness?

This section reviews the evidence on personal budgets, focusing in turn on their impact on: (1) choice and control, (2) health outcomes, (3) quality of life and well-being, and (4) costs and cost-effectiveness.

Do personal budgets enhance choice and control?

Webber et al. (2014) examined the literature on the impact of personal budgets for individuals with mental health problems. In five of the 15 studies included in the review the impact of personal budgets on choice and control was reported, with four studies (Eost-Telling, 2010; Hatton & Waters, 2011; Spandler & Vick, 2004; Teague & Boaz, 2003) observing an increase in the levels of perceived control and choice. Conversely, a survey by Cheshire West and Chester Council in England in 2010 found that individuals receiving a personal budget felt less in control of their care and support compared to other social care groups (Cheshire West & Chester Council, 2010). Davidson et al. (2013), referred to earlier, examined the experiences of 58 patients with long-term conditions of the effect of personal health budgets using a qualitative study design. The majority of interviewees reported increased choice and control, while only a minority commented that the personal health budget had no impact on perceived choice and control. The latter generally reflected a lack of understanding or lack of information about the nature and purpose of the budget. The majority of the budget-holders did not know whether their budget was adequate or not because they did not know the initial budget allocation or how much money was left. Nine months after receiving the money, about 50% of respondents felt that the level of the budget was adequate for their needs. This was mainly because a part of the budget was still available or because all services had already been purchased.

Welch et al. (2016) examined the perceptions of 10 organizational representatives in implementing personal health budgets for people with substance misuse problems in England. The interviewees reported that choice and control were likely to increase through the option of selecting providers who were not available within conventional health care delivery. It was also felt that providers had become more responsive to the needs of clients and that patients had increased responsibility for their own care. However, a number of challenges and concerns were identified. First, it was reported that increased choice and control had resulted in increased stress and anxiety, rather than empowering individuals. A second concern was related to the types of services that could be purchased. Study participants commented that more guidance was required. About 80% of the budgets were managed notionally and it was felt that direct payments would ensure more flexibility because such payments were considered as the only option allowing individuals absolute control over their budget. Moreover, direct payments were perceived as the only option that would allow individuals absolute control over their budget. The representatives responsible for implementing personal health budgets also expressed concerns about the inappropriate use of funds, particularly if the requested support did not conform with professional or evidence-based knowledge. Glendinning et al. (2008) evaluated the individual budget pilot programme from 13 local authority sites in England. The target population included adults and seniors with physical, cognitive and psychiatric disabilities who were eligible for long-term care and other disability support services. They found that patients continued to purchase traditional services such as home care; however, greater choice and control was experienced.

Larsen et al. (2015) evaluated the experiences with personal budgets of 47 psychiatric patients receiving care from integrated teams. Only four respondents reported a perceived loss of choice. Spandler & Vick (2006) examined the views of 58 mental health service users receiving direct payments. They identified improved levels of choice, control and independence. Breda et al. (2004) evaluated the impact of personal assistance budgets in the Flanders region (Belgium) three years after implementation. The introduction of this type of personal budget scheme resulted in an increased degree of choice. However, a discrepancy was observed between the needs and the available services, particularly for services for which only limited alternatives in formal care were available. Personal assistance budgets were also associated with a considerable administrative burden.

Do personal budgets improve health outcomes?

A comprehensive analysis by Forder et al. (2012) examined the impact of the personal health budget pilot programme in England. Their findings suggest that the programme did not result in a significant impact on health status (assessed as blood glucose in diabetes patients and lung function in chronic obstructive pulmonary disease patients) or on mortality. Gadsby et al. (2013) evaluated the impact of personal budgets in 11 OECD countries and concluded that improvements in health are possible but more evidence is needed.

In examining the perceptions of patients with long-term conditions, Davidson et al. (2013) found that the majority of respondents reported improvements in health across a range of domains that was far wider than the condition for which the money was given, including better care arrangements and better relationships with health professionals. In an evaluation of the 'Cash and Counseling' programme in the USA, 6700 older adults and younger people with disability-related needs were randomized to a self-directed programme or to a traditional agency-based programme. In the 'Cash and Counseling' arm, similar or better health outcomes were achieved compared with the agency-based programme (Boston College, 2017). Jones et al. (2013) compared the introduction of personal budgets in the UK to conventional health care delivery. The aim of the introduction of the personal budgets was to secure a series of services and support such as home-based care, transport or therapies, but no significant associations between group changes in health outcomes and mortality were found.

Do personal budgets improve quality of life and well-being?

Evaluations of personal budget programmes in Australia, England and the USA suggest that such schemes may improve satisfaction, well-being and some aspects of quality of life (Gadsby et al., 2013). A literature review examining the impact of personal budgets for individuals with mental health problems reported mixed findings. Some evidence related to the impact of personal budgets on quality of life, satisfaction and mental health was found, but this was not unequivocal (Webber et al., 2014).

Welch et al. (2016) identified a number of benefits associated with personal health budgets, including increased self-confidence and self-esteem and the potential to rebuild shattered lives. Larsen et al. (2015) described the most commonly reported positive outcomes as including mental and emotional well-being (reported by 34 of 47 participants), and confidence and skills (reported by 28 participants). Only four participants also reported negative outcomes such as stress and bureaucracy. Spandler & Vick (2006) found improved well-being in a sample of mental health service users receiving direct payments. Jones et al. (2013) and Forder et al. (2012) both evaluated the personal health budget pilot programme in England as noted earlier. Jones et al. (2013) found no significant differences between an intervention group receiving personal budgets (n=1171) and a control group receiving conventional health care delivery (n=1064) in health-related quality of life. In contrast, psychological well-being significantly improved in the intervention group compared to the control. Mixed results were also observed by Forder et al. (2012), such that for health-related quality of life no significant improvements were found, while the use of personal health budgets was associated with a significant improvement in care-related quality of life and psychological well-being.

Do personal budgets reduce costs and and provide value for money?

Gadsby et al. (2013) reported mixed findings on the impact of personal budgets on costs. On the one hand, personal budget schemes can result in short-term cost savings at an individual level. On the other hand, costs may rise if people purchase care for services previously bought out-of-pocket (substitution effect). The aforementioned review by Webber et al. (2014) of the impact of personal budgets for people with mental health problems identified two studies that reported on cost-effectiveness. These found personal budgets to be either cost-neutral (Glendinning et al., 2008) or cost-effective (Forder et al., 2012). In the latter study the change from baseline to follow-up (at 12 months) in costs of inpatient care were found to be significantly higher in the personal health budget group compared to the control group (–£2150 vs. –£830, P=0.040). No significant between-group differences in changes in total costs were observed (intervention vs. controls: £800 vs. £1920, P=0.319). The personal health budget group showed greater benefit (0.057 vs. 0.018)[1] and lower total costs (£800 vs. £1920) compared to the control group. The authors noted that the findings of their study must be cautiously interpreted due to a number of methodological problems.

In summary, there is at present no conclusive answer to the question 'What is the impact of personal budgets and similar schemes on the outcomes of choice and control', 'health', 'quality of life and well-being', and 'cost and cost-effectiveness'. The available evidence suggests that personal budgets may have a positive impact on choice, control, quality of life and well-being, and to some extent on costs and cost-effectiveness, but this is far from unequivocal. Studies were characterized by heterogeneity in study designs. For example, only a small number of studies used a controlled design. It is clear that more research based on sound methodological principles is required. Such studies could examine both the effectiveness and cost-effectiveness of personal budget programmes in order to help inform policy development. Future research should also address the long-term consequences of such programmes and the development of a general framework for the evaluation of personal budget programmes and initiatives. This would enable better cross-country comparisons, while being mindful that it remains important to take country-specific contexts into account.

Conclusions

Personal budgets and similar schemes are an alternative way of purchasing elements of health and social care services, enabling individuals to shift from a passive recipient of care role to an active purchaser role. They can thus be considered as a mechanism towards more personalization in health and social care delivery. Originating from the independent living and disability rights movements, personal budget programmes have

---

1   Measured by the ASCOT (Adult Social Care Outcomes Toolkit). This measure is designed to capture information about an individual's social care-related quality of life.

been introduced in a number of countries. In general, they are aimed at promoting choice, control and independence for the service users by involving them in the planning and purchasing of health and/or social care. Considerable differences across countries persist in terms of eligible target populations, accounting mechanisms and budget deployments. This means that in some countries cash payments are provided to individuals directly while in other countries organizations retain responsibility for making payments in conjunction with the patients. The international evidence about personal budgets and similar schemes is rather limited. Some evidence was found that personal budgets can improve choice, control, well-being and quality of life. Evidence related to their impact on health outcomes, costs and value for money is scarce. For whom and how personal budget schemes could best be implemented and the related consequences of these choices remains inconclusive.

Recommendations

We provide some recommendations for policy and further research below. These are presented in an integrated way such that both sets of recommendations are combined. The reason for this approach is that the information derived from scientific research can serve as input for policy decisions.

It is important to clearly define the types of care and support services that can be purchased using personal budgets. Choices need to be made as to whether or not to limit the available options to only those for which there is an evidence base. As a starting point, one could consider excluding options for which there is no evidence or that are considered to be harmful. It is, however, important that there are appropriate options to meet the needs of individuals. Thoughtful consideration must go into the design of these programmes in order to minimize the risk of unintended consequences and counter the barriers hampering successful implementation. The information derived from scientific research can serve as a guiding tool to help determine which services can be purchased with personal budgets. Thus, further research should examine both the effectiveness and cost-effectiveness of personal budget programmes. Evidence about the effectiveness of strategies – i.e. which strategies work best for whom and under what circumstances – is currently insufficient to inform policy-making. Since governments face the challenge of priority setting in the allocation of scarce health care resources, health economic evaluations of such payment schemes can provide payers and governments with improved insights on how to spend the available resources in the most efficient way.

'Informed choice' requires the availability of accessible and accurate information. This should include clear information about the amount of funds being allocated, the types of services that can be purchased with the personal budget, and related accounting requirements. Special attention should be given to target populations with limited ability or lack of capacity to enable them to participate fully in personal budget programmes. Financial support through personal budgets is only one approach towards more personalization in health and social care delivery. Personal budget schemes must be embedded in wider policies aimed at people with health and social care needs.

The origin of personal budgets lies in the independent living and disability rights movements of the 1970s that argued for greater self-determination and the right of disabled people to make decisions about the services that affect their lives. More recently, personal (health) budgets have also been discussed in the movement towards more integrated health and social care delivery for people with chronic conditions. In this context, personal (health) budgets are considered 'financial incentives'. Other incentives that may be more appropriate for integrated care include pay-for-performance, pay-for-coordination and all-inclusive payments (global budget and bundled payment). Therefore, the role of personal budgets in the movement towards greater integration of health and social care should be viewed within the larger picture of integrating (elements from) other financial incentives.

References

Alakeson V (2010). International developments in self-directed care. *Issue Brief (Commonwealth Fund)*, 78:1–11.

Alakeson V et al. (2016). Debating personal health budgets. *BJPsych Bulletin*, 40:34–7.

American Elder Care Research Organization (2017). Receive payment as a caregiver: Cash and Counseling and other options. Available at: https://www.payingforseniorcare.com/longtermcare/resources/cash-and-counseling-program.html (accessed 2 October 2017).

Appleby J, Harrison A, Devlin N (2003). *What is the real cost of more patient choice?* London: King's Fund.

Auerbach SM (2001). Do patients want control over their own health care? A review of measures, findings and research issues. *Journal of Health Psychology*, 6:191–203.

Bennett S (2016). *Integrated Personal Commissioning: Emerging framework.* London: NHS England & Local Government Association.

Boston College (2017). *An environmental scan of self-direction in behavioral health.* Boston: Boston College, National Resource Center for Participant-Directed Services, University of Maryland.

Breda J et al. (2004). *Three years later: Evaluation of the personal assistance budget use. Final Report.* Antwerp: Department of Sociology, University of Antwerp.

Cheshire West & Chester Council (2010). *Findings from the personal budgets survey.* Cheshire: Cheshire West & Chester Council.

Davidson J et al. (2013). Choosing health: qualitative evidence from the experiences of personal health budget holders. *Journal of Health Services Research & Policy*, 18:50–8.

Department of Health (2012). Personal health budgets to be rolled out. Available at: https://www.gov.uk/government/news/personal-health-budgets-to-be-rolled-out (accessed 14 February 2017).

Department of Health (2014). Care and support statutory guidance: issued under the Care Act 2014. Available at: https://www.gov.uk/government/publications/care-act-2014-statutory-guidance-for-implementation (accessed 24 January 2017).

Department of Health (2015). The Care Bill – Personalising care and support planning. Factsheet 4. Available at: https://www.gov.uk/government/uploads/system/uploads/attachment_data/file/268681/Factsheet_4_update.pdf (accessed 16 January 2017).

Doty P, Mahoney KJ, Simon-Rusinowitz L (2007). Designing the Cash and Counseling demonstration and evaluation. *Health Services Research*, 42:378–96.

Eost-Telling C (2010). *Stockport Self Directed Support Pilot in Mental Health: Final report of the evaluation of the Self Directed Support Pilot.* Chester: University of Chester.

European Platform for Rehabilitation (2013). *Personal budgets. A new way to finance disability services.* Brussels: European Platform for Rehabilitation (EPR).

Flemish Agency for People with a Disability (2017). Personal budgets. Available at: https://www.vlaanderen.be/nl/gezin-welzijn-en-gezondheid/handicap/persoonsvolgende-financiering-pvf-basisondersteuningsbudget-bob-en-persoonsvolgende-budget-pvb-voor (accessed 18 January 2017).

Flemish Government (2013). *Draft note on personal budgets for people with a disability*. Brussels: Flemish Government, Cabinet of the Flemish Minister of Welfare, Public Health and Family.

Flemish Government (2015). Flemish policy for disabled people: introduction of the personal budgets decree. Available at: http://www.jovandeurzen.be/sites/jvandeurzen/files/Meerjarenplanfinaal_VR6feb2015_0.pdf (accessed 18 January 2017).

Forder J et al. (2012). *Evaluation of the personal health budget pilot programme*. London: Department of Health.

Gadsby EW (2013). *Personal budgets and health: a review of the evidence*. Kent: University of Kent, Centre for Health Services Studies.

Gadsby EW et al. (2013). Personal budgets, choice and health: a review of international evidence from 11 OECD countries. *International Journal of Public and Private Healthcare Management and Economics*, 3:15–28.

Galpin D, Bates N (2009). *Social work practice with adults*. Exeter: Learning Matters.

Glendinning C et al. (2008). *Evaluation of the individual budgets pilot programme: Final report*. York: Social Policy Research Unit, University of York.

Government of the Netherlands (2015). European code of social security. National report submitted in conformity with Article 74 of the European Code of social security.

Government of the United Kingdom (2007). Putting people first: A shared vision and commitment to the transformation of adult social care. Available at: http://webarchive.nationalarchives.gov.uk/20130107105354/http:/www.dh.gov.uk/prod_consum_dh/groups/dh_digitalassets/@dh/@en/documents/digitalasset/dh_081119.pdf (accessed 15 January 2017).

Hatton C, Waters J (2011). *The National Personal Budget Survey*. Lancaster: In Control/Lancaster University.

Health Foundation (2010). *Evidence scan: Personal health budgets*. London: Health Foundation.

Hsu J (2010). *Medical Savings Accounts: What is at risk?* World Health Organization Report, background paper 17. Geneva: World Health Organization.

Independent Living Institute (2010). *Personal Assistance in Sweden*. Gentbrugge: Independent Living Institute.

Jones K et al. (2013). Personalization in the health care system: do personal health budgets have an impact on outcomes and cost? *Journal of Health Services Research & Policy*, 18(Suppl. 2):59–67.

Kaambwa B et al. (2015). Investigating consumers' and informal carers' views and preferences for consumer directed care: a discrete choice experiment. *Social Science & Medicine*, 140:81–94.

Kodner DL (2003). Consumer-directed services: lessons and implications for integrated systems of care. *International Journal of Integrated Care*, 3:e12.

Larsen J et al. (2015). Outcomes from personal budgets in mental health: service users' experiences in three English local authorities. *Journal of Mental Health*, 24:219–24.

NHS England (2015). The forward view into action: new care models: update and initial support. Available at: https://www.england.nhs.uk/wp-content/uploads/2015/07/ncm-support-package.pdf (accessed 17 January 2017).

O'Shea L, Bindman AB (2016). Personal health budgets for patients with complex needs. *New England Journal of Medicine*, 375:1815–17.

Pike B, O'Nolan G, Farragher L (2016). *Individualised budgeting for social care services for people with a disability: International approaches and evidence on financial sustainability*. Dublin: Health Research Board.

Productivity Commission (2011). Disability Care and Support. Productivity Commission Inquiry Report. Available at: http://www.pc.gov.au/inquiries/completed/disability-support/report/disability-support-volume2.pdf (accessed 17 January 2017).

Ridley J et al. (2011). *Evaluation of self-directed support test sites in Scotland*. Edinburgh: Scottish Government Social Research.

Scottish Government (2010). *Self-directed support: a National Strategy for Scotland*. Edinburgh: Scottish Government.

Scottish Government (2014). *Statutory Guidance to accompany the Social Care (Self-Directed Support) (Scotland) Act 2013*. Edinburgh: Scottish Government.

Spandler H, Vick N (2004). *Direct payments, independent living and mental health: an evaluation*. London: Health and Social Care Advisory Service.

Spandler H, Vick N (2006). Opportunities for independent living using direct payments in mental health. *Health and Social Care in the Community*, 14:107–15.

Teague GB, Boaz TL (2003). *Evaluation of the adult mental health self-directed care project*. Florida: Florida Department of Children and Families.

Tilly J, Wiener JM (2001). *Consumer-directed home and community services: policy issues*. Washington DC: Urban Institute.

Ungerson C (2004). Whose empowerment and independence? A cross-national perspective on 'cash-for-care' schemes. *Ageing and Society*, 24:189–212.

Webber M et al. (2014). The effectiveness of personal budgets for people with mental health problems: a systematic review. *Journal of Mental Health*, 23:146–55.

Welch E et al. (2016). Implementing personal health budgets in England: a user-led approach to substance misuse. *Health and Social Care in the Community*, 10.

Wise J (2016). MPs question whether adults with personal care budgets get best care. *BMJ*, 353:i3224.

11 | Choosing treatments and the role of shared decision-making

FRANCE LÉGARÉ, MARTIN HÄRTER, ANNE M.
STIGGELBOUT, RICHARD THOMSON, DAWN
STACEY

Introduction

In 2015 people in OECD countries consulted a medical practitioner between two and sixteen times (OECD, 2015). These care-seekers were once expected to go along with whatever the doctor decided was best, but this has been slowly changing since the 1970s. As highlighted in Chapter 2 of this book, growing awareness of the limits of medical interventions and of the lack of control over decisions about one's own care (Illich, 1975) led to calls for equality between the patient and the health professional towards establishing a partnership for making decisions and determining the direction of care.

The notion of a more participatory approach to informed decision-making was first proposed by Robert Veatch in 1972, who suggested the idea of "sharing of decision-making" (Veatch, 1972). Evidence was accumulating that where doctors and patients agreed on the problem, outcomes were better (Starfield et al., 1979). In 1982 a US presidential commission noted that while health care systems were increasingly effective at addressing disease, there was a "diminished capacity and inclination to care for the patient in more human terms" (President's Commission for the Study of Ethical Problems in Medicine and Biomedical and Behavioral Research, 1982, p. 33). These observations came at a time when there was increasing recognition of practice variations (Wennberg & Gittelsohn, 1973) and of unnecessary surgery (Leape, 1989) across the USA. Neither of these could be explained by variation in the burden of disease or medical need, while evidence pointed to widespread overuse, underuse and misuse of tests and treatments. Policy-makers finally began to take note, and shared decision-making was proposed as one potential solution. The US Presidential Commission stated that "[p]ractitioners should seek not only to understand each

283

patient's needs and develop reasonable alternatives to meet those needs but also . . . present the alternatives in a way that enables patients to choose one they prefer. To participate in this process, patients must engage in a dialogue with the practitioner and make their views on well-being clear" (President's Commission for the Study of Ethical Problems in Medicine and Biomedical and Behavioral Research, 1982, p. 44). Shared decision-making (SDM) was seen to be especially appropriate with regard to 'preference-sensitive' conditions (Weinstein, 2000; Weinstein, Clay & Morgan, 2007). It began to take root as a core approach in primary care and to be considered the crux of person-centred care (Weston, 2001; Charles, Gafni & Whelan, 1997).

Along with supported self-management (Effing et al., 2007), SDM has now entered government policy and legislation in several countries. Since 1968 more than 6000 articles have been published about the theory and practice of SDM, and as of 2013 over 500 per year (Koster, 2016), indicating an exponential growth of scientific research in this area (Blanc et al., 2014). Much research has focused on studying the impacts of SDM tools (such as decision aids) but there remains a dearth of evidence that takes into account the full complexity of SDM and, more importantly, its implementation in clinical practice (Coulter, 2017), and physicians have been slow to adopt it (Couet et al., 2015).

With the notion of the relationship at its core, SDM can be defined as an interpersonal, interdependent process in which health professionals, patients and their caregivers relate to and influence each other as they collaborate in making decisions about a patient's health care (Légaré & Witteman, 2013). Together they consider the scientific evidence and the patient's preferences and values before making a treatment choice. The information transfer is two-way, and the health professional may not be the only, or even the main, source of information for patients. Patients' own unique experiences and preferences are equally important for informing the decision, acting as experts in their own right (Charles, Gafni & Whelan, 1997). It can involve the patient and their family and caregivers (Légaré, Stacey & Pouliot, 2011), along with one or more health professionals (often working in teams with patients who have chronic illnesses), as well as other health care workers, for example in the context of community-based primary care and home care (Légaré et al., 2015).

This chapter begins by setting out the challenges of arriving at a consensual definition of SDM. It discusses how SDM has entered policy debate and legislation and the possible drivers behind this. We examine the empirical evidence for its impact on outcomes at the individual, organizational and system levels, and discuss barriers to its implementation. We discuss models of SDM and how it can be measured, as well as current research trends, and finally propose a framework for a way forward.

How do we define SDM?

SDM is thought to involve three main steps. First, the clinician and the patient recognize and acknowledge that a decision is required, such as making a choice about starting, continuing, stopping or postponing treatment for a given condition. This is called the decision point (Coulter, 2011), not to be confused with a single point in time, as decisions can be an ongoing event (Rapley, 2008). Second, both parties understand the best available evidence concerning the risks, benefits and consequences of available options, including the option of doing nothing (watchful waiting). Third, the treatment decision reflects the patient's informed values and preferences about the outcomes of options. For example, a woman with breast cancer may prefer to have conservative breast surgery rather than a mastectomy in the knowledge that survival rates are equivalent (Fisher et al., 2002). Or a patient may not want to be prescribed medication, preferring to cope with the condition rather than live with the side-effects of the medication (Weiss et al., 2015). Such decisions can be supported by specifically designed patient decision aids, such as leaflets, videos or web-based tools. Tailored to a person's health condition, decision aids present the evidence and help clinicians and patients clarify their preferences and values (Stacey et al., 2017). Collections of decision aids can be found at the A to Z Inventory of Decision Aids (Ottawa Hospital Research Institute, 2015) and at the Med-Decs database (Stalmeier, 2012).

However, as noted, at its core SDM is about relationships and values, and as such it is difficult to define. Charles, Gafni & Whelan (1997) identified four key components: the patient and the clinician are involved in all phases; both parties share information; both parties take steps to build a consensus about the preferred treatment; and an agreement is reached about the treatment to be implemented. These components have since been renamed, further divided and redefined. However, most definitions still revolve around information exchange, deliberation, making the decision, and follow-up (Makoul & Clayman,

2006; Stacey et al., 2010; Elwyn et al., 2012; Stiggelbout, Pieterse & De Haes, 2015). The single defining feature of SDM remains what Ian McWhinney called the "exchange and synthesis of meanings" (Stewart, 2003) that take place in the clinical encounter.

When SDM entered clinical practice, it was typically in the context of 'professional equipoise' (Pauker & Kassirer, 1997; Elwyn et al., 2000), that is, in situations where the doctor had no clear preference about the best treatment choice. However, more recently SDM has been recognized as desirable in all situations where there is more than one reasonable approach to managing or treating a given condition (including watchful waiting). It is also seen to be useful for eliciting patients' values, namely what matters to the patients or their family members about the decision, such as efficacy, side-effects and cost, as well as life philosophies, priorities and life circumstances (Weinstein, Clay & Morgan, 2007; Lee, Low & Ng, 2013). Even where probabilities of risks and benefits of a given treatment are known for the population as a whole, these do not automatically translate to the individual, and the importance attached to risks and benefits may differ among individual patients, depending on their values and preferences.

While SDM is widely seen to be core to person-centred care (Coulter, 2017), some authors have taken a more cautious approach. For example, some authors have noted that SDM has been used to make patients uniquely responsible for their health (care) choices, with health professionals no longer being held accountable for decisions (Tobias & Souhami, 1993; Buetow & Kenealy, 2007; Sandman, Gustavsson & Munthe, 2016). Others noted that patients do not necessarily want to involve clinicians in decisions (Degner & Sloan, 1992) or prefer that the clinician makes treatment decisions on their behalf (Woolf, 2001; Schattner, 2002). Yet others argued that SDM can make patients feel anxious and insecure (Levy et al., 1989; Caldon et al., 2011; West & West, 2002) and there have been concerns that SDM might inadvertently favour those with higher education and disadvantage those who are already marginalized, thus reinforcing health inequities (Thomson, Murtagh & Khaw, 2005). We shall come back to these concerns later.

How has SDM entered law and policy?

There is now increasing consensus that there is an ethical imperative for health professionals to share important decisions with patients

(Salzburg Global Seminar, 2011). In recognition, many countries in Europe, North America and Australia (Härter, van der Weijden & Elwyn, 2011) have put in place formal recognition of SDM in the form of policy and regulatory frameworks as part of a wider move towards more person-centred systems. Elsewhere, the importance of SDM is increasingly being considered, with a small number of countries in South America and south-east Asia slowly introducing related policies (Härter et al., 2017b). Their rationale ranges from respect for consumer and patient rights and democratic public engagement to more instrumental arguments such as that it might increase efficiency and help control health care costs (Gibson, Britten & Lynch, 2012).

Most European countries are legislating on informed consent and patients' right to information using civil law (e.g. the Netherlands) or public law (e.g. Finland) (*see* Chapter 13). Other countries have dedicated elements of their national or regional legislation specifically to their interpretations of SDM. These include France (2002 Act on Patients' Rights and Quality of Care) (République Française, 2002), Chile (2006 Law on Rights and Responsibilities of People when Engaging in their Healthcare) (Bravo et al., 2011), Norway (1999 Patients' Rights Act) (Ringard et al., 2013), Sweden (2015 Patient Act) (Riksdag, 2014) (Box 11.1), Germany (Patients' Rights Act) (Bundesministerium für Gesundheit, 2013), the UK (2012 Health and Social Care Act) (Government of the

---

Box 11.1 Excerpt from the 2015 Patient Act, Sweden

"Caregivers are required to provide you with all necessary information no matter who you are or what background you have . . . The information must be adapted to your particular circumstances and capabilities . . . You must always have the chance to explain what you want to happen – then it is up to you to decide how much you want to take advantage of that opportunity. Once you are familiar with the options that are available, you can give your consent or otherwise indicate your preferences. You are always entitled to turn down any care that is offered to you. You can also change your mind after you have approved a certain kind of care."

Source: 1177 Vårdguiden, 2016

United Kingdom, 2012), and the United States (2010 Patient Protection and Affordable Care Act) (US Congress, 2010). Elsewhere, patients' rights to information and participation in their own care are recognized across a broad diversity of legislation, such as in Italy and Denmark (Tragakes et al., 2008; Dahl Steffensen, Hjelholt Baker & Vinter, 2017).

SDM legislation facilitates the appropriate application of the so-called 'reasonable patient standard'. The standard for informed consent is typically physician-based. This means that clinicians must provide patients with the information that a so-called 'responsible body of physicians' would consider appropriate under similar circumstances (Moulton et al., 2013). However, this is slowly changing, with for example approximately half of the states in the USA having adopted 'the reasonable patient standard' instead (Spatz, Krumholz & Moulton, 2016). This views the informed consent communication process from the patient's perspective, that is, clinicians must provide patients with all the information that a 'reasonable patient' would want under similar circumstances. Case law based on this standard has also been applied in Australia, Canada, the Netherlands and the United Kingdom (Box 11.2), whereas elsewhere

---

Box 11.2 A reasonable patient

Montgomery v Lanarkshire Health Board, 2015, UK. A woman with insulin-dependent diabetes claimed that her obstetrician failed to communicate the risk of shoulder dystocia during vaginal delivery (a complication associated with foetal macrosomia) that ultimately resulted in severe foetal brain anoxia. She claimed that had she received full information about the risks, she would have opted for a caesarean delivery. Yet the treating obstetrician (and other expert physicians called to trial) claimed that the ensuing risk was very small and thus appropriately not communicated, because a caesarean delivery is not in the maternal interest. The UK Supreme Court ruled that the standard for what physicians should inform patients about the risks, benefits and alternatives of treatment '*will no longer be determined by what a responsible body of physicians deems important but rather by what a reasonable patient deems important*'.

Source: Spatz, Krumholz & Moulton, 2016

in Europe the notion of the 'reasonable body of physicians' standard prevails. The importance of establishing the 'reasonable patient' as the standard in the context of SDM can be illustrated by Washington State in the USA. Washington State is among the US states where informed consent has been patient-based since a key court case in 1999 (King & Moulton, 2006). In 2007 it introduced legislation that supports the use of SDM and it also provided that if a clinician uses a 'certified decision aid' as part of the informed consent process, there is a presumption that informed consent has been given (Washington State Health Care Authority, 2016). Thus, the context of the 'reasonable patient' as the norm facilitated the introduction of explicit SDM legislation. This suggests that a similar move would be necessary in Europe if SDM is to be implemented on a large scale.

However, available evidence suggests that while countries in Europe are engaging in a variety of activities conducive to the wider implementation of SDM, system-wide approaches to translating SDM into routine practice are as yet lacking. Coulter et al. (2015) assessed the readiness for SDM in five European countries by examining clinical policies and the availability of various SDM support services in France, Germany, the Netherlands, Spain and the UK in 2015. They found that while SDM was receiving growing attention, it was not yet as high on the policy agenda as it was in the USA at the time. There was evidence of research activity around SDM, increasing advocacy by patient groups on patient rights and SDM, and the incorporation of SDM in ethical and professional standards. But there was a lack of professional leadership and of institutional support. Furthermore, countries varied greatly with regard to the development and availability of SDM tools. Some had been developed and tested with patients locally but mostly in the context of research, with little institutional support or strategic planning for wider dissemination.

Coulter et al. (2015) further highlighted that the training infrastructure necessary for clinical staff to acquire SDM skills was patchy in the countries studied. While SDM was beginning to be included in basic communication skills training, it was not yet implemented as a core component of health professional education and training. This situation is now changing in some countries, such as in the Netherlands and Germany, where SDM is taught and examined in most medical schools, although on a limited scale (van der Weijden et al., 2017; Härter et al., 2017a). In Switzerland, all five medical schools (Basel, Bern, Geneva,

Lausanne and Zürich) have formally integrated SDM into both under-graduate and postgraduate training (general internal medicine) (Selby, Auer & Cornuz, 2017).

SDM is a fast-moving field and, in addition to educational progress, efforts to develop strategic policy frameworks for SDM are under way across Europe. Thus the Netherlands has seen a range of policy moves to a more systematic implementation of SDM at the national level, as exemplified by a 2015 letter to Parliament from the Minister of Health (Rijksoverheid, 2015). The Ministry of Health is introducing a specific registration code to finance additional time needed for SDM, and forthcoming amendments to the Medical Treatment Agreement Act will require physicians to inform the patient about risks and benefits and discuss treatment options (van der Weijden et al., 2017). In addition, the national associations of medical specialists and of patients and consumers are campaigning together to promote nationwide implementation of SDM (Federatie Medisch Specialisten, 2015).

Similarly, SDM is now firmly on the policy agenda in the UK, with policy-makers, professional regulators and societies, and patient organizations, as well as the courts, committed to ensuring that SDM becomes the norm throughout the National Health Service (NHS) (Coulter et al., 2017). A key challenge has been the coordination of various activities and initiatives and in 2015 over 40 organizations came together to form the SDM Collaborative, led by the National Institute for Health and Care Excellence (NICE). The Collaborative has published an SDM consensus statement and an action plan which sets out actions taken by individual partners in the short- and medium term (National Institute for Health and Care Excellence, 2016).

Progress has been somewhat slower in France, despite having the legal foundations in place for system-wide strengthening of SDM, in particular through the aforementioned 2002 Act on Patients' Rights and Quality of Care. The 2016 health reform provided for the introduction of a public information service which seeks to disseminate information on health, and especially on treatment, care and support offered to the public (Moumjid et al., 2017). Under the responsibility of the Minister for Health, the information should be in simple language and accessible for people with disabilities.

Finally, a number of countries, including the UK, the Netherlands, Germany and Norway, have invested in initiatives to make patient decision aids available to some extent (Coulter et al., 2017; van der Weijden et al., 2017; Härter et al., 2017a; Ringard et al., 2013). For example, in the UK NICE hosts 27 (as of August 2017) short-form patient decision aids to help patients have informed conversations about their condition with their health care provider (NHS RightCare, 2017; NHS England, n/d). In the Netherlands, the national associations of medical specialists and of patients host publicly available patient decision aids on national patient portals (van der Weijden et al., 2017). In Germany, the Institute for Quality and Efficiency in Health Care (IQWiG) recently developed three decision aids for the national breast, colon and cervical cancer screening programmes in response to requests from the Federal Joint Committee, the highest decision-making body in the German statutory health insurance system (Härter et al., 2017a).

Despite this progress in implementing SDM in European countries, considerable barriers remain. For SDM to become a standard approach in the clinical encounter, there is a need for professional organizations to incorporate patient decision support tools in clinical practice guidelines and, more broadly, for policy-makers and institutions to support local clinicians in the routine implementation of SDM (Coulter et al., 2015). We will return to the issue of what needs to be done later.

What does SDM achieve?

Shared decision-making has been associated with a number of expectations, ranging from improving population health outcomes, reducing health inequalities, optimizing health care costs, improving patient experiences, and increasing patient knowledge or engagement in their own care, to reducing litigation. Whether SDM is likely to achieve any of these expected outcomes depends on a range of factors, which we review here.

Overall, the principal conviction underlying SDM is that clinicians must both honour the patient's self-determination and offer a relationship of support, that is, SDM recognizes both autonomy and interdependence as key motivators. It also recognizes the importance of sharing the probabilistic nature of evidence and it recognizes that both emotional and cognitive factors play a role. These 'dualities' are reflected in many studies of SDM. Early evidence found that a relationship of mutual respect or equality between the patient and doctor during the decision-making process increases patient satisfaction (Menzel, Coleman & Katz, 1959). These early findings have been replicated elsewhere, with recent systematic review evidence demonstrating that SDM may have a positive impact on affective-cognitive patient outcomes, such as knowledge, satisfaction with care, and concerns/anxieties about the illness (Shay & Lafata, 2015). Compared to patients who did not reach agreement with their health professionals on certain key components of the clinical encounter, those who did reach an agreement felt more satisfied with the clinical encounter (Krupat et al., 2001).

These kinds of outcome are important. Research on decision-making has shown that personal decision-making involves a negotiation process with the 'outside world' which encompasses more than cognition. However, much SDM work has focused on cognition (e.g. knowledge, understanding) rather than emotion. Emotional factors such as trust, reassurance and comfort influence intermediate outcomes including adherence (Sewitch et al., 2003) and self-care skills, which in turn influence health outcomes (Street et al., 2009). These factors could also, in part, explain differences between decisions made in natural contexts and those made in experimental contexts (Rapley et al., 2006).

There is a fundamental ethical argument for involving patients in decisions about their own care and treatment, since it is their body and their illness, and so it is their aspirations, values and preferences that should be addressed. Evidence suggests that patients generally want more information about their health condition and would like to take an active role in decisions about their care (Alston et al., 2012; Kiesler & Auerbach, 2006). However, the degree to which a decision is shared varies widely in terms of the underlying health problem, the treatment or care options and the actors involved, including the patients themselves (Hagbaghery, Salsali & Ahmadi, 2004; Joseph-Williams, Edwards & Elwyn, 2014).

In terms of reducing health inequalities, systematic review evidence suggests that SDM significantly increases knowledge among disadvantaged groups, as well as their clarity about their values and preferences, although evidence is less clear on impacts on adherence levels, anxiety and health outcomes, as well as on screening/treatment preferences, intentions or uptake (Durand et al., 2014). Others observed that reducing the patient/clinician power differential is essential before most patients feel comfortable or competent to engage in SDM (Joseph-Williams, Edwards & Elwyn, 2014).

In some countries litigation is a major concern, and Durand et al. (2015) found that poor communication is strongly correlated with medical malpractice litigation. However, based on a synthesis of five studies, they concluded that there is insufficient evidence to determine whether SDM reduces medical malpractice litigation. Nevertheless, effective decision support can lead to decreased decisional conflict (i.e. personal uncertainty regarding one's choice) and some evidence suggests that if SDM is applied, patients appear to be more satisfied and more compliant with the treatment they have agreed upon, which is likely to reduce the risk of litigation (Ubbink, Santema & Lapid, 2016).

Among health professionals in particular, there is widespread concern about the time required for implementing SDM in routine clinical care (Légaré et al., 2008). The belief that it will lengthen consultations is so pervasive that the Dutch government proposes to compensate clinicians for the additional time they perceive they would need to implement it, as noted above. Yet although consultation lengths vary depending on the context, there is no definitive evidence that SDM systematically requires more time than usual care (Légaré et al., 2012b; Légaré et al., 2018) except in palliative care contexts (Stacey et al., 2017). Furthermore, any additional time spent on SDM may be recouped if patients return less frequently.

Among policy-makers another prime concern is the effective use of scarce resources. There are inherent challenges in assessing the cost-effectiveness of SDM, and robust evidence that SDM may lead to system-wide savings is lacking (Walsh et al., 2014; Trenaman, Bryan & Bansback, 2014). A systematic review of the effects of decision aids for people facing treatment or screening decisions found that patients who were better informed and had been given an opportunity to weigh up the risks of treatment options tended to choose more conservative options (Stacey et al., 2017). Based on such observations, there is an expectation among policy-makers that decision support tools can reduce overuse of costly services and treatments (Elwyn, Tilburt & Montori, 2013). There is indeed a persuasive argument that providing care that is informed and consistent with people's values can lead to more appropriate use of resources (Mulley, Trimble & Elwyn, 2012). However, if SDM is an ethical imperative (Box 11.3), and patients value being involved in the decision-making process, the promise of significant savings should not be a condition for its implementation, and indeed could jeopardize implementation efforts (Walsh et al., 2014; Sandman, Gustavsson & Munthe, 2016).

Box 11.3 The ethical imperative for shared decision-making

"The benefits of shared decision-making to Society will accrue by the accumulated trust that the profession engenders through daily interactions that demonstrate unequivocal fidelity to the dignity and values of informed patients. We do not advocate the abrogation of professional roles: it will remain necessary for physicians to disagree, even argue, respectfully, with patients, provided patients' views are taken seriously. But, as clinicians invite and welcome patient involvement, it is also essential to share in the work of making difficult decisions, not to abandon patients at the fork in the road."

Source: Elwyn, Tilburt & Montori, 2013

What practical tools support SDM?

Patient decision aids are the principal tool used to support SDM. In a review of 105 studies involving 31 043 patients, Stacey et al. (2017) showed that those who engaged in SDM and received a decision aid (either written, electronic, audio-visual or web-based tool formats) had greater knowledge of the evidence, felt clearer about what mattered to them, had more accurate expectations about the risks and benefits, and participated more in the decision-making process compared to those receiving usual care. Yet as noted earlier in this chapter, while there has been tremendous progress in the development of patient decision aids, including a generic decision aid (Ottawa Hospital Research Institute, 2015) that can be adapted to any health-related or social decision (Arimori, 2006; Saarimaki, 2013), it is unlikely that decision aids will be created for every decision and in every language. Also, their implementation remains challenging, in particular where the process is disconnected from the routine workflow or from the wider system context (Elwyn, Frosch & Kobrin, 2016). The fundamental need is still for skilled clinicians to have the right conversations with patients (Kunneman & Montori, 2016). Patient decision aids and other tools can facilitate the conversation, but they cannot replace it.

A significant body of work has focused on training health professionals in SDM. While there remains lack of consensus on the precise components of SDM (Shay & Lafata, 2014; Légaré et al., 2013; Légaré

& Witteman, 2013), there is agreement that risk communication skills can be learned by clinicians, both in their professional training and continuing professional education. Such training programmes for practitioners are becoming increasingly common (Diouf et al., 2016), with their effectiveness often measured in terms of changes in clinicians' behaviours and patient experiences (Al-Janabi, Flynn & Coast, 2012).

A 2018 Cochrane review of the effectiveness of interventions to improve health professionals' adoption of SDM found the overall evidence to be of low quality, with uncertainty about what type of intervention works best or what their key components should be (Légaré et al., 2018). It did suggest that interventions that simultaneously target both the health professional (e.g. training) and the patient (e.g. decision aids) are likely to be more effective than each on their own. Légaré et al. (2013) identified the range of core competencies clinicians should acquire for effectively involving patients in health-related decisions. These include being aware of patients' information needs, knowing how to communicate relevant information, nondirective interviewing, risk communication, eliciting patients' preferences, personalized care planning, and self-management support. They also include learning to use patient decision aids (Stacey et al., 2013) or clinical tools such as SURE to screen for decisional comfort (Légaré et al., 2010).

In summary, while promising, the existing evidence base on the effectiveness of SDM remains somewhat ambiguous or, with respect to certain outcomes such as cost savings, in need of more research. Evidence points to positive outcomes at the individual level but there are large gaps in the evidence about outcomes at the clinical, organizational and systems level, largely because of a lack of implementation at these levels (Elwyn, Frosch & Kobrin, 2016). Existing measures are still under development, as we discuss below. Perhaps a more fundamental and still unresolved question is what and who defines a 'good decision', and how to evaluate it (Hamilton et al., 2017), an issue discussed in some detail in Chapter 4 of this book.

What are the barriers to implementing SDM?

We established earlier that SDM is recognized as the core of person-centred care and is increasingly present in health care policy and legislation worldwide. Yet widespread implementation of SDM in routine practice (Couet et al., 2015) or at a system level (Elwyn et al., 2013) remains the exception. We have also noted that patient decision aids are a helpful tool in SDM, and numerous accredited patient decision aids are available (Volk et al., 2013). Yet patient decision aids are not widely used in clinical practice and few people are even aware they exist (Lepine et al., 2016).

The evidence points to a number of barriers that hamper the routine implementation of SDM in clinical practice. We have highlighted the many real or perceived barriers noted by health care providers, such as time constraints to actively engage in SDM, or attitudes, such as the belief that patients want decisions made for them, or not being in the habit of engaging their patients in SDM (Légaré et al., 2006; Godolphin, Towle & McKendry, 2001; Makoul, Arntson & Schofield, 1995). Perhaps clinicians are reluctant because they were trained to relieve and protect patients from anxiety-provoking information (Tudiver et al., 2002). Further, patients might ask for a treatment option that the clinician does not consider beneficial and the clinician may be concerned about potential malpractice litigation (Zikmund-Fisher et al., 2016), although there is no conclusive evidence about the latter, as noted earlier (Durand et al., 2015).

There are also barriers on the part of the patient, who may not want to engage in SDM. The evidence on patient preferences about participating in decision-making is very mixed, for reasons we do not yet fully understand (Chewning et al., 2012). The role patients wish to play in the decision may depend on the type of health problem, on personal characteristics (Thompson, 2007), or on the level of trust between the patient and the physician: the lower the trust, the less the patient feels comfortable in engaging in the process (Kraetschmer et al., 2004). Also, attitudes and behaviours are slow to change. Thus even where clinicians wish to implement SDM, their communication skills may be inadequate (Stiggelbout, Pieterse & De Haes, 2015). In addition, patients are often reluctant to question their doctors because they worry this will be perceived as challenging the clinician's expertise ('being difficult'), which might, in turn, negatively impact the quality of care the patient will receive in the future (Adams et al., 2012; Frosch et al., 2012).

The inconsistent evidence base about the benefits and risks of SDM and consequent lack of confidence in SDM interventions might also reduce decision-makers' support for relevant strategies, as might the overlap in terminology between patient engagement and SDM and the conceptual vagueness surrounding its key concepts (Légaré et al., 2013; Légaré & Witteman, 2013). Moreover, a set of best practices for SDM has yet to be agreed upon, and many of the underlying barriers themselves, such as clinician indifference, remain under-investigated (Elwyn et al., 2013).

Perhaps a more fundamental challenge relates to the issue of power, a challenge highlighted elsewhere in this volume (*see* Chapters 4, 5, 6 and 12). SDM requires an explicit sharing of power and knowledge in a relationship that has traditionally been characterized by an imbalance of power in favour of the clinician (Joseph-Williams, Edwards & Elwyn, 2014). In many cultures there is a strong hierarchy of authority which is not openly challenged, at personal, institutional or political levels (Rahimi, Alizadeh & Légaré, 2017), and this also applies to significant subcultures in western liberal societies (Coleman-Brueckheimer, Spitzer & Koffman, 2009; Mead et al., 2013). There is a need for researchers to develop patient decision aids and models that are flexible enough to be adapted to a variety of cultures, involving stakeholders from diverse backgrounds and paying particular attention to categories of patients who find risk–benefit information challenging. SDM training should also include considerations of health literacy and cultural competencies, and should increase awareness of variation in patient preferences (Hawley & Morris, 2016; Alden et al., 2014).

Much of the work on SDM has focused on patients' and clinicians' attitudes to and engagement in SDM. Conversely, little is known about policy-makers' views on and understanding of SDM, despite their key role in developing strategies necessary for its widespread implementation. Little is known, too, about the views of health care organizations, which might be reluctant to invest in SDM as it may involve changing established work patterns or provider tasks (Elwyn, Frosch & Kobrin, 2016). Some countries have changed financial incentives for providers towards value-based payment methods that seek to optimize health outcomes for the patient per dollar spent (Porter, 2010). There is increasing experimentation with, for example, pay-for-performance schemes, capitation and bundled payment arrangements or accountable care organizations to strengthen care coordination and hold health care providers to account for delivering high quality care (Anell & Glenngård, 2014; Nolte, Knai & Saltman, 2014; Kronick, Casalino & Bindman, 2015), and SDM could at least theoretically be built into such payment systems. However, such approaches are highly complex, requiring careful design, relevant measures and indicators, and consideration of the context in which the payment system is introduced. The risk is that such systems can be distorted by uncontrollable factors such as patients' socioeconomic status, or measures that are inadequate for the task. For example, attribution (which doctors are responsible for which patient outcomes?) must factor in risk-adjustment and randomness or else physicians will be incentivized to avoid patients with multi-morbidities, who are exceptionally high users of hospital services (Anell & Glenngård, 2014). Without institutional consensus on what constitutes value and quality in health care, measurement might simply reflect what physicians, politicians or accountants value, rather than what patients value (Mannion & Braithwaite, 2012).

How should we measure SDM?

Many reviews have shown that SDM processes and outcomes are difficult to quantify (Elwyn et al., 2001; Dy, 2007; Légaré et al., 2007; Simon, Loh & Harter, 2007; Kryworuchko et al., 2008; Scholl et al., 2011; Sepucha & Scholl, 2014). Identifying relevant theoretical models for SDM, evaluating interventions in clinical practice and measuring their impact (including cost-effectiveness) remain the subject of ongoing research in this relatively young field.

The kinds of outcome researchers seek primarily reflect the expectations of those assessing SDM. Where patient engagement is built into legislation (such as the Affordable Care Act in the USA), health care administrators seek reliable and valid system level measures that allow conclusions about the impacts of SDM strategies on population health. A major impediment to the more rapid spread of SDM may be that there are not yet enough system measures that can be effectively and efficiently tracked by health care organizations. Much research has explored more process-oriented outcomes, for example measures of the patient's role in decision-making (Conway, Mostashari & Clancy, 2013).

Those who are interested in clinical practice may focus their research on the creation of brief tools, such as the three-question CollaboRATE (Box 11.4), which measures efforts made by the clinical team to engage them in decision-making as reported by patients (Barr et al., 2014).

Several conceptual frameworks have been proposed for measuring SDM. The most comprehensive and commonly used model was designed

---

Box 11.4 The CollaboRATE tool: a three-item patient-reported measure of SDM

The CollaboRATE tool consists of three items.
   Thinking about the appointment you have just had:

1. How much effort was made to help you understand your health issues?
2. How much effort was made to listen to the things that matter most to you about your health issues?
3. How much effort was made to include what matters most to you in choosing what to do next?

Responses to each item can range from 0 (No effort was made) to 9 (Every effort was made) for a maximum total of 27.

Source: Barr et al., 2017

---

by Makoul & Clayman, and it identifies nine essential constructs that describe the observable features of SDM in a consultation (Makoul & Clayman, 2006; Clayman et al., 2012). Using this framework, Bouniols, Leclère & Moret (2016) reviewed and mapped validated SDM measurement tools and found that none of the identified tools mapped on all the nine elements described by Makoul & Clayman, although all measured three of the elements ('define/explain problem', 'patient values/ preferences', and 'check/clarify understanding'). The MAPPIN' SDM instrument and SDM'Mass developed by Kasper and colleagues (Kasper et al., 2012; Geiger & Kasper, 2012) cover eight of the components.

Elwyn, Frosch & Kobrin (2016) developed a conceptual framework that hypothesizes a set of outcomes of SDM (or 'collaborative deliberation') that considers the 'reach' of its consequences. Proximal effects are immediate, for example informed preferences; distal effects are more enduring, such as modified relationships; and distant effects may change service utilization or institutional norms. A different approach was taken by Sepucha and colleagues, whose model for decision-making distinguishes three general constructs across the continuum of the decision-making process (Sepucha & Mulley, 2009; Sepucha & Scholl, 2014):

• Decision antecedents, or the features of the patient, provider or organization that may influence the decision-making process;

- Decision-making process or behaviour in the consultation, such as patient involvement in the decision, decisional conflict or the use of patient decision aids; and
- Decision outcomes, including knowledge, decision regret, decision quality and patient's experience of care.

Tools to measure decision antecedents at the patient level include the Control Preferences Scale, which evaluates the preferred role of a patient in decision-making (Degner & Sloan, 1992); the Autonomy Preference Index, which measures patient preferences about their role in decision-making and their desire to be informed; and tools that assess broader patient characteristics such as health literacy (Aboumatar et al., 2013) and the culture and history of the physician/patient power imbalance. Each of these instruments has its strengths and weaknesses.

Decision-making processes are commonly assessed using the Observing Patient Involvement Scale, or OPTION (Elwyn et al., 2005); two 9-item SDM questionnaires (patient and clinician versions) (Kriston et al., 2010; Scholl et al., 2012); or the Decisional Conflict Scale (DCS) (O'Connor, 1995). Few process measures adequately capture implementation, and different stakeholders have different perceptions as to whether SDM has occurred (Rodenburg-Vandenbussche et al., 2015; Shay & Lafata, 2014). Interestingly, only studies in which the patient reported that SDM had occurred (rather than reported by the doctor, or a third observer) found a significant association with improved patient outcomes (Stewart, 2001). This finding suggests that the patient's perspective is critical to the science of measuring SDM.

Decision outcomes are assessed by measuring decision quality, decision satisfaction or decision regret (Sepucha, Fowler & Mulley, 2004; Brehaut et al., 2003). Many of these scales have good reliability statistics, but the validity of most tools remains undetermined, especially as far as diverse populations are concerned. In addition, there are important ceiling effects (high-level scores with little variability in both patient-reported outcomes and other process measures). Very few measures are sensitive to changes in outcomes over time (Kirwan et al., 2016; Barr & Elwyn, 2015). Finally, there is still a gap between measuring SDM for research purposes and measurement for clinical and policy-oriented purposes.

Some researchers use measurement frameworks to explain the mechanisms underlying SDM behaviours and explore the relationships between the different constructs of sociocognitive models. Many such models posit that behaviour is driven by intention, and that intention has measurable and modifiable determinants (Frosch et al., 2009; Desroches et al., 2011).

New theoretical frameworks are expanding our understanding of decision-making but they have yet to demonstrate their applicability. Measures need to be practical, valid and reliable, and developed in consultation with patients. There is a need for wider testing with both exploratory and confirmatory factor analyses, and for revising existing instruments. Scales should be tested for responsiveness before being used in intervention studies. Further work on discriminant validity would enable us to assess if a scale can distinguish between a decision-making process that is unilateral and one that is truly shared. In the best of all possible worlds, a standardization of outcome measures would allow more meaningful cross-study comparisons (Scholl et al., 2011; Decary et al., 2017).

What are the research trends in SDM?

Research on SDM has gone beyond decisions about medical diagnostics and treatments. For example, in the era of personalized medicine SDM is clearly called for concerning decisions about, and follow-up of, genetic tests for predispositions for which data and treatments are not yet available (Katz, Kurian & Morrow, 2015). Dyadic SDM research now takes into account the mutual influence of the patient and the physician in the consultation (Melbourne et al., 2011; Couet et al., 2015; Légaré et al., 2012a; LeBlanc et al., 2009). Research has also moved beyond conceptualizing SDM as a single encounter to broadening research beyond the consultation (Rapley, 2008). SDM has been incorporated into many more decision contexts, such as around loss of functional autonomy (Hanson et al., 2011), palliative care (Belanger, Rodriguez & Groleau, 2011) and mental illness (Coffey et al., 2016).

A key development has been the involvement of a wider range of actors in SDM research, such as family caregivers who are closely involved in decisions about the care of relatives, and a wider group of health professionals and social care workers (Garvelink et al., 2016; DeKeyser Ganz et al., 2016). Researchers are developing models, assessment tools, interventions and decision support tools that take into account decisions shared between all these actors (Laidsaar-Powell et al., 2013; Stacey et al., 2010; Garvelink et al., 2016). A growing team consciousness of SDM could improve resource use and other group-level performance scores (Sorbero et al., 2008), as well as bringing about change in the cultural norms of health care organizations and systems (Elwyn, Frosch & Kobrin, 2016), with an increasing volume of work looking specifically at the impact of SDM at the meso and macro levels (Ballard-Barbash, 2012).

Identifying better measures for SDM remains a core research area, as demonstrated by the recent application call for measures of SDM by the US-based Agency for Healthcare Research and Quality (Agency for Healthcare Research and Quality, 2016). Much research has been devoted to exploring the relationships between the constructs of various behavioural models and proposing tools that are sensitive to the less rational and more affective aspects of behaviour change (Sniehotta, 2009; Kelders et al., 2016). Considerable research is also being devoted to developing and measuring the impact of patient decision aids (Volk et al., 2016). Lastly, the contribution of SDM to reducing waste in health care is gaining attention as most industrialized countries face increasing financial constraints (Morgan et al., 2016).

How can we move SDM forward?

Frosch & Carman (2016) propose a framework of 'patient and family engagement' for moving ahead with interventions and policies to implement SDM. Their model envisages a continuum of patient engagement that is applicable to direct patient care, organizational governance and policy development, and yet remains flexible enough to match the capabilities, interests and goals of individual patients (Dy & Purnell, 2012). It posits that patient values influence not only clinical decisions but also decisions about hospital design, recruitment, quality improvement strategies and policy priorities. The continuum structure of this framework is also responsive to the accumulation of evidence about what works and what does not.

Facilitators for developing such a culture of engagement at the policy level are social and cultural norms that are open to public influence, as well as institutions that are open to public participation, as demonstrated, for example, by state policies responding to public pressure to control the tobacco market (World Health Organization, 2017). The organization, financing and governance of health care systems play a key role (Korda & Eldridge, 2011). Legislation can also facilitate patient engagement by, for example, mandating public advisory councils in hospitals (Carman et al., 2013).

SDM is only one of the many facets of greater engagement of patients and the wider public in health care at the different tiers of the system. As several contributions to this volume have shown, fostering an engagement culture at all levels and including civil society is essential if equal partnerships and effective relationships between patients and professionals are to be translated into a reality. SDM is mostly applicable at the clinical level (Carman et al., 2013), and its effective translation into routine practice will require a change in the status quo, which in turn will require greater investment in educating the public about health and health care, and the acquisition of skills and competencies to ask questions, express values and preferences, and understand risks. This transformation is necessary more than ever, at both the individual and system level, for ethical, financial, social, political and legal (in some countries) reasons. Finally, it forms a core element of health care quality, with more responsive services likely to lead to better outcomes, improved patient experiences and more effective self-management.

Conclusion

In summary, health care decisions that will lead to improved population health, patient experience and cost-effectiveness depend on an understanding of the best available scientific evidence and on patients' informed values and preferences. SDM is an approach that has the potential to improve population health by reducing harms of treatments that are not beneficial for all and increasing the benefits of those that are. It also has the potential to improve patient experience by engaging them in the decision-making process. In addition, although the evidence remains patchy, it has the potential to ensure a more appropriate use of limited resources and thus increase the cost-effectiveness and sustainability of health systems. There are effective interventions for facilitating SDM, including training health care professionals and patient decision aids. However, SDM is not yet widely implemented in routine clinical practice, with various barriers obstructing its adoption at the individual patient and provider level and, more importantly perhaps, at organizational and system levels. These barriers can be overcome by establishing a culture of patient engagement at all levels of the health care system, from individual decisions and programme development to research and health policy.

Note

We would like to acknowledge Louisa Blair who edited the manuscript. Funding was provided by the Canada Research Chair in Shared Decision Making and Knowledge Translation.

References

1177 Vårdguiden (2016). Patient Act. Sweden: Skane. Available at: https://www.1177.se/Other-languages/Engelska/Regler-och-rattigheter/ Patientlagen/ (accessed 27 September 2017).

Aboumatar HJ et al. (2013). The impact of health literacy on desire for participation in healthcare, medical visit communication, and patient reported outcomes among patients with hypertension. *Journal of General Internal Medicine*, 28:1469–76.

Adams JR et al. (2012). Communicating With Physicians About Medical Decisions: A Reluctance to Disagree. *Archives of Internal Medicine*, 172:1184–6.

Agency for Healthcare Research and Quality (2016). *Developing Measures of Shared Decision Making (R01)*. Available at: https://grants.nih.gov/grants/ guide/pa-files/PA-16-424.html (accessed 29 September 2017).

Al-Janabi H, Flynn TN, Coast J (2012). Development of a self-report measure of capability wellbeing for adults: the ICECAP-A. *Quality of Life Research*, 21:167–76.

Alden DL et al. (2014). Cultural targeting and tailoring of shared decision making technology: a theoretical framework for improving the effectiveness of patient decision aids in culturally diverse groups. *Social Science & Medicine*, 105:1–8.

Alston C et al. (2012). *Communicating with patients on health care evidence*. Washington, DC: Institute of Medicine of the National Academies.

Anell A, Glenngård A (2014). The use of outcome and process indicators to incentivize integrated care for frail older people: a case study of primary care services in Sweden. *International Journal of Integrated Care*, 14:e038.

Arimori N (2006). Randomized controlled trial of decision aids for women considering prenatal testing: the effect of the Ottawa personal decision guide on decisional conflict. *Japan Journal of Nursing Science*, 3:119–30.

Ballard-Barbash R (2012). Multilevel intervention research applications in cancer care delivery. *Journal of the National Cancer Institute Monograph*, 44:121–2.

Barr PJ, Elwyn G (2015). Measurement challenges in shared decision making: putting the 'patient' in patient-reported measures. *Health Expectations*, 19(5):993–1001.

Barr PJ et al. (2014). The psychometric properties of CollaboRATE: a fast and frugal patient-reported measure of the shared decision-making process. *Journal of Medical Internet Research*, 16:e2.

Barr PJ et al. (2017). Evaluating CollaboRATE in a clinical setting: analysis of mode effects on scores, response rates and costs of data collection. *BMJ Open*, 7:e014681.

Belanger E, Rodriguez C, Groleau D (2011). Shared decision-making in palliative care: a systematic mixed studies review using narrative synthesis. *Palliative Medicine*, 25:242–61.

Blanc X et al. (2014). Publication trends of shared decision making in 15 high impact medical journals: a full-text review with bibliometric analysis. *BMC Medical Informatics and Decision Making*, 14:1–9.

Bouniols N, Leclère B, Moret L (2016). Evaluating the quality of shared decision making during the patient-carer encounter: a systematic review of tools. *BMC Research Notes*, 9:382.

Bravo P et al. (2011). Shared decision making in Chile: supportive policies and research initiatives. *Zeitschrift für Evidenz, Fortbildung und Qualität im Gesundheitswesen*, 105:254–8.

Brehaut JC et al. (2003). Validation of a decision regret scale. *Medical Decision Making*, 23:281–92.

Buetow S, Kenealy T (2007). *Ideological debates in family medicine*. New York: Biomedical Books.

Bundesministerium für Gesundheit (2013). Gesetz zur Verbesserung der Rechte von Patientinnen und Patienten. Berlin, Germany: Bundesministerium für Gesundheit.

Caldon LJ et al. (2011). Clinicians' concerns about decision support interventions for patients facing breast cancer surgery options: understanding the challenge of implementing shared decision-making. *Health Expectations*, 14:133–46.

Carman KL et al. (2013). Patient and family engagement: a framework for understanding the elements and developing interventions and policies. *Health Affairs (Millwood)*, 32:223–31.

Charles C, Gafni A, Whelan T (1997). Shared decision-making in the medical encounter: what does it mean? (or it takes at least two to tango). *Social Science & Medicine*, 44:681–92.

Chewning B et al. (2012). Patient preferences for shared decisions: a systematic review. *Patient Education and Counseling*, 86:9–18.

Clayman ML et al. (2012). Development of a shared decision making coding system for analysis of patient-healthcare provider encounters. *Patient Education and Counseling*, 88:367–72.

Coffey M et al. (2016). Study protocol: a mixed methods study to assess mental health recovery, shared decision-making and quality of life (Plan4Recovery). *BMC Health Services Research*, 16:392.

Coleman-Brueckheimer K, Spitzer J, Koffman J (2009). Involvement of Rabbinic and communal authorities in decision-making by haredi Jews in the UK with breast cancer: an interpretative phenomenological analysis. *Social Science & Medicine*, 68:323–33.

Conway PH, Mostashari F, Clancy C (2013). The future of quality measurement for improvement and accountability. *JAMA*, 309:2215–16.

Couet N et al. (2015). Assessments of the extent to which healthcare providers involve patients in decision making: a systematic review of studies using the OPTION instrument. *Health Expectations*, 18:542–61.

Coulter A (2011). *Making Shared Decision-Making a Reality*. London: King's Fund.

Coulter A (2017). Shared decision making: everyone wants it, so why isn't it happening? *World Psychiatry*, 16:117–18.

Coulter A et al. (2015). European experience with shared decision making. *International Journal of Person Centered Medicine*, 5(1):6.

Coulter A et al. (2017). Shared decision making in the UK: moving towards wider uptake. *Zeitschrift für Evidenz, Fortbildung und Qualität im Gesundheitswesen*, 123:99–103.

Dahl Steffensen K, Hjelholt Baker V, Vinter MM (2017). Implementing shared decision making in Denmark: first steps and future focus areas. *Zeitschrift für Evidenz, Fortbildung und Qualität im Gesundheitswesen*, 123:36–40.

Decary S et al. (2017). Decisional conflict screening for a diversity of primary care decisions. Are we SURE yet? *Journal of Clinical Epidemiology* 89: 238–9.

Degner LF, Sloan JA (1992). Decision making during serious illness: what role do patients really want to play? *Journal of Clinical Epidemiology*, 45:941–50.

DeKeyser Ganz F et al. (2016). Development of a Model of Interprofessional Shared Clinical Decision Making in the ICU: a Mixed-Methods Study. *Critical Care Medicine*, 44:680–9.

Desroches S et al. (2011). Exploring dietitians' salient beliefs about shared decision-making behaviors. *Implementation Science*, 6:57.

Diouf NT et al. (2016). Training health professionals in shared decision making: update of an international environmental scan. *Patient Education and Counseling*, 99(11):1753–8.

Durand MA et al. (2014). Do interventions designed to support shared decision-making reduce health inequalities? A systematic review and meta-analysis. *PLoS One*, 9:e94670.

Durand MA et al. (2015). Can shared decision-making reduce medical malpractice litigation? A systematic review. *BMC Health Services Research*, 15:167.

Dy SM (2007). Instruments for Evaluating Shared Medical Decision Making: a Structured Literature Review. *Medical Care Research and Review*, 64(6):623–49.

Dy SM, Purnell TS (2012). Key concepts relevant to quality of complex and shared decision-making in health care: a literature review. *Social Science & Medicine*, 74:582–7.

Effing T et al. (2007). Self-management education for patients with chronic obstructive pulmonary disease. *Cochrane Database of Systematic Reviews*, CD002990.

Elwyn G, Frosch DL, Kobrin S (2016). Implementing shared decision-making: consider all the consequences. *Implementation Science*, 11:114.

Elwyn G, Tilburt J, Montori V (2013). The ethical imperative for shared decision-making. *European Journal for Person Centered Healthcare*, 14:129–31.

Elwyn G et al. (2000). Shared decision making and the concept of equipoise: the competences of involving patients in healthcare choices. *British Journal of General Practice*, 50:892–9.

Elwyn G et al. (2001). Measuring the involvement of patients in shared decision-making: a systematic review of instruments. *Patient Education and Counseling*, 43:5–22.

Elwyn G et al. (2005). *Shared decision making measurement using the OPTION instrument*. Cardiff: Cardiff University. Available at: http://www.glynelwyn.com/uploads/2/4/0/4/24040341/option_12_book.pdf (accessed 28 June 2018).

Elwyn G et al. (2012). Shared decision making: a model for clinical practice. *Journal of General Internal Medicine*, 27:1361–7.

Elwyn G et al. (2013). "Many miles to go . . .": a systematic review of the implementation of patient decision support interventions into routine clinical practice. *BMC Medical Informatics and Decision Making*, 13.

Federatie Medisch Specialisten (2015). *Onderwerp: Samen beslissen*. Utrecht, Netherlands. Available at: http://www.demedischspecialist.nl/samen-beslissen (accessed 29 September 2016).

Fisher B et al. (2002). Twenty-year follow-up of a randomized trial comparing total mastectomy, lumpectomy, and lumpectomy plus irradiation for the treatment of invasive breast cancer. *New England Journal of Medicine*, 347:1233–41.

Frosch DL, Carman KL (2016). Embracing patient and family engagement to advance shared decision making. In: Elwyn G, Edwards A, Thompson R (eds). *Shared Decision Making in Health Care: Achieving evidence-based patient choice*. Oxford: Oxford University Press, 13–18.

Frosch DL et al. (2009). Adjuncts or adversaries to shared decision-making? Applying the Integrative Model of behavior to the role and design of decision support interventions in healthcare interactions. *Implementation Science*, 4:73.

Frosch DL et al. (2012). Authoritarian physicians and patients' fear of being labeled 'difficult' among key obstacles to shared decision making. *Health Affairs*, 31:1030.

Garvelink MM et al. (2016). Development of a decision guide to support the elderly in decision making about location of care: an iterative, user-centered design. *Research Involvement and Engagement*, 2:1–16.

Geiger F, Kasper J (2012). Of blind men and elephants: suggesting SDM-MASS as a compound measure for shared decision making integrating patient, physician and observer views. *Zeitschrift für Evidenz, Fortbildung und Qualität im Gesundheitswesen*, 106:284–9.

Gibson A, Britten N, Lynch J (2012). Theoretical directions for an emancipatory concept of patient and public involvement. *Health*, 16:531–47.

Godolphin W, Towle A, McKendry R (2001). Challenges in family practice related to informed and shared decision-making: a survey of preceptors of medical students. *JAMC*, 165:434–5.

Government of the United Kingdom (2012). Health and Social Care Act 2012, c.7.

Hagbaghery MA, Salsali M, Ahmadi F (2004). The factors facilitating and inhibiting effective clinical decision-making in nursing: a qualitative study. *BMC Nursing*, 3:1–11.

Hamilton JG et al. (2017). What is a good medical decision? A research agenda guided by perspectives from multiple stakeholders. *Journal of Behavioral Medicine*, 40(1):52–68.

Hanson LC et al. (2011). Improving Decision-Making for Feeding Options in Advanced Dementia: a Randomized, Controlled Trial. *Journal of the American Geriatrics Society,* 59:2009–16.

Härter M, van der Weijden T, Elwyn G (2011). Policy and practice developments in the implementation of shared decision making: an international perspective. *Zeitschrift für Evidenz, Fortbildung und Qualität im Gesundheitswesen,* 105:229–33.

Härter M et al. (2017a). The long way of implementing patient-centered care and shared decision making in Germany. *Zeitschrift für Evidenz, Fortbildung und Qualität im Gesundheitswesen,* 123:46–51.

Härter M et al. (2017b). Shared decision making in 2017: international accomplishments in policy, research and implementation. *Zeitschrift für Evidenz, Fortbildung und Qualität im Gesundheitswesen,* 123:1–5.

Hawley ST, Morris AM (2017). Cultural challenges to engaging patients in shared decision making. *Patient Education and Counseling,* 100(1):18–24.

Illich I (1975). *Limits to Medicine: Medical Nemesis: the Expropriation of Health.* London: Marion Boyards Publishers Ltd.

Joseph-Williams N, Edwards A, Elwyn G (2014). Power imbalance prevents shared decision making. *BMJ,* 348:g3178.

Kasper J et al. (2012). MAPPIN' SDM–the multifocal approach to sharing in shared decision making. *PLoS One,* 7:e34849.

Katz SJ, Kurian AW, Morrow M (2015). Treatment decision making and genetic testing for breast cancer: mainstreaming mutations. *JAMA,* 314:997–8.

Kelders SM et al. (2016). Health Behavior Change Support Systems as a research discipline. A viewpoint. *International Journal of Medical Informatics,* 93:3–10.

Kiesler DJ, Auerbach SM (2006). Optimal matches of patient preferences for information, decision-making and interpersonal behavior: evidence, models and interventions. *Patient Education and Counseling,* 61:319–41.

King JS, Moulton BW (2006). Rethinking informed consent: the case for shared medical decision-making. *American Journal of Law & Medicine,* 32:429–501.

Kirwan JR et al. (2016). Commentary: Patients as Partners. Building on the Experience of Outcome Measures in Rheumatology. *Arthritis & Rheumatology,* 68:1334–6.

Korda H, Eldridge GN (2011). Payment incentives and integrated care delivery: levers for health system reform and cost containment. *Inquiry,* 48:277–87.

Koster J (2016). Pubmed PubReMiner. 1.14 ed. Amsterdam: Department of Oncogenomics, AMC.

Kraetschmer N et al. (2004). How does trust affect patient preferences for participation in decision-making? *Health Expectations*, 7:317–26.

Kriston L et al. (2010). The 9-item Shared Decision Making Questionnaire (SDM-Q-9). Development and psychometric properties in a primary care sample. *Patient Education and Counseling*, 80:94–9.

Kronick R, Casalino LP, Bindman AB (2015). Apple pickers or federal judges: strong versus weak incentives in physician payment. *Health Services Research*, 50:2049–56.

Krupat E et al. (2001). When physicians and patients think alike: patient-centered beliefs and their impact on satisfaction and trust. *Journal of Family Practice*, 50:1057–62.

Kryworuchko J et al. (2008). Appraisal of primary outcome measures used in trials of patient decision support. *Patient Education and Counseling*, 73:497–503.

Kunneman M, Montori VM (2016). When patient-centred care is worth doing well: informed consent or shared decision-making. *BMJ Quality & Safety*, 26(7):522–4.

Laidsaar-Powell RC et al. (2013). Physician–patient–companion communication and decision-making: a systematic review of triadic medical consultations. *Patient Education and Counseling*, 91:3–13.

Leape LL (1989). Unnecessary surgery. *Health Services Research*, 24:351–407.

LeBlanc A et al. (2009). Decisional conflict in patients and their physicians: a dyadic approach to shared decision making. *Medical Decision Making*, 29:61–8.

Lee YK, Low WY, Ng CJ (2013). Exploring patient values in medical decision making: a qualitative study. *PLoS One*, 8:e80051.

Légaré F, Witteman HO (2013). Interventions for increasing the use of shared decision making by healthcare professionals. *Health Affairs (Millwood)*, 32:276–84.

Légaré F, Stacey D, Pouliot S (2011). Interprofessionalism and shared decision-making in primary care: a stepwise approach towards a new model. *Journal of Interprofessional Care*, 25.

Légaré F et al. (2006). Primary health care professionals' views on barriers and facilitators to the implementation of the Ottawa Decision Support Framework in practice. *Patient Education and Counseling*, 63:380–90.

Légaré F et al. (2007). Instruments to assess the perception of physicians in the decision-making process of specific clinical encounters: a systematic review. *BMC Medical Informatics and Decision Making*, 7:30.

Légaré F et al. (2008). Barriers and facilitators to implementing shared decision-making in clinical practice: update of a systematic review of health professionals' perceptions. *Patient Education and Counseling*, 73:526–35.

Légaré F et al. (2010). Are you SURE?: assessing patient decisional conflict with a 4-item screening test. *Canadian Family Physician*, 56:e308–14.

Légaré F et al. (2012a). Some but not all dyadic measures in shared decision making research have satisfactory psychometric properties. *Journal of Clinical Epidemiology*, 65:1310–20.

Légaré F et al. (2012b). Patients' Perceptions of Sharing in Decisions. *Patient*, 5:1–19.

Légaré F et al. (2013). Core competencies for shared decision making training programs: insights from an international, interdisciplinary working group. *Journal of Continuing Education in the Health Professions*, 33:267–73.

Légaré F et al. (2014). Interventions for improving the adoption of shared decision making by healthcare professionals. *Cochrane Database of Systematic Reviews*, CD006732.

Légaré F et al. (2015). Improving Decision making On Location of Care with the frail Elderly and their caregivers (the DOLCE study): study protocol for a cluster randomized controlled trial. *Trials*, 16:50.

Lepine J et al. (2016). What factors influence health professionals to use decision aids for Down syndrome prenatal screening? *BMC Pregnancy and Childbirth*, 16:262.

Levy SM et al. (1989). Breast conservation versus mastectomy: distress sequelae as a function of choice. *Journal of Clinical Oncology:* 7:367.

Makoul G, Clayman ML (2006). An integrative model of shared decision making in medical encounters. *Patient Education and Counseling*, 60:301–12.

Makoul G, Arntson P, Schofield T (1995). Health promotion in primary care: physician–patient communication and decision making about prescription medications. *Social Science & Medicine*, 41:1241–54.

Mannion R, Braithwaite J (2012). Unintended consequences of performance measurement in healthcare: 20 salutary lessons from the English National Health Service. *Internal Medicine Journal*, 42:569.

Mead EL et al. (2013). Shared decision-making for cancer care among racial and ethnic minorities: a systematic review. *American Journal of Public Health*, 103:e15–29.

Melbourne E et al. (2011). Dyadic OPTION: measuring perceptions of shared decision-making in practice. *Patient Education and Counseling*, 83:55–7.

Menzel H, Coleman J, Katz E (1959). Dimensions of being "Modern" in medical practice. *Journal of Chronic Diseases*, 9:20–40.

Morgan DJ et al. (2016). 2016 Update on Medical Overuse: a systematic review. *JAMA Internal Medicine*, 176(11):1687–92.

Moulton B et al. (2013). From informed consent to informed request: do we need a new gold standard? *Journal of the Royal Society of Medicine*, 106:391–4.

Moumjid N et al. (2017). Moving towards shared decision making in the physician–patient encounter in France: state of the art and future prospects. *Zeitschrift für Evidenz, Fortbildung und Qualität im Gesundheitswesen*, 123:41–5.

Mulley AG, Trimble C, Elwyn G (2012). Stop the silent misdiagnosis: patients' preferences matter. *BMJ*, 345:e6572.

National Institute for Health and Care Excellence (2016). *Shared Decision Making Collaborative – An Action Plan*. Available at: https://www.nice.org.uk/Media/Default/About/what-we-do/shared-decision-making-collaborative-action-plan.pdf (accessed 28 June 2018).

NHS England (n/d). Shared Decision Making. Available at: https://www.england.nhs.uk/shared-decision-making/ (accessed 28 June 2018).

NHS Rightcare (2017). *Evidence Search*. London: National Institute for Health and Care Excellence.

Nolte E, Knai C, Saltman RB (eds) (2014). *Assessing chronic disease management in European health systems*. Copenhagen: WHO Regional Office for Europe on behalf of the European Observatory on Health Systems and Policies.

O'Connor AM (1995). Validation of a decisional conflict scale. *Medical Decision Making*, 15:25–30.

OECD (2015). Doctors' consultations. Available at: https://data.oecd.org/healthcare/doctors-consultations.htm (accessed 16 August 2017).

Ottawa Hospital Research Institute (2015). *Patient Decision Aids*. Ottawa, Canada: Ottawa Hospital Research Institute. Available at: decisionaid.ohri.ca/index.html (accessed 28 June 2018).

Pauker SG, Kassirer JP (1997). Contentious screening decisions: does the choice matter? *New England Journal of Medicine*, 336:1243–4.

Porter ME (2010). What Is Value in Health Care? *New England Journal of Medicine*, 363:2477–81.

President's Commission for the Study of Ethical Problems in Medicine and Biomedical and Behavioral Research (1982). Making Health Care Decisions. The Ethical and Legal Implications of Informed Consent in the Patient–Practitioner Relationship. Washington, DC: U.S. Government Printing Office.

Rahimi SA, Alizadeh M, Légaré F (2017). Shared decision making in Iran: Current and future trends. *Zeitschrift für Evidenz, Fortbildung und Qualität im Gesundheitswesen*, 123:52–5.

Rapley T (2008). Distributed decision making: the anatomy of decisions-in-action. *Sociology of Health & Illness*, 30:429–44.

Rapley T et al. (2006). Doctor–patient interaction in a randomised controlled trial of decision-support tools. *Social Science & Medicine*, 62:2267–78.

République Française (2002). Loi n 2002-303 du 4 mars 2002 relative aux droits des malades et à la qualité du système de santé. Available at: https://www.legifrance.gouv.fr/affichTexte.do?cidTexte=JORFTEXT000000227015 (accessed 28 June 2018).

Rijksoverheid (2015). *Kamerbrief over Samen beslissen*. Available at: https://www.rijksoverheid.nl/documenten/kamerstukken/2015/10/29/kamerbrief-over-samen-beslissen (accessed 29 September 2016).

Riksdag (2014). Patientlag (2014:821). Available at: https://www.riksdagen.se/sv/dokument-lagar/dokument/svensk-forfattningssamling/patientlag-2014821_sfs-2014-821 (accessed 28 June 2018).

Ringard A et al. (2013). Norway: health system review. *Health Systems in Transition*, 15:1–162.

Rodenburg-Vandenbussche S et al. (2015). Dutch Translation and Psychometric Testing of the 9-Item Shared Decision Making Questionnaire (SDM-Q-9) and Shared Decision Making Questionnaire-Physician Version (SDM-Q-Doc) in Primary and Secondary Care. *PLoS One*, 10:e0132158.

Saarimaki ASD (2013). Are you using effective tools to support patients facing tough cancer-related decisions? *Canadian Oncology Nursing Journal*, 23:137–44.

Salzburg Global Seminar (2011). Salzburg statement on shared decision making. *BMJ*, 342:d1745.

Sandman L, Gustavsson E, Munthe C (2016). Individual responsibility as ground for priority setting in shared decision-making. *Journal of Medical Ethics*, 42(10):653–8.

Schattner A (2002). What do patients really want to know? *QJM*, 95:135–6.

Scholl I et al. (2011). Measurement of shared decision making – a review of instruments. *Zeitschrift für Evidenz, Fortbildung und Qualität im Gesundheitswesen*, 105:313–24.

Scholl I et al. (2012). Development and psychometric properties of the Shared Decision Making Questionnaire – physician version (SDM-Q-Doc). *Patient Education and Counseling*, 88:284–90.

Selby K, Auer R, Cornuz J (2017). Shared decision making in preventive care in Switzerland: from theory to action. *Zeitschrift für Evidenz, Fortbildung und Qualität im Gesundheitswesen*, 123:91–4.

Sepucha K, Mulley AG jr (2009). A perspective on the patient's role in treatment decisions. *Medical Care Research and Review*, 66:53S–74S.

Sepucha KR, Scholl I (2014). Measuring shared decision making: a review of constructs, measures, and opportunities for cardiovascular care. *Circulation: Cardiovascular Quality and Outcomes*, 7:620–6.

Sepucha KR, Fowler FJ jr, Mulley AG jr (2004). Policy support for patient-centered care: the need for measurable improvements in decision quality. *Health Affairs (Millwood)*, Suppl Variation, VAR54–62.

Sewitch MJ et al. (2003). Patient nonadherence to medication in inflammatory bowel disease. *American Journal of Gastroenterology*, 98:1535–44.

Shay LA, Lafata JE (2014). Understanding patient perceptions of shared decision making. *Patient Education and Counseling*, 96:295–301.

Shay LA, Lafata JE (2015). Where is the Evidence? A Systematic Review of Shared Decision Making and Patient Outcomes. *Medical Decision Making*, 35:114–31.

Simon D, Loh A, Harter M (2007). Measuring (shared) decision-making – a review of psychometric instruments. *Zeitschrift fur arztliche Fortbildung und Qualitatssicherung*, 101:259–67.

Sniehotta F (2009). An Experimental Test of the Theory of Planned Behavior. *Applied Psychology: Health and Well-Being*, 1:257–70.

Sorbero ME et al. (2008). *Outcome Measures for Effective Teamwork in Inpatient Care. Final Report*. Santa Monica: RAND Corporation.

Spatz ES, Krumholz HM, Moulton BW (2016). The new era of informed consent: getting to a reasonable-patient standard through shared decision making. *JAMA*, 315:2063–4.

Stacey D et al. (2010). Shared decision making models to inform an interprofessional perspective on decision making: a theory analysis. *Patient Education and Counseling*, 80:164–72.

Stacey D et al. (2013). Coaching and guidance with patient decision aids: a review of theoretical and empirical evidence. *BMC Medical Informatics and Decision Making*, 13:S11.

Stacey D et al. (2017). Decision aids for people facing health treatment or screening decisions. *Cochrane Database of Systematic Reviews*, 4, CD001431.

Stalmeier P (2012). *Med-Decs International Database for Support on Medical Choices*. Available at: http://www.med-decs.org/en (accessed 28 June 2018).

Starfield B et al. (1979). Patient-doctor agreement about problems needing follow-up visit. *JAMA*, 242:344-6.

Stewart M (2001). Towards a global definition of patient centred care. *BMJ*, 322:444-5.

Stewart M (2003). *Patient-centered medicine: transforming the clinical method*. Abingdon: Radcliffe Med Press.

Stiggelbout AM, Pieterse AH, De Haes JC (2015). Shared decision making: concepts, evidence, and practice. *Patient Education and Counseling*, 98:1172-9.

Street RL et al. (2009). How does communication heal? Pathways linking clinician–patient communication to health outcomes. *Patient Education and Counseling*, 74:295-301.

Thompson AG (2007). The meaning of patient involvement and participation in health care consultations: a taxonomy. *Social Science & Medicine*, 64:1297-310.

Thomson R, Murtagh M, Khaw F (2005). Tensions in public health policy: patient engagement, evidence-based public health and health inequalities. *Quality & Safety in Health Care*, 14:398-400.

Tobias JS, Souhami RL (1993). Fully informed consent can be needlessly cruel. *BMJ*, 307:1199-201.

Tragakes E et al. (2008). Latvia: health system review. Health systems in transition, 10(2): 1-253.

Trenaman L, Bryan S, Bansback N (2014). The cost-effectiveness of patient decision aids: a systematic review. *Healthcare (Amsterdam)*, 2:251-7.

Tudiver F et al. (2002). What influences family physicians' cancer screening decisions when practice guidelines are unclear or conflicting? *Journal of Family Practice*, 51:760.

Ubbink DT, Santema TB, Lapid O (2016). Shared Decision-Making in Cosmetic Medicine and Aesthetic Surgery. *Aesthetic Surgery Journal*, 36:NP14–NP19.

US Congress (2010). Patient Protection and Affordable Care Act. Library of Congress.

van der Weijden T et al. (2017). Shared decision making, a buzz-word in the Netherlands, the pace quickens towards nationwide implementation.

Zeitschrift für Evidenz, Fortbildung und Qualität im Gesundheitswesen, 123:69–74.

Veatch R (1972). Models for Ethical Medicine in a Revolutionary Age. *Hastings Center Report,* 2:5–7.

Volk RJ et al. (2013). Ten years of the International Patient Decision Aid Standards Collaboration: evolution of the core dimensions for assessing the quality of patient decision aids. *BMC Medical Informatics and Decision Making,* 13 Suppl 2:S1.

Volk RJ et al. (2016). Patient Decision Aids for Colorectal Cancer Screening: A Systematic Review and Meta-analysis. *American Journal of Preventive Medicine,* 51(5):779–91.

Walsh T et al. (2014). Undetermined impact of patient decision support interventions on healthcare costs and savings: a systematic review. *BMJ,* 348:g188.

Washington State Health Care Authority (2016). Engaging health consumers through Shared Decision Making (SDM). Washington: Washington State Health Care Authority.

Weinstein JN (2000). The missing piece: embracing shared decision making to reform health care. *Spine,* 25:1–4.

Weinstein JN, Clay K, Morgan TS (2007). Informed patient choice: patient-centered valuing of surgical risks and benefits. *Health Affairs (Millwood),* 26:726–30.

Weiss MC et al. (2015). Medication decision making and patient outcomes in GP, nurse and pharmacist prescriber consultations. *Primary Health Care Research & Development,* 16:513–27.

Wennberg J, Gittelsohn (1973). Small area variations in health care delivery. *Science,* 182:1102–8.

West AF, West RR (2002). Clinical decision-making: coping with uncertainty. *Postgraduate Medical Journal,* 78:319–21.

Weston WW (2001). Informed and shared decision-making: the crux of patient-centered care. *CMAJ,* 165:438–9.

Woolf SH (2001). Editorial: the Logic and Limits of Shared Decision Making. *Journal of Urology,* 166:244–245.

World Health Organization (2017). *Case Studies on Enforcement of Tobacco Control Legislation.* Available at: http://www.who.int/tobacco/research/legislation/case_studies_index/en/ (accessed 29 September 2017).

Zikmund-Fisher BJ et al. (2016). Perceived Barriers to Implementing Individual Choosing Wisely(R) Recommendations in Two National Surveys of Primary Care Providers. *Journal of General Internal Medicine,* 32(2): 210–17.

12 The person at the centre? The role of self-management and self-management support

ELLEN NOLTE, ANDERS ANELL

Introduction

Overcoming care fragmentation remains among the key challenges facing health systems globally (Nolte & McKee, 2008; Saini et al., 2017; Schoen et al., 2011). This has become particularly acute against the background of a changing disease burden and the rising number of people with multiple health problems. Policy-makers have recognized this challenge and countries are exploring new approaches to health care delivery to enhance the coordination of care and so better meet the needs of those with chronic and multiple health problems and optimize service use (Nolte, Knai & Saltman, 2014; Wodchis et al., 2015; World Health Organization Regional Office for Europe, 2016). The focus has tended to be on the service provider side, with the introduction of innovative care models such as through strengthening multidisciplinary team work, the use of care coordinators or case managers, co-location of different providers, and shared pathways, among other developments (Nolte & Knai, 2015). The need for involving the individual and their family is widely recognized, although more often than not the focus tends to be on educational elements emphasizing knowledge and adherence to expert advice.

Yet individuals have an important role to play in protecting and promoting their own health, deciding on appropriate approaches to maintain health and managing chronic conditions and the impacts they have on life and well-being (National Voices, 2014). There is a range of ways by which people take an active role in their own care, including through shared decision-making, care planning and self-management (*see* Chapter 11). While conceptually different (Lhussier et al., 2015), the fundamental notion underpinning each is their aim to engage patients in decisions about their care (Coulter & Collins, 2011; Coulter et al., 2015) and that service users and their carers should form an integral part of the care process (Health Foundation, 2014). This is seen to be of particular relevance in the context of chronic disease, which confronts those affected with a spectrum of needs and requires them to manage the impact of the illness on physical, psychological and social functioning, to interact with health care providers and implement treatment regimens, to monitor their health status and make associated care decisions, to alter their behaviour and to engage in activities that promote physical and psychological well-being (Clark, 2003). Service users inevitably become a major caretaker and thus a core part of the 'workforce' in chronic care (Dubois, Singh & Jiwani, 2008).

This chapter focuses on self-management and self-management support, which are considered to be core components of person-centred care (International Alliance for Patients' Organizations, 2006; National Voices, 2014; Health Foundation, 2014). Self-management support is seen to be key to enable service users to move from passive recipients to active partners in care (World Health Organization Regional Office for Europe, 2016). Most often conceptualized in the context of chronic, long-term health problems, it features as one of the four interacting components of the Chronic Care Model that are considered to be essential to providing high-quality care for those with chronic disease (Wagner, 1998). Many countries in Europe and elsewhere have included self-management support as an integral component of national, regional or local strategies, and approaches to service delivery that aim to better meet the needs of people with long-term health problems (Nolte & Knai, 2015; Nolte, Knai & Saltman, 2014; World Health Organization Regional Office for Europe, 2016).

A range of expectations has been associated with self-management and support interventions and policies in this context. For example, it is anticipated that supporting service users recognizes their own knowledge and capacity, that it increases their confidence, strengthens preventive activities and ensures appropriate use of services, and will thus reduce costs and make service delivery more sustainable. There is also an expectation that it will improve service users' experiences of health care, and give people more control over their lives, empower them as partners and improve health outcomes and well-being. Yet, as Morgan et al. (2016) argued, it remains unclear "how all these promising ideas hang together" (p. 2), or whether (and how) these ambitions can be achieved simultaneously (Entwistle, Cribb & Owens, 2016). There is evidence that some forms of support for self-management can impact positively on some of these anticipated outcomes for some service user groups (Franek, 2013; Taylor et al., 2014), but not all aims have been met. In particular, robust evidence that self-management efforts will reduce service utilization has so far been established for selected (hospital) services and selected conditions only (National Voices, 2014; Taylor et al., 2014). Entwistle, Cribb & Owens (2016) also contended that practices seeking to support self-management can, at times, undermine rather than enhance people's experiences of health care.

This chapter explores some of the key issues pertaining to contemporary policy and practice around self-management and support in the context of wider efforts to enhance care coordination in a move to more person-centred systems. It begins by summarizing common definitions of self-management and self-management support and a brief description of what we know about the availability of self-management support strategies in European settings. We then discuss key insights from the evidence base on the impact of self-management interventions. We examine in greater detail some of the challenges facing service users, practitioners and policy-makers in conceptualizing and implementing relevant strategies and discuss policy implications.

Defining self-management and self-management support

Kendall et al. (2011) traced the emergence of self-management in the health field to the self-care and self-help movements that evolved from the 1970s in particular, although early accounts date at least to the 18th century. A focus has been on achieving equality between the provider and service user in terms of making decisions and the capacity to determine the direction of their own care. Mirroring the wider discussion around person-centredness (Chapter 2), interpretations of self-management have since developed in different ways, largely reflecting different disciplinary and professional perspectives and expectations in the context of a changing health care environment, which involves technological advances, the rising burden of chronic disease and the increasing need for cost-containment.

Against this background, it is not surprising that there is no single, universally accepted definition of self-management and self-management support, and the scope of what is considered varies. In an early review, Clark et al. (1991) distinguished between self-care and self-management, with the former referring to a wide range of preventive behaviours and actions taken by those who are healthy or are at risk of ill-health.

Self-management, in contrast, was interpreted in the context of chronic disease and was seen to refer more specifically to the active participation of people in their own treatment, undertaking related tasks and activities with the collaboration and guidance of the individual's physician and other health care providers (Clark et al., 1991; Lorig, 1993). However, although self-care and self-management (and indeed self-management support) form distinct multidimensional constructs (Jones et al., 2011), boundaries between concepts have increasingly blurred and related terms are now often used interchangeably in health policy and research literature (Sadler, Wolfe & McKevitt, 2014).

As noted, self-management is most often conceptualized in the context of chronic disease, and this is further illustrated by a widely used definition proposed by the Institute of Medicine. It describes self-management as "the tasks that individuals must undertake to live well with one or more chronic conditions. These tasks include having the confidence to deal with medical management, role management, and emotional management of their conditions" (Adams, Greiner & Corrigan, 2004, p. 57). One other widely cited definition is that proposed by Barlow et al. (2002), suggesting a broader conceptualization that also takes account of the wider psychosocial context within which people live. Accordingly, self-management includes "the individual's ability to manage the symptoms, treatment, physical and psychosocial consequences and lifestyle changes inherent in living with a chronic condition" (p. 178). Vassilev et al. (2011) further highlighted the role of social networks in the management of long-term health problems.

Corbin & Strauss (1985) identified, based on in-depth interviews with middle-aged and older couples in the USA, three types of 'work' that those with chronic illness have to undertake when managing their condition/s at home: illness work (medical management of the condition), everyday life work (maintaining, changing and creating new meaningful behaviours or life roles), and biographical work (managing the emotional impacts of having a chronic condition and its consequences). Building on this framework, Lorig & Holman (2003) distinguished six core self-management skills: problem solving, decision-making, resource utilization, the formation of a patient–provider partnership, action planning and self-tailoring. These tasks form key components of the Chronic Disease Self-Management Programme (CDSMP) (Stanford Medical School, 2017), developed by the same authors (Lorig et al.,

2001; Lorig et al., 1999) and implemented widely since; we will discuss this programme below.

Self-management *support* has been defined as "the systematic provision of education and supportive interventions by health care staff to increase patients' skills and confidence in managing their health problems, including regular assessment of progress and problems, goal setting, and problem-solving support" (Adams, Greiner & Corrigan, 2004, p. 57). This definition is reflective of the IOM's more health-care-centred definition of self-management mentioned above. Yet support interventions and approaches extend further, as shown by Taylor et al. (2014), who developed a taxonomy for self-management support. It considers four dimensions: (i) the recipient (patients, carers, health professionals, organizations); (ii) self-management components; (iii) modes of delivery (face to face, remote, telehealth care, web based); and (iv) people delivering the support (lay, professionals), with identified components summarized in Box 12.1.

Box 12.1 Taxonomy of self-management support as proposed by Taylor et al. (2014)

Reviewing the evidence from 30 qualitative systematic reviews (covering 515 unique studies) and 102 quantitative systematic reviews (covering 969 RTCs), Taylor et al. (2014) identified 14 types of component of self-management support, which may be directed at the patient or carer. These include: education about condition and management, information about available resources (financial, social), personalized action plan, regular clinical review, monitoring with feedback, practical support with adherence (medicine reviews, dosette boxes, prompts, reminder checklists), equipment, safety netting (e.g. specialist telephone advice), training to communicate with health professionals, training for activities of daily living (e.g. occupational therapy), training for practical self-management activities (e.g. inhaler technique instructions), training for psychological strategies (problem solving, action planning, goal setting, distraction, relaxation, etc.), social support (e.g. befriending, peer support or mentoring), and lifestyle advice and support (diet, physical activity, smoking cessation, handling life stresses).

Box 12.1 (cont.)

Indirect components were those delivered to health professionals such as education and training (e.g. adult learning and communication skills), equipment (e.g. clinical information systems, protocols for disease assessment), prompts (e.g. reminders to discuss action plan), feedback and review (e.g. review from managers, on-site mentoring, monthly reports) and financial incentives, as well as those delivered at an organizational level such as training in implementing self-management, equipment including telehealth care tools, protocols for disease assessment, prompts incorporated into the clinical record system, audit and feedback at organizational level, and financial incentives.

What is happening across Europe?

Decision-makers across Europe have recognized the need for implementing policies and strategies to support self-management mainly in the context of chronic diseases (Elissen et al., 2013; Nolte & Knai, 2015). Available overviews of best practice cases highlight that supporting the active participation of patients in their care is seen as a priority to optimally respond to patient needs and improve health outcomes (European Commission, 2017; World Health Organization Regional Office for Europe, 2016).

However, approaches to self-management support vary widely between and within countries in terms of content, format, provider and availability (Elissen et al., 2013). For example, Kousoulis et al. (2014) carried out a review of the literature on diabetes self-management arrangements in place in six European countries (Bulgaria, Greece, the Netherlands, Norway, Spain and the UK). Covering the period 2000–2013, the review included 56 studies that reported on 21 interventions and programmes for diabetes and chronic disease self-management. Two-thirds (*n*=13) of programmes and interventions were set in the UK, five in the Netherlands, one each in Norway, Spain and Bulgaria and none in Greece (where initial discussions and approaches had only started to emerge at the time of the study), typically located in primary care settings. The majority of approaches comprised educational or training programmes, typically, although not always, emphasizing behavioural change as an important goal while the mode and duration of related interventions varied. Other models included technological support tools, often web-based, that sought to strengthen self-monitoring abilities and individual responsibility, again with considerable variation in terms of focus and content.

Similar variation in the levels of support provided was demonstrated by Nolte, Knai & Saltman (2014) in a review of some 50 coordinated care approaches across 13 countries in Europe. The large majority of these approaches provided some form of patient self-management support, typically involving education for self-management, frequently delivered in a group-based context or on a one-to-one basis and most often in the context of disease management programmes. Education offered within the reviewed approaches tended to focus on disease control through the provision of information about the disease, healthy behaviours and practical instructions concerning, for instance, blood glucose monitoring, foot examination or insulin injection. Most approaches also sought to involve patients in the development of a care or treatment plan and goal setting, and provided regular assessment of patient needs and problems. They typically used support materials in the form of information brochures to complement patient education programmes, with a smaller number using interactive web sites or telephone-based support services to provide patients with personalized information on how to manage their disease. In the majority of cases, self-management support was provided by health professionals including physicians, or, more frequently, by trained nurses within primary care settings. Self-management support programmes provided by others, including lay people, were uncommon, but one well-known example includes the Expert Patient Programme in England (*see* below). Overall, the review found that while approaches to patient support for self-management had moved beyond the mere distribution of information materials, approaches in place tend to reflect service-driven programmes aimed at disease control rather than more general support strategies targeting the wider social context within which people live and drawing on a wider potential support network including other patients, peers or volunteers, among others.

Clearly, reviews such as those presented here risk overlooking examples of innovative practices locally (World Health Organization Regional Office for Europe, 2016). At the same time, it is also clear, in particular in the context of chronic diseases, that while countries are exploring a range of novel approaches to enhance care coordination and integration, and transform service delivery more broadly, strategic programmes and initiatives to strengthen self-management support appear to have remained relatively underdeveloped. We will return to the challenges of systematically implementing self-management support strategies later in this chapter.

What is the evidence?

Reviews of self-management support interventions have described improvements in selected health outcomes among people with chronic disease, including health-related quality of life and healthy behaviours (Franek, 2013; Panagioti et al., 2014). There is also some evidence for the potential of such interventions to reduce health service utilization without compromising patient health outcomes, but observed effects tend to be small and the evidence was found to be strongest for respiratory and cardiovascular problems (Panagioti et al., 2014). Focusing specifically on self-monitoring as one component of self-management, McBain, Shipley & Newman (2015) found, in a review of systematic reviews, evidence of significant reductions in hospitalizations and readmissions to hospital, specifically for heart failure and chronic obstructive pulmonary disease (COPD). At the same time, their review also reported evidence suggesting that observed reductions in (re-)admissions may lead to increases in service use elsewhere in the health care system.

Taylor et al. (2014), based on a review of the qualitative and quantitative evidence (*see also* Box 12.1), concluded that "overall, there appears to be a great deal of evidence, much of it favourable, relating to self-management support across most of the [chronic conditions] studied, but it is clear that not everything works" (p. 418). The authors found no one component to be superior to any other and the most effective interventions were multifaceted and multidisciplinary. They identified a set of core components common to self-management support that are applicable to most chronic conditions, for example education and the provision of knowledge and information about the condition, while noting that interactive learning was likely to be more effective than passive education and education provided in isolation. Some selected components were associated with specific characteristics of a given condition, such as support for activities of daily living for those with disabling conditions (e.g. stroke, lower back pain, progressive neurological disorders, COPD), action plans for those with conditions that are at risk of marked exacerbations (e.g. asthma, COPD), or intensive disease-specific training to enable self-management of specific clinical tasks (e.g. type 1 diabetes, home dialysis for people with chronic kidney disease). Importantly, they found that supported self-management needed to be tailored to the individual, their culture and beliefs, as well as taking account of the natural progression of the condition in order to be effective.

A number of studies and reviews have specifically focused on the effectiveness of the aforementioned CDSMP (Lorig et al., 2001) and related strategies and found the evidence to be somewhat mixed (Foster et al., 2007). For example, Brady et al. (2013) conducted a meta-analysis of 23 studies of the CDSMP delivered in small English-speaking group mode. They demonstrated small to moderate improvements in psychological health and selected health behaviours such as exercise and cognitive symptom management that remained after 12 months. But they did not find robust evidence that the programme reduced health care utilization. This latter finding was confirmed in two Canadian studies that were also unable to demonstrate robust evidence for CDSMP reducing health service use (Jaglal et al., 2014; Liddy et al., 2015).

Kendall et al. (2012) highlighted the importance of the group context within which the CDSMP is being delivered. Based on insights from a focus group study of participants and peer leaders in Australia, they found that positive impacts such as increased knowledge, which led to an increased sense of confidence, perceptions of greater control and a positive attitude to their disease, crucially depended on the "social aspect of the group" (p. 7). Noting that self-management is at its core a social concept, their work pointed to the role of social processes including social engagement, the development of a collective identity, collaborative coping and shared learning in determining the outcomes achieved through CDSMP courses. This observation of the key role of the group context is further supported by Brady et al. (2013), who found that alternative delivery modes of the CDSMP (e.g. internet) had fewer significant improvements than the small English-speaking group mode. A recent scoping review of evidence of benefits and challenges from participating in group-based patient education programmes by Stenberg et al. (2016) also supports this conclusion. However, that review was unable to disentangle the effects of different types of intervention and it remains unclear whether the nature of the intervention or its mode of delivery is more important in enhancing self-reported outcomes such as reduced symptom distress or improved self-management skills.

What are the challenges?

We have seen above that there is evidence that some forms of support for self-management have impacted positively on some outcomes for some service user groups, but overall the evidence remains inconsistent. In particular, robust evidence that self-management efforts will reduce service utilization, and thus health care costs, remains weak. There are a number of reasons why this might be the case. For example, Panagioti et al. (2014) suggested that strategies for self-management support vary in the way in which they explicitly seek to reduce service use, for example those specifically targeting the control of exacerbations in COPD. Others might aim to enhance patient empowerment more broadly, and the outcomes are therefore likely to vary. Targeting service use implicitly assumes that utilization is always user-led, which may, however, not be the case. Also, many self-management interventions have fairly limited impacts, and there is little robust data on long-term outcomes (Taylor et al., 2014).

Nolte & Osborne (2013) noted that part of the challenge lies in the use of outcome measures that do not adequately capture the intended impacts of self-management interventions, and measures are frequently developed without appropriate service user input (Boger et al., 2015). Others have highlighted concerns around the appropriateness of certain interventions, poor design or theoretical assumptions (or lack thereof) underlying the intervention. For example, a strong focus has so far been on psychological mechanisms around concepts such as self-efficacy and patient activation (Hibbard et al., 2004; Lorig & Holman, 2003), which is also reflected in the frequency by which these mechanisms are represented in the literature (Lu, Li & Arthur, 2014), while socioeconomic considerations have been incorporated less frequently. Interventions that are solely based on psychological models of self-management have been criticized "for their individualistic, biomedical and prescriptive focus on disease management" (Sadler, Wolfe & McKevitt, 2014, p. 2). Such an approach, it is argued, failed to address lay understandings of self-management and the social context within which people live and which in turn shapes self-management practices (Ong et al., 2014). Pickard & Rogers (2012) also noted that programmes based on the CDSMP, such as the aforementioned Expert Patient Programme in England and similar approaches elsewhere (Liddy et al., 2015; Haslbeck et al., 2015; Contel et al., 2015; Expert Patients Programme, 2012), aimed to train an "ideal typical, late-modern patient: responsible, self-directed and managing her own health" (p. 102). Such an approach, it is contended, involved an implicit shift in responsibility from the professional to the (lay) service user with regard to managing the disease and its psychosocial impacts (Sadler, Wolfe & McKevitt, 2014). Related programmes are thus likely to benefit only that part of the population that is capable of taking up these roles, which, in turn, might increase health inequities (Kendall et al., 2011).

Health care providers are increasingly encouraged to support people with chronic conditions to learn self-management skills. Indeed, education and training of health professionals in implementing self-management has been identified as an important component of self-management support interventions (Taylor et al., 2014). Yet, as argued by Sadler, Wolfe & McKevitt (2014), such an approach implies a shared understanding of self-management between service users and providers, and this may not be a given. Using a systematic review and narrative synthesis of qualitative studies (*n*=55), the authors found important differences between lay and health professionals' understandings of self-management. They also showed that these understandings differed from the dominant model of self-management that draws on the concept of self-efficacy underpinning approaches such as the CDSMP or the Expert Patients Programme. For example, health professionals tended to interpret self-management as a tool to promote compliance with expert advice and treatment, to monitor and control symptoms and engage in healthy behaviours, or what Morgan et al. (2016) referred to as 'narrow approaches' to self-management support (Box 12.2).

Box 12.2 Managing conditions well vs. managing (or living) well with conditions

Based on a synthesis of the evidence on health and social care professionals' approaches to self-management support for people with chronic disease, Morgan et al. (2016) distinguished those

---

Box 12.2 (cont.)

which focus on supporting people to *manage their condition(s) well* in biomedical or disease-control terms (narrow approaches) from those that emphasize supporting people to *managing well (or living well) with their condition(s)* (broad approaches). In this interpretation, narrow approaches tend to focus on improving the control of symptoms and to reduce the risk of disease progression, exacerbations or complications. Forms of support are often limited to didactic education and motivation, and success is typically assessed using biomedical indicators, such as blood sugar levels in people with diabetes, or intermediate indicators such as behaviour change that will lead to changes in the biomedical indicators. Narrow approaches might take account of emotional issues, but this mostly seeks to encourage behaviour change to achieve disease control rather than to engage with patients' lived experiences.

Conversely, the broader approach to self-management support was seen to be oriented towards supporting people to achieve a better quality of life, while also supporting the development of patients' autonomy and self-determination. Measures of 'success' tend to consider progress in different domains such as people's ability to adapt to and cope with their condition(s), their sense of control, and their ability to develop their own solutions to health-related problems. Forms of support are often characterized by a considerable degree of flexibility on the part of the practitioner, seeking to incorporate individuals' circumstances and lived experiences, and creating scope for individuals to shape the agenda for discussion and action with their practitioners. The approach tends to be characterized by more "equitable and mutually respectful professional–patient relations" (p. 8) whereas the narrow approach was seen to underpin the more (traditional) hierarchical practitioner–patient model of communication.

The authors highlighted that broader approaches tend to be less evident in practice, which they linked, in part, to the challenges of implementing them within existing service delivery frameworks. Importantly, a considerable proportion of reviewed studies had concerned diabetes (~ 40%) and this could have impacted the wider focus on 'narrower' approaches to self-management support

---

Box 12.2 (cont.)

interventions in practice. This is mainly because in diabetes, disease-control measures (such as diet, exercise, monitoring and medication management) are particularly relevant in terms of their impact on the longer-term trajectory of the condition (complications such as blindness, neuropathy and vascular problems) and thus quality of life. These efforts are more easily measured through biomedical indicators such as HbA1c and they incentivize a narrow approach (or disincentivize a move away from it). Such a focus will be less suitable for other conditions such as, for example, cancers or dementias where people can do less to control the disease and its progression.

According to Sadler, Wolfe & McKevitt (2014), such a 'narrow' view was at times also taken by lay people, in particular among those with certain characteristics such as emotional difficulties, low educational attainment or cultural beliefs that place trust in professional expertise and knowledge. Health professionals tended to expect that patients take increased responsibility to manage their own health, but this view was not necessarily shared by all service users. Importantly, lay views about self-management placed particular value on the quality of the relationship between the professional and the service user, seeing self-management as a collaborative partnership. But this understanding was less commonly expressed by providers. Overall, self-management appeared to form part of what Sadler, Wolfe & McKevitt (2014) described as "lay construction of illness narratives" (p. 15) that enabled people to make sense of and cope with their condition(s), and adapt to them in their everyday lives as a 'social practice', which involves the ability to mobilize social support from family and friends. These themes again tended to be less commonly reflected upon by health professionals.

This apparent disjoint between service users' and health professionals' understandings of self-management is further illustrated by Boger et al. (2015), who synthesized the evidence of different stakeholders' views on self-management outcomes, including patients, their families, health professionals, purchasers of services and policy-makers. Focusing on three exemplar conditions (diabetes, stroke, colorectal

cancer), the review found that much of the evidence was from studies
of the experience of self-management rather than actual views on
desired outcomes. Importantly, several themes that were identified to
be relevant by patients were not mentioned by health professionals,
such as maintaining independence and a desire that the condition
or illness should not define people's lives ('being me') (Table 12.1).

Table 12.1 *Self-management outcomes described as important by*
stakeholder group

Theme	Outcome	Patient	Family and friends	Health professional
Applicable knowledge				
	Patient knowledge about the condition	×	×	×
	Having trustworthy and accessible information and resources	×		
Independence				
	Physical independence/not being a burden to family	×		
	Feeling in control of the condition and having confidence to manage it	×		
	Independence from health professionals	×		
	Equity of power with professionals	×		
	Feeling holistically supported by health services	×		
Positive network				
	Positive relationships with professionals	×		

Table 12.1 *(cont.)*

Theme	Outcome	Patient	Family and friends	Health professional
	Involving family members in self-management			×
Being me				
	Feeling 'normal'	×		
	Maintaining social identity	×		
	Managing condition within the context of own life	×		
	Having choices and options over management strategies	×		
Self-management skills				
	Managing consequences of treatment	×		
	Managing emotions		×	
	Managing stress	×	×	
	Patients who are motivated to self-manage			×
	Patients who are empowered			×
Optimal bio-psychosocial health				
Emotional	Improved confidence/ self-efficacy			×
	Feeling good and well	×		
	Improved patient quality of life			×
Physical	Improved health	×	×	
	Improved biomedical markers			×
	Preventing deterioration	×	×	×
	Staying alive	×		
Social	Meeting family expectations and being 'useful' to family	×		

Table 12.1 *(cont.)*

Theme	Outcome	Patient	Family and friends	Health professional
	Improved relationships with family member with chronic condition		×	
	Improved communication with family member with chronic condition		×	

Source: adapted from Boger et al., 2015

Where there were overlaps, different stakeholder groups tended to conceptualize related outcomes in different ways. For example, while applicable knowledge was seen to be important, health professionals tended to interpret this outcome as knowledge about the disease process ('knowing that') while patients and their families focused on knowledge that was personally relevant and tailored to their specific situation ('knowing how'; *see* Greenhalgh et al. (2011)). Similarly, patients and professionals considered gaining self-management skills to be important, yet only health professionals identified motivation or goal-setting as core outcomes while patients emphasized managing emotions and stress (Table 12.1). Reflecting the findings by Sadler, Wolfe & McKevitt (2014), Boger et al. (2015) also highlighted the importance that patients attached to the quality of the relationship with the health professional (*see* Box 12.3), an issue that was not brought up by health professionals. Boger et al. (2015) were unable to identify evidence about how purchasers of services or policy-makers conceptualize self-management and desired outcomes, an issue also highlighted by Harvey et al. (2015), and which we will return to later in this chapter.

Box 12.3 The value of different aspects of self-management support

Of course, identifying the range of outcomes different stakeholders view as relevant does not necessarily mean that all outcomes are valued as equally important. Burton et al. (2017) demonstrated in

Box 12.3 (cont.)

a study of preferences of people with chronic pain or with breathlessness because of chronic respiratory disease that respondents consistently placed a high value on support services that take account of their personal situation and that were oriented to what matters to them for living well. Conversely, more personally relevant information was valued less highly while a friendly and communicative style was valued least. At the same time, respondents varied in the value they placed on different aspects, with a substantial minority rating the provision of personally relevant information highest, and these differences were not associated with broader social or demographic characteristics. Overall these findings suggest that a 'one-size-fits-all' approach to self-management is unlikely to meet people's diverse needs, and strategies need to take account of this diversity.

As noted, differing interpretations of outcomes by different stakeholders likely reflect diversity in conceptualizations of self-management and self-management support, which further influence, or are influenced by, understandings of responsibility for self-management, along with what would be seen to qualify as 'good' self-management. For example, from a service perspective 'goodness' may be more closely linked to strict adherence to advice from health professionals, while from a user perspective it may mean adapting advice and modifying adherence in order to live well (Boger et al., 2015). Differing views on 'goodness' can create tensions between service users and health professionals, especially where user wants and preferences do not align with what the professional considers as the 'right' course of action (Carr et al., 2014), or where user choices are associated with increased costs to the system (Harvey et al., 2015).

The notion of 'responsibility' in and for self-management was further explored by Mudge, Kayes & McPherson (2016), who carried out a metasynthesis of 14 qualitative studies of clinicians' (nurses, physicians, allied health professionals) views on their role in delivering self-management approaches. The theme of 'control' dominated reported perceptions: exercising authority over the patient (clinician control) (mainly) through education and instruction to help patients to control their condition (disease control) by adopting appropriate behaviours (patient control). This view concurs with what Morgan et al. (2016) described as a narrow approach to self-management support (*see* Box 12.2), which relies to a great extent on clinical markers to monitor progress; those not successfully managing their condition were often labelled as non-compliant (shifting responsibility to the patient). Mudge, Kayes & McPherson (2016) highlighted that there appeared to be an (implicit) assumption that clinicians owned the control and would 'grant' it to patients to take on control themselves. At the same time, their review also showed that (some) clinicians recognized a paradigm shift away from the traditional expert-dominated, paternalistic relationship to one that values patient expertise and input, and that acknowledged patients' lived experiences. Those experiencing the shift highlighted the challenges involved, such as sharing or 'letting go' of control. They also reiterated the tensions that are inherent in accepting the patients' expertise as a legitimate input, and which might override the clinician's perspective on a given issue and required professionals to reflect on their role as 'experts' (Carr et al., 2014).

Specifically focusing on patients' accounts of formal and informal self-management support for type 2 diabetes, Foss et al. (2016), based on a metasynthesis of the qualitative evidence (29 studies set in European countries), confirmed that, among people with diabetes, perceptions of self-management go beyond compliance and control. Indeed, self-management practices were seen to be the result of a range of interrelated factors that operate at micro and macro levels and "that exist not as part of the lives of patients but as actually founding or constituting their lives" (p. 681). Understandings of self-management centred around a sense of agency and identity and how environmental factors were connected to everyday lives and behaviours; a desire to achieve minimal disruption of everyday life; the significance and meaning of social networks both influencing and constituting self-management; the role of economic hardship in negotiating priorities in self-management; the challenges created by an emphasis on individual responsibility in encounters with the health service but also at the wider societal level as expressed by a need to 'keep up appearances', and feelings of guilt and shame when failing to comply with treatments or advice; and structural influences of the (primary) care system such as lack of adequate support structures including information, competencies and knowledge, alongside perceived lack of communication and collaboration, and of biopsychosocial approaches in practice.

The findings by Foss et al. (2016) echo those by Burton et al. (2017), Morgan et al. (2016) and Sadler, Wolfe & McKevitt (2014) in that the lay or service user perspectives on self-management and support go beyond those constructed in contemporary policy and practice. The authors note how their review "paints a picture of individuals struggling with social, emotional and economic challenges" (p. 681). They found that people would feel supported by the health service at times, but that this encounter was periodically experienced as 'yet another demand in their lives' and that personal circumstances could stand in the way of 'doing the right thing' (p. 681). Based on these observations, and in line with other accounts (Entwistle, Cribb & Owens, 2016; Kendall et al., 2011; Mudge, Kayes & McPherson, 2016; Sadler, Wolfe & McKevitt, 2014; Vassilev et al., 2011), the authors suggest that the contemporary conceptualization of self-management as an 'individual ability' misses the reality of patients' experiences of and capacity for self-management that is shaped by their social and material resources and the local context within which they live. Sadler, Wolfe & McKevitt (2014) further emphasized the need for self-management support strategies to be based on social models to address differences in lay expectations and abilities to take responsibility in terms of learning self-management skills and to tailor professional support accordingly. This suggests that self-management support efforts should be targeted at all levels, from the individual (micro) to the societal (macro) level in order to be effective (Hinder & Greenhalgh, 2012; Rogers et al., 2015).

There is also a need to address the broader societal understanding of chronic conditions and of presenting a 'public story' that can positively impact people's help-seeking behaviour and public perceptions of need (Taylor et al., 2014). Particular issues arise for those where there is little public understanding of the nature of the health problem and the potential for being stigmatized and seen as 'half a person' because of loss of capacity, the (apparent) failure to take responsibility, or being seen as posing a burden to society (Bratzke et al., 2015; Rogers et al., 2015; Vassilev et al., 2016). Rogers et al. (2015) further highlighted the importance of creating supportive social and policy environments that help people to better self-manage. In the context of diabetes, they draw attention to the role of, for example, the media in reinforcing negative stereotypes in relation to individual responsibility for the development of diabetes through poor lifestyle choices, alongside wider food policies that may (implicitly) promote diabetogenic environments and the production of unhealthy foods. Context matters, however, with people in different countries experiencing different challenges, as shown in a comparative study of people with diabetes in Bulgaria and the UK (Vassilev et al., 2016). This demonstrated how respondents in Bulgaria faced actual lack of resources, access to good quality food and medicines to enable self-management of their condition, pointing to the need for policy solutions that take account of local context.

Moving forward

Morgan et al. (2016) proposed that self-management support should "enable people to live (and die) well with their long-term condition(s)" (p. 11), suggesting that approaches to self-management support that draw on concepts such as empowerment and involvement should prompt questions about the scope of what people are actually empowered to do. Living with long-term health problems challenges individuals on many levels, of which interacting with the health service is only one, if an important one (May et al., 2014). This chapter has explored some of the key issues pertaining to contemporary policy and practice around self-management and support and how existing approaches that focus on care coordination may fall short of taking account of the wider social context within which people live. There may be a risk that strategies and approaches continue to emphasize the 'narrow' focus as exemplified by a recent analysis by Jonkman et al. (2016), who proposed a 'new operational definition' of self-management interventions, which stresses individual responsibility for management and behavioural change "in order to function optimally" (p. 34). Indeed, observations from the review of support efforts in Europe described above suggest a continued focus on medical and behavioural management (Elissen et al., 2013), whereas less emphasis appears to be placed on the wider social context within which people live.

   This may, in part, reflect a wider political context that emphasizes individual responsibility over more collective and regulatory efforts, for example promoting behavioural change interventions over structural solutions to create the necessary physical and social infrastructure (for example, transport) (Rogers et al., 2015). However, it also highlights the challenges involved in taking a comprehensive, system-wide approach in devising policies to address the rising burden of chronic disease more broadly, which requires the capacity for multi- and intersectoral collaboration that extends beyond the immediate health sector (Richardson, Zaletel & Nolte, 2016) and the ability (and willingness) to confront stakeholders that prioritize the interests of business and industry that run counter to wider public health goals.

The chapter has explored the challenges facing service users and health care providers in conceptualizing and implementing relevant strategies. There is so far little robust evidence about how managers and policy-makers view self-management in terms of strategies and desired outcomes (Boger et al., 2015; Harvey et al., 2015). Yet given their role in developing and funding services that support self-management, and in promoting a move of health systems towards supporting self-management more broadly, it will be important to better understand how their priorities map with the stakeholders they aim to support (Boger et al., 2015). There is a particular need to understand the aims and objectives policy-makers seek to achieve in pursuing self-management support strategies to help inform the nature and scope of relevant interventions and approaches and their likelihood of success. Kendall et al. (2011), in a review of policy documents and interview data in Australia, noted that one conception of self-management saw it as a cost-cutting mechanism that 'works' through reducing risk behaviour and improving health and thus reduces the use of costly health services. Yet as we have seen, the available evidence that existing approaches to self-management support will indeed reduce utilization (and health care costs) has so far remained weak (Panagioti et al., 2014). This highlights the need for a better understanding of the causal pathways by which such (intermediary) goals can be realistically achieved in practice.

We have also seen that different interpretations of self-management by different stakeholders may create tensions, such as between service users and health professionals in terms of judging the appropriateness of a particular course of self-management activity (Carr et al., 2014; Harvey et al., 2015). There may also be tensions between service users and their families and wider social networks, which could constrain efforts to self-manage effectively (Foss et al., 2016; Sadler, Wolfe & McKevitt, 2014). Tensions may further arise within and between health professionals tasked with actively engaging patients in their own care although Mudge, Kayes & McPherson (2016), in their analysis of clinicians' views on their role in self-management, did not identify substantive evidence that there would be important differences in the clinicians' views in this respect. Instead, what appeared to be more important was the challenges clinicians faced when actively incorporating self-management into their daily practice, requiring them to 'let go' of being the expert, 'holding back' and talking less and listening more.

Harvey et al. (2015) suggested that there will likely be tensions between professionals and managers or decision-makers also. For example, as part of a wider move to evidence-based practice, there may be a requirement for standardization of care processes at the organizational level. Yet, as Taylor et al. (2014) have shown, for self-management support to be effective, practitioners need to tailor their practice to individual service users' needs and preferences, and this may run counter to standardized approaches. Challenges will also arise from the wider health care policy environment, for example as it relates to the provision of sustainable funding for self-management support interventions to enable firm embedding of relevant programmes in daily practice. This can be especially challenging in resource-constrained settings (Rogers et al., 2015). But even where the wider policy context is supportive *in principle*, tensions may arise where national or macro-level priorities are not aligned and other (potentially competing) goals dominate service delivery priorities locally. This can be illustrated by evidence from England, which found that implementation of comprehensive self-management support strategies at local level was hampered by a continued emphasis on a biomedical model of chronic disease management, with measurement and payment linked to biomedical outcomes, most prominently within the system-wide pay-for-performance scheme in primary care (Kennedy et al., 2014; Reidy et al., 2016) (*see also* Box 12.4). Reinforcement of a focus on the biomedical model was also noted in other system contexts where pharmaceutical companies have taken a greater role in the funding and delivery of self-management support programmes in the absence of national funding sources (Rogers et al., 2015).

Box 12.4 Implementing self-management support at the local level in the English NHS

In England, Clinical Commissioning Groups (CCGs; the purchasers of most health care in the English NHS) are encouraged to use a 'House of Care' model to service provision, which focuses on

Box 12.4 (cont.)

the integration of service users' experiences and resources (NHS England, 2017). Building on experiences in the UK and the Chronic Care Model developed by Wagner and colleagues in the United States, it considers four core interdependent components to realize person-centred coordinated care (Coulter, Roberts & Dixon, 2013). These are: engaged, informed individuals and carers (left wall of the house); health and care professionals committed to partnership working (right wall); commissioning including 'more than medicine' (floor); and organizational and supporting processes (roof). Self-management support is seen to be among the core strategies commissioners are asked to consider for supporting the delivery of person-centred care (Coalition for Collaborative Care and NHS England, 2016).

Reidy et al. (2016) examined the way CCGs consider and conceptualize self-management support and the extent to which this was reflected in the strategic planning and commissioning of services. Drawing on an analysis of planning documents of nine CCGs and interviews, the authors found that commissioners' conceptualization of self-management support tended to reflect the national agenda or 'official terminology', which focused on support strategies as a means to reduce service utilization against the need for cost containment. While self-management support was generally seen to form an important component of culture change in service delivery, the operationalization of relevant strategies in practice was seen to be challenging unless guided by a top-down initiative. There was a reported lack of capacity to engage with the public for developing and implementing self-management support strategies, where these were not linked to traditional, nationally driven outcome measures and payments relating to biomedical outcomes.

Conclusions

The evidence presented in this chapter highlights that there is still a long way to go for health systems that seek to strengthen self-management support as part of a wider strategy of moving towards more coordinated, person-centred health systems. We have seen that any such strategy needs to consider the wider context within which people live and efforts should be targeted at the micro, that is the individual level, the organizational level and the macro or system level. Strategies also need to go beyond the immediate health care context in order to take full account of the broader influences that impact self-management activities at the individual level, of which the encounter with service providers is only one, albeit key, factor. Rather than supporting people to *manage their condition(s) well* in biomedical or disease-control terms (narrow approaches), the emphasis should be on supporting people to *manage well (or live well) with their condition(s)* (broad approaches). There are implications for the training of health and care professionals and how this needs to be adapted to enable providers engaging in a true partnership with the individual service user that provides the support appropriate to the individual's preferences and needs. Managers need to consider approaches of how to best support their staff in providing self-management support, which will involve making relevant activities a priority, and which in turn requires the ability of organizations to do so against the background of demands placed upon them by the wider system context. This also highlights the need for the wider policy framework to be alert to the potential tensions and unintended consequences of policies that are not consistent, and to create a policy environment that provides the means for those who are asked to implement change to acquire the actual capacity and competence to do so, which will be critical for success.

References

Adams K, Greiner A, Corrigan J (eds.) (2004). *The 1st Annual Crossing the Quality Chasm Summit: A Focus on Communities*. Washington DC: National Academies Press.

Barlow J et al. (2002). Self-management approaches for people with chronic conditions: a review. *Patient Education and Counseling*, 48:177–87.

Boger E et al. (2015). Self-management and self-management support outcomes: a systematic review and mixed research synthesis of stakeholder views. *PLoS One*, 10:e0130990.

Brady T et al. (2013). A meta-analysis of health status, health behaviors, and healthcare utilization outcomes of the Chronic Disease Self-Management Program. *Preventing Chronic Disease*, 10: 120112.

Bratzke L et al. (2015). Self-management priority setting and decision-making in adults with multimorbidity: a narrative review of literature. *International Journal of Nursing Studies*, 52:744–55.

Burton C et al. (2017). The value of different aspects of person-centred care: a series of discrete choice experiments in people with long-term conditions. *BMJ Open*, 7:e015689.

Carr S et al. (2014). Looking after yourself: clinical understandings of chronic-care self-management strategies in rural and urban contexts of the United Kingdom and Australia. *SAGE Open Medicine*, 2:2050312114532636.

Clark N (2003). Management of chronic disease by patients. *Annual Review of Public Health*, 24:289–313.

Clark N et al. (1991). Self-management of chronic disease by older adults. *Journal of Aging and Health*, 3:3–27.

Coalition for Collaborative Care & NHS England (2016). Delivering personalised care and support planning: the journey to person-centred care. Available at: https://www.england.nhs.uk/wp-content/uploads/2016/04/info-commissioners-care-support-planning.pdf (accessed 14 August 2017).

Contel J et al. (2015). Chronic and integrated care in Catalonia. *International Journal of Integrated Care*, 15:e025.

Corbin J, Strauss A (1985). Managing chronic illness at home: three lines of work. *Qualitative Sociology*, 8:224–47.

Coulter A, Collins A (2011). Making shared decision-making a reality. No decision about me, without me. London: King's Fund.

Coulter A, Roberts S, Dixon A (2013). *Delivering better services for people with long-term conditions. Building the house of care.* London: King's Fund.

Coulter A et al. (2015). Personalised care planning for adults with chronic or long-term health conditions. *Cochrane Database of Systematic Reviews*, 3:CD010523.

Dubois C, Singh D, Jiwani I (2008). The human resource challenge in chronic care. In: Nolte E, McKee M (eds.) *Caring for people with chronic conditions. A health system perspective.* Maidenhead: Open University Press.

Elissen A et al. (2013). Is Europe putting theory into practice? A qualitative study of the level of self-management support in chronic care management approaches. *BMC Health Services Research*, 13:117.

Entwistle V, Cribb A, Owens J (2016). Why health and social care support for people with long-term conditions should be oriented towards enabling them to live well. *Health Care Analysis*, 26:48–65.

European Commission (2017). Blocks. Tools and methodologies to assess integrated care in Europe. Report by the Expert Group on Health Systems Performance Assessment. Luxembourg: Publications Office of the European Union.

Expert Patients Programme (2012). Expert Patients Programme Self-Management Courses. Available at: https://www.selfmanagementuk.org/ (accessed 9 March 2017).

Foss C et al. (2016). Connectivity, contest and the ties of self-management support for type 2 diabetes: a meta-synthesis of qualitative literature. *Health and Social Care in the Community*, 24:672–86.

Foster G et al. (2007). Self-management education programmes by lay leaders for people with chronic conditions. *Cochrane Database of Systematic Reviews*, 4, CD005108.

Franek J (2013). Self-management support interventions for persons with chronic disease: an evidence-based analysis. *Ontario Health Technology Assessment Series*, 13:1–60.

Greenhalgh T et al. (2011). Storylines of self-management: narratives of people with diabetes from a multiethnic inner city population. *Journal of Health Services Research & Policy*, 16:37–43.

Harvey J et al. (2015). Factors influencing the adoption of self-management solutions: an interpretive synthesis of the literature on stakeholder experiences. *Implementation Science*, 10:159.

Haslbeck J et al. (2015). Introducing the chronic disease self-management program in Switzerland and other German-speaking countries: findings of a cross-border adaptation using a multiple-methods approach. *BMC Health Services Research*, 15:576.

Health Foundation (2014). Person-centred care made simple. What everyone should know about person-centred care. London: Health Foundation.

Hibbard J et al. (2004). Development and testing of a short form of the Patient Activation Measure. *Health Services Research*, 40:1918–30.

Hinder S, Greenhalgh T (2012). "This does my head in". Ethnographic study of self-management by people with diabetes. *BMC Health Services Research*, 12:83.

International Alliance for Patients' Organizations (2006). Declaration on: Patient-centred healthcare. Available at: https://www.iapo.org.uk/ sites/default/files/files/IAPO_declaration_ENG_2016.pdf (accessed 12 September 2016).

Jaglal S et al. (2014). Impact of a chronic disease self-management program on health care utilization in rural communities: a retrospective cohort study using linked administrative data. *BMC Health Services Research*, 14:198.

Jones M et al. (2011). A thematic analysis of the conceptualisation of self-care, self-management and self-management support in the long-term conditions management literature. *Journal of Nursing and Healthcare of Chronic Illness*, 3:174–85.

Jonkman N et al. (2016). Self-management interventions: proposal and validation of a new operational definition. *Journal of Clinical Epidemiology*, 80:34–42.

Kendall E et al. (2011). Self-managing versus self-management: reinvigorating the socio-political dimensions of self-management. *Chronic Illness*, 7:87–98.

Kendall E et al. (2012). Social processes that can facilitate and sustain individual self-management for people with chronic conditions. *Nursing Research and Practice*, 282671.

Kennedy A et al. (2014). Implementation of a self-management support approach (WISE) across a health system: a process evaluation explaining what did and did not work for organisations, clinicians and patients. *Implementation Science*, 9:129.

Kousoulis A et al. (2014). Diabetes self-management arrangements in Europe: a realist review to facilitate a project implemented in six countries. *BMC Health Services Research*, 14:453.

Lhussier M et al. (2015). Care planning for long-term conditions – a concept mapping. *Health Expectations*, 18:605–24.

Liddy C et al. (2015). Impact of a chronic disease self-management program on healthcare utilization in eastern Ontario, Canada. *Preventive Medicine Reports*, 2:586–90.

Lorig K (1993). Self-management of chronic illness: a model for the future. *Generations*, 17:11–4.

Lorig K, Holman H (2003). Self-management education: history, definition, outcomes, and mechanisms. *Annals of Behavioral Medicine*, 26:1–7.

Lorig K et al. (1999). Evidence suggesting that a chronic disease self-management program can improve health status while reducing hospitalization: a randomized trial. *Medical Care*, 37:5–14.

Lorig K et al. (2001). Chronic disease self-management program: 2-year health status and health care utilization outcomes. *Medical Care*, 39:1217–23.

Lu Y, Li Z, Arthur D (2014). Mapping publication status and exploring hotspots in a research field: chronic disease self-management. *Journal of Advanced Nursing*, 70:1837–44.

May C et al. (2014). Rethinking the patient: using Burden of Treatment Theory to understand the changing dynamic of illness. *BMC Health Services Research*, 14:281.

McBain H, Shipley M, Newman S (2015). The impact of self-monitoring in chronic illness on healthcare utilisation: a systematic review of reviews. *BMC Health Services Research*, 15:565.

Morgan DJ et al. (2016). We need to talk about purpose: a critical interpretive synthesis of health and social care professionals' approaches to self-management support for people with long-term conditions. *Health Expectations* [Epub ahead of print].

Mudge S, Kayes N, McPherson K (2016). Who is in control? Clinicians' view on their role in self-management approaches: a qualitative metasynthesis. *BMJ Open*, 5:e007413.

National Voices (2014). *Supporting self-management*. London: National Voices.

NHS England (2017). House of Care – a framework for long term condition care. Available at: https://www.england.nhs.uk/ourwork/ltc-op-eolc/ltc-eolc/house-of-care/#sol (accessed 14 August 2017).

Nolte E, Knai C (eds.) (2015). *Assessing chronic disease management in European health systems. Country reports.* Copenhagen: WHO Regional Office for Europe on behalf of the European Observatory on Health Systems and Policies.

Nolte E, McKee M (eds.) (2008). *Caring for people with chronic conditions: a health system perspective.* Maidenhead: Open University Press.

Nolte S, Osborne R (2013). A systematic review of outcomes of chronic disease self-management interventions. *Quality of Life Research*, 22:1805–16.

Ong B et al. (2014). Behaviour change and social blinkers? The role of sociology in trials of self-management behaviour in chronic conditions. *Sociology of Health & Illness*, 36:226–38.

Panagioti M et al. (2014). Self-management support interventions to reduce health care utilisation without compromising outcomes: a systematic review and meta-analysis. *BMC Health Services Research*, 14:356.

Pickard S, Rogers A (2012). Knowing as practice: self-care in the case of chronic multimorbidities. *Social Theory & Health*, 10:101–20.

Reidy C et al. (2016). Commissioning of self-management support for people with long-term conditions: an exploration of commissioning aspirations and processes. *BMJ Open*, 6:e010853.

Richardson E, Zaletel J, Nolte E (2016). National diabetes plans in Europe. What lessons are there for the prevention and control of chronic diseases in Europe? Copenhagen: WHO Regional Office for Europe on behalf of the European Observatory on Health Systems and Policies.

Rogers A et al. (2015). Meso level influences on long-term condition self-management: stakeholder accounts of commonalities and differences across six European countries. *BMC Public Health*, 15:622.

Sadler E, Wolfe C, McKevitt C (2014). Lay and health care professional understandings of self-management: a systematic review and narrative synthesis. *SAGE Open Medicine*, 2:2050312114544493.

Saini V et al. (2017). Drivers of poor medical care. *Lancet* , 390:178–90.

Schoen C et al. (2011). New 2011 survey of patients with complex care needs in eleven countries finds that care is often poorly coordinated. *Health Affairs (Millwood)*, 30:2437–48.

Stanford Medical School (2017). Stanford Patient Education Research Center. Available at: http://patienteducation.stanford.edu/ (accessed 3 May 2017).

Stenberg U et al. (2016). A scoping review of the literature on benefits and challenges of participating in patient education programs aimed at promoting self-management for people living with chronic illness. *Patient Education and Counseling*, 99:1759–71.

Taylor S et al. (2014). A rapid synthesis of the evidence on interventions supporting self-management for people with long-term conditions: PRISMS – Practical systematic Review of Self-Management Support for long-term conditions. *Health Services and Delivery Research*, 2.

Vassilev I et al. (2011). Social networks, social capital and chronic illness self-management: a realist review. *Chronic Illness*, 7:60–86.

Vassilev I et al. (2016). The articulation of neoliberalism: narratives of experience of chronic illness management in Bulgaria and the UK. *Sociology of Health & Illness*, 39:349–64.

Wagner E (1998). Chronic disease management: what will it take to improve care for chronic illness. *Effective Clinical Practice*, 1:2–4.

Wodchis W et al. (2015). Integrating care for older people with complex needs: key insights and lessons from a seven-country cross-case analysis. *International Journal of Integrated Care*, 15:e021.

World Health Organization Regional Office for Europe (2016). Lessons from transforming health services delivery: compendium of initiatives in the WHO European Region. Copenhagen: World Health Organization Regional Office for Europe.

13 | Patients' rights: from recognition to implementation

WILLY PALM, HERMAN NYS, DAVID TOWNEND,
DAVID SHAW, TIMO CLEMENS, HELMUT BRAND

Introduction

Patients' rights can be seen as a precondition to empowering people and moving to health systems that are more person-centred. They provide a foundation for citizens to be considered as actors in control of their own health care delivery process.

Increasingly, the challenges and potential solutions that health systems are facing are explored through a patients' rights lens. Changes, such as the rapid ageing of the population and the rising burden of chronic conditions (including mental health problems), along with scientific and technological developments as well as cultural preferences, are creating new questions that are often debated within the context of fundamental rights, including self-determination, dignity and equality. The growing complexity of health care together with innovations in the fields of medicine (e.g. precision medicine) and of information and communication technology (ICT) (e.g. e-health), along with an increased focus on quality and safety, are likely to impact patients' rights, especially with regard to privacy and equity. These elements require the development of coherent strategies around citizens' involvement and patients' rights with respect to health and social care. The notion of patients' rights reflects a shift towards a more equal relationship between the individual service user and the provider, such that the provider acts as a clinical expert in support of a more active patient, based on increased patient autonomy and better communication (Emanuel and Emanuel, 1992) (*see* Chapter 2).

The formulation of patients' rights can also help to grow awareness. For patients, this includes a more active role in their own care, while for providers it involves greater understanding of the impact of interventions on patients. It can also guide and steer policy-makers in reforming health systems by recognizing the potentially vulnerable position of patients due to information asymmetry, but also due to the sometimes critical and intimate context, which requires a great deal of trust between patients and caregivers.

This chapter analyses the relevance and usefulness of patients' rights for achieving broader health system objectives of person-centredness and patient empowerment. It begins by presenting a conceptual framework looking at different aspects of patients' rights, followed by an assessment of the state of patients' rights and their enforcement systems in various countries. This also highlights some national examples of good practice. Drawing on the existing evidence about the actual use of patients' rights and their impacts on outcomes at individual, organizational and system levels it then develops some policy lessons for further promoting, defining and implementing patients' rights.

The chapter draws on a mapping exercise that was conducted in 2015 and funded under the EU health programme. The project explored the situation in 30 European countries (28 EU Member States plus Norway and Iceland) using a survey of national patients' rights experts (European Commission, 2018).

Defining patients' rights

Historically, the notion of patients' rights is firmly rooted in the recognition of the inherent dignity of all human beings and their equal and unalienable rights, such as the Universal Declaration of Human Rights (UDHR) and other sources of international law. Given the particularly vulnerable position of people when seeking health care, it was considered important to specify these basic rights in the care setting. Clearly, basic rights such as the right to be free from cruel, inhuman or degrading treatment (Article 5 UDHR) or the right to privacy (Article 12 UDHR) have a special meaning when transferred to a care context. Patients' rights are primarily addressed to health professionals (and caregivers more generally), who have a duty to respect the basic human rights of the people they treat or care for in all circumstances. This is essentially based on bioethical principles as expressed in the Hippocratic Oath (Will, 2011). However, patients' rights also cover more systemic factors and state responsibilities in the organization and delivery of care. State parties have three types of obligation: to respect human rights themselves, to protect against violations by third parties, and to fulfil the conditions for their realization

(Office of the United Nations High Commissioner for Human Rights, the World Health Organization, 2008).

Some commentators distinguish individual rights 'as a patient' from the collective and social rights 'to become a patient'; the latter refer to issues of coverage, access and entitlements (Nys & Goffin, 2011). Individual patients' rights and social rights are considered to be different in nature, although the right to medical care is also enshrined as a fundamental human right (Article 25 UDHR). Individual rights aim at protecting the individual sphere, whereas social rights, such as the right to health care, are to safeguard the participation of people in social benefits (Leenen, 1994). Patients' rights prevent society from unlawfully intruding into a person's private sphere, while access rights to health care require governments to work towards their full realization in accordance with resource constraints.

In a similar way, patients' rights are distinguished from the concepts of patient safety and quality of care. Indeed, the right to medical treatment that is safe and of high quality is seen to be part of a consumer protection framework. Some argue that violations of standards of quality and safety should be interpreted differently from a breach of human rights, the only exception being where maltreatment by a health care provider is systemic (Ezer & Cohen, 2013).

The need for better legal protection of patients was prompted by evidence demonstrating variation in medical practice associated with variations in health outcomes, along with evidence of adverse events and medical errors. It also highlighted the importance of informational and procedural rights, often referred to as consumer-oriented rights, although they clearly have a human rights component as well.

While human rights are universal, indivisible, interdependent and interrelated, social and consumer rights leave more room for national variation, determined by social, economic and cultural factors. However, even if social and consumer-oriented patients' rights have different origins and address different needs and expectations, they cannot be completely separated from the human rights framework. This is illustrated by the fundamental right to "the enjoyment of the highest attainable standard of physical and mental health", which was first internationally recognized by the 1946 Constitution of the World Health Organization (WHO). This human right to health is generally defined in broad terms, ranging from rights related to broader health determinants to the right to medical care and access to health services. It also includes more typical patients' rights, such as the right to be free from non-consensual medical treatment, the right to seek, receive and impart information and ideas concerning health issues, or the right to have personal health data treated with confidentiality (Office of the High Commissioner for Human Rights, 2000). It also includes collective citizens' rights such as the participation in health-related decision-making at national and community levels. The involvement of citizens at a systems level is expected to help reduce the gap between theory and practice in individual patients' rights (Hart, 2004).

Overall, then, these rights are complementary and interdependent (Roscam Abbing, 2014). Patients' rights can only be fully accomplished in an environment that ensures that the care provided meets high standards of quality and safety, and that has put mechanisms in place for redress or compensation where standards are not being met. A strong patient voice and the promotion of patients' rights are also considered important for maintaining a focus on quality, especially in times of increased financial pressures (OECD, 2017).

European frameworks for patients' rights

Patients' rights are mainly determined at the national level and to some extent reflect differences in national contexts, especially where this concerns ethical questions, such as around the beginning and end of life. However, supra-national frameworks, such as the aforementioned UDHR and, within Europe, the European Convention on Human Rights (1950), play a role in influencing national legislation, as do more recent policy concerns, such as growing migration, increased mobility of patients and the need for cross-national cooperation in health care as well as the internationalization of medical research (Roscam Abbing, 2004).

Within the European context, several developments have contributed significantly to promoting patients' rights legislation in European countries (Leenen, Gevers & Pinet, 1993). These include the 1994 Amsterdam Declaration on the promotion of the rights of patients in Europe. It was a first attempt to formulate a consistent set of patients' rights that should apply irrespective of the characteristics of a country's health system or specific circumstances of patients. The Declaration sought to enhance awareness among citizens about their (active) role in health care, to strengthen collaboration and trust between patients and providers, and to support policy-makers in developing patient-centred policies (Table 13.1). This vision of strengthening citizens' voice and choice in health care was later reasserted in the Ljubljana Charter on Reforming Health Care (1996).

This was followed, in 1997, by the European Convention on Human Rights and Biomedicine (Oviedo Convention) (Council of Europe, 1997). While primarily intended to protect human dignity against misuse of biological and medical advances, it also contains general patients' rights (Table 13.1). These rights can be directly invoked in countries that have ratified this convention, provided they are unconditional and sufficiently precise (Nys & Goffin, 2011).

Within the EU, the issue of patients' rights in the context of EU integration was pursued as early as 1984, when the European Parliament adopted a Resolution inviting the European Commission to submit a proposal for a "European Charter on the Rights of Patients", taking into account the freedom of establishment for doctors and practitioners of paramedical professions. In 2002 the Active Citizenship Network, a group of European civic organizations, launched a European Charter of Patients' Rights, which contains 14 specific patients' rights and three additional active citizenship rights (Box 13.1). This initiative was inspired by the Charter of Fundamental Rights of the EU that was adopted in Nice in 2000. Mainly drawing on the right to health care (Article 35 of the Charter of Fundamental Rights of the EU), the focus was on access to high quality health care, which was seen to be of particular importance in the context of EU enlargement and increasing mobility in health care. Since 2007 an annual European Patients' Rights Day has been organized to increase awareness about the importance of patients' rights.

Another example of a voluntary arrangement developed by civil society is the European Cancer Patients' Bill of Rights that was launched by the European Cancer Concord initiative in 2014. Motivated by the substantial differences in cancer incidence and mortality between countries in Europe, the charter provides three main rights: the right to accurate information and pro-active involvement, the right to timely and appropriate specialized care underpinned by research and innovation, and the right to be treated in health systems that ensure improved outcomes, patient rehabilitation, best quality of life and affordable health care (Lawler et al., 2014).

Box 13.1 The European Charter of Patients' Rights

1. Right to preventive measures
2. Right of access
3. Right to information
4. Right to consent
5. Right to free choice
6. Right to privacy and confidentiality
7. Right to respect of patients' time
8. Right to the observance of quality standards
9. Right to safety
10. Right to innovation
11. Right to avoid unnecessary suffering and pain
12. Right to personalized treatment
13. Right to complain
14. Right to compensation

Rights of active citizenship

- Right to perform general interest activities
- Right to perform advocacy activities
- Right to participate in policy-making in the area of health

Source: Active Citizenship Network, 2002

In 2011 the EU adopted and implemented the Directive on the application of patients' rights in cross-border health care, which essentially focuses on social and consumer patients' rights in the context of cross-border health care (Table 13.1).

Among the four frameworks reviewed here, only the Biomedicine Convention and the EU Directive are legally binding. Yet all four influenced the promotion and development of patients' rights in Europe, as noted earlier. While there are slight differences in the formulation of these rights, with an emphasis on certain dimensions, there is relative consensus on the core elements of patients' rights. Specific patients' rights that are aimed at protecting specific patient groups (e.g. minors, those with disabilities or those with mental health problems) or people in specific circumstances (e.g. clinical trials, genetic testing) are omitted from the assessment presented in Table 13.1.

Table 13.1 *Patients' rights as defined under four different European frameworks*

Human rights categories	WHO/Europe Amsterdam Declaration (1994)	Council of Europe Biomedicine Convention (1997)	Active Citizenship Network European Charter of Patients' Rights (2002)	EU Directive on the application of patients' rights in cross-border health care (2011)
Right to respect, dignity, integrity and non-discrimination	Respect (1.1) Integrity and protection (1.3) Respect of values, convictions and culture (1.5, 1.8) Dignity in treatment and dying (1.8, 5.11) Support of family, relatives and friends (5.9) Non-discrimination (6.2)	Protection of dignity and identity, non-discrimination, respect of integrity (1) Primacy of the interest and welfare of the human being (2)		Non-discrimination with regard to nationality (4.3)
Right to privacy and confidentiality	Respect of privacy (1.4, 4.6–8) Confidentiality and protection of personal information (4.1) Access to medical file (4.4) and control over personal and medical data (4.5)	Respect for private life in relation to personal health information (10.1)	Confidentiality of personal information and protection of privacy (6)	Union provisions on the protection of personal data (4.2.e) Access to (written or electronic) medical record (4.2.f and 5.d)

Table 13.1 (cont.)

Human rights categories	WHO/Europe Amsterdam Declaration (1994)	Council of Europe Biomedicine Convention (1997)	Active Citizenship Network European Charter of Patients' Rights (2002)	EU Directive on the application of patients' rights in cross-border health care (2011)
Right to liberty and self-determination	Self-determination (1.2) Information (2) • Health services (2.1) • Health status (2.2) • Treatment options (2.2) • Second opinion (2.7) • Health providers (2.8) Informed consent (3.1)	Free and informed consent (5) Information about health (10.2)	Information regarding health status, health services (3), treatment options (4) Informed consent (4) Free choice (5)	Information • on quality and safety standards and guidelines (4.2.a) • on providers (incl. availability, quality and safety, prices, authorization or registration status, professional liability protection (4.2.b and 6.3) • on treatment options (4.2.b) • on rights and entitlements to cross-border care (5.b and 5.4) • on patients' rights, complaints procedures and mechanisms for seeking remedies, dispute settlement (6.3)

Right to health			
Protection of health and pursuit of highest attainable level (1.6) Access to health services (5.1)	Equitable access to health care of appropriate quality (3) Observance of relevant professional obligations and standards (4)	Preventive measures (1) Equal access to health services (2)	Care in accordance with the standards and guidelines on quality and safety laid down by the Member State of treatment (4.1.b) Non-discrimination
• Equity and non-discrimination (5.1, 5.5) • Quality of care (5.3) • Continuity and cooperation (5.4) • Choice (5.6) • Social care (5.7) • Relief of suffering (5.10) and humane terminal care (5.11)		• Respect of patients' time (7) • Observance of quality standards (8) • Safety (9) • Access to innovation (10) • Avoidance of unnecessary suffering and pain (11) • Personalized treatment (12)	• scale of fees (4.4) • medical follow-up (5.c) Reimbursement of cross-border health care (7–9) • same level of reimbursement (7.2.4) and transparent mechanism for calculation (7.2.6) • applicable limitations, conditions, eligibility criteria, formalities can only apply if justified by overriding reasons of general interest (7.2.7–9) • prior authorization cannot be refused if treatment cannot be provided domestically within a medically justifiable time-limit (8.5) • fair, transparent and swift administrative procedures (9)

Table 13.1 (cont.)

Human rights categories	WHO/Europe Amsterdam Declaration (1994)	Council of Europe Biomedicine Convention (1997)	Active Citizenship Network European Charter of Patients' Rights (2002)	EU Directive on the application of patients' rights in cross-border health care (2011)
Right to remedy		Judicial protection against unlawful infringement (23) Fair compensation for undue damage (24) Application of appropriate sanctions (25)	Complain and receive feedback (13) Sufficient and swift compensation in case of harm caused by treatment (14)	Transparent complaints procedures and mechanisms to seek remedies in case of harm (4.2.c) Systems of professional liability insurance, or equivalent (4.2.d) Procedures for appeal and redress in case of non-respect of entitlement rights (5.b)
Right to participation, representation and collective action	Representation at each level of the health system (5.2)		Perform general interest and advocacy activities for the protection of patients' rights (part III) Participate in health policy-making (part III)	

Types of patients' rights

Drawing on the comparison of patients' rights frameworks in the preceding section, we identify 13 core patients' rights that can be clustered into six categories: self-determination, confidentiality, access to health care, choice, information and redress (Table 13.2). These rights require specific action or measures for implementation, while others, such as the right to respect a patient's integrity, do not necessarily require a particular translation but are more reliant on attitudes within health care settings. Similarly, the right to collective participation and action is not included in this list as it is considered a fundamental citizens' right that transcends the position of a particular individual, although it plays an important role in helping to implement individual patients' rights (Hart, 2004).

Table 13.2 *Clusters of core patients' rights as identified from four patients' rights frameworks*

Self-determination	1. The right to (informed) consent
	2. The right to participate in (clinical) decision-making/to choose treatment options
Confidentiality	3. The right to data confidentiality
	4. The right to access one's medical record
Access to health care	5. The right to benefit from medical treatment according to needs
	6. The right to safe and high-quality treatment received in a timely manner
Choice	7. The right to choose a health care provider
	8. The right to a second opinion
Information	9. The right to information about one's health
	10. The right to information about health care providers
	11. The right to information about rights and entitlements
Redress	12. The right to complain
	13. The right to compensation

Several of these rights are interconnected. Thus, informational and procedural rights ('information' and 'redress') cut across the various clusters as they support the implementation and protection of other rights.

For example, the right to information about one's health is intrinsically connected to the right to informed consent. Informed consent is also linked to the right to a second opinion, which at the same time can be considered as a right 'derived' from the right to choose one's provider. Provider choice in turn is supported by the right to information about health care providers. The right to access medical records can also be seen as an informational right. While it serves as a way to control confidentiality and accuracy of personal data, it is also an important lever to evaluate if the right to safe and high-quality treatment was violated and to exercise the procedural right to complain or to claim compensation in case of any harm. Finally, the right to participate in clinical decision-making is perhaps seen less as a traditional right but rather as an extension of the right to informed consent.

Mapping the implementation of patients' rights in EU Member States

EU Member States have taken different approaches to implementing patients' rights, reflecting differences in health systems as well as countries' legislative traditions (Roscam Abbing, 2014). Most European countries have brought together all general patients' rights into one dedicated law (Hart, 2004). Finland, the Netherlands and Hungary were among the first to develop such a unified law, followed by a second group of countries which were inspired by the Council of Europe's Biomedicine Convention. More recently, countries such as Germany and Denmark have consolidated or coordinated their existing framework, while others introduced relevant legislation following public pressure (e.g. Portugal) or examples from neighbouring countries (e.g. Luxembourg). At the time of writing, Bulgaria and Italy were the only countries that had yet to implement a special law or charter on patients' rights.

The most important initial driver of the development of patients' rights legislation was the fundamental rights movements of the 1970s, which was accompanied, in some countries, by the development of health law as a separate legal discipline (e.g. the Netherlands, Norway, Slovenia). Among countries in central and eastern Europe, the political transition of the early 1990s promoted patients' rights legislation (den Exter, 2002). As noted earlier, civil society, especially patients' organizations, also played an important part in placing patients' rights on the political agenda (e.g. France, Romania), while more recently media coverage of patients' rights violations has helped to increase awareness of this issue.

The adoption of special patients' rights laws typically meant an important shift towards a more patient-oriented approach, not only with respect to formulating more detailed rights but also in terms of improving transparency and enhancing awareness. At the same time, other legislation (such as civil, criminal, disciplinary or administrative law) will still apply, in particular as far as procedural patients' rights are concerned, such as the right to compensation, which is often enforced through traditional legislation governing breach of duty of care or negligence.

As countries pursue different routes, and do so at a different pace, any attempt to classify or map approaches will intrinsically be limited (Nys & Goffin, 2011). Concerning special patients' rights laws, countries use different approaches to enforcement: legal, quasi-legal and moral rights (Fallberg, 2000) (Table 13.3).

- *Legal patients' rights* are well-defined, actionable rights based on the (horizontal) relationship between the provider and the user of health services. Taking the contractual nature of this relationship as the legal basis, some countries have formalized this as a specific 'sui generis' contract to distinguish it from other contractual forms; examples include the Netherlands (Table 13.3). Other countries have also taken a private law approach to adopting directly enforceable patients' rights laws, with countries such as Germany, Portugal and Spain classifying it as a generic service contract (Barendrecht et al., 2007).
- *Quasi-legal patients' rights* refer to (vertical) obligations imposed on health care providers by public or administrative law or legally binding codes of medical duty. Finland led the way with an act rooted in the Nordic legal tradition of obligations (rather than rights) defined in the context of the 'social contract' between the state and its citizens (Fallberg, 2000). Elsewhere, enforcement relies more on public sector regulation, such as in France and Greece (Table 13.3). In contrast to the legal patients' rights approach, quasi-legal rights imply that any direct civil action taken by the individual in case of violation of rights would be subject to a prior sanction taken against the provider. Also, in countries that have implemented a legal patients' rights framework, but where this framework does not contain specific sanctions or enforcement mechanisms, then these rights could be classified as quasi-legal by nature. This is, for example, the case in Scotland.

Table 13.3 *Mapping national approaches according to their enforceable character and type of legislation*

	Legal patients' rights				Quasi-legal patients' rights	Moral patients' rights
	horizontal / private				*vertical / public*	
	'Sui generis' private contracts		*Generic private contracts*			
Special patients' rights law	Netherlands (1994) Estonia (2001) Lithuania (2001) Slovakia (2004)		Hungary (1997) Belgium (2002) Spain (2002) Poland (2009) Latvia (2010) Czech Republic (2011) Germany (2013) Luxembourg (2014)		Finland (1992) Iceland (1997) Norway (1999) France (2002) Romania (2003) Croatia (2004) Greece (2005) Slovenia (2008) Cyprus (2005) Portugal (2014) Denmark (2014) Sweden (2015)	Austria (2002) United Kingdom (England) (2009) Ireland (2012) Malta (2016)
Patients' rights split across different pieces of legislation	Bulgaria, Italy					

Source: adapted from Nys & Goffin, 2011

- *Moral patients' rights* rely on soft law, non-legally binding documents such as patient charters or codes of conduct. This is mostly the case in countries that operate a public health service as the concrete realization of the state's duty to provide medical treatment to its citizens. Here, patients' rights tend to be included in non-binding charters and they tend to have a 'declaratory' function through formulating citizens' legitimate expectations vis-à-vis the state and its agents, and they are aimed mainly at preventing any violation through raising awareness among patients and providers. At the same time, in some countries such charters can have quasi-legal power, such as the NHS Constitution in England, or in Austria agreements between the federation and individual states that establish patients' rights charters. These are, however, not legally binding on health care providers.

Table 13.3 summarizes national approaches to patients' rights legislation across 30 countries in the EU and the European Economic Area. Further detail on individual countries' approaches is provided in the Should this be cited as Appendix 13.1?.

The inclusion of countries in a particular category does not reflect the strength of patients' rights enforcement. In practice, legal rights are not necessarily more enforceable than quasi-legal or moral rights. Several countries with quasi-legal approaches, such as the Nordic countries, have elaborate dispute settlement mechanisms in place, including no-fault patient injury compensation schemes. Also, the NHS Constitution in England is enforced through the regulation of fundamental standards set out in the health and social care legislation. Here, the Care Quality Commission, the independent regulator of all health and social care services in England, can sanction any breaches of the requirements through NHS staff (Care Quality Commission, 2015).

The nature of individual patients' rights

If patients' rights are to contribute to more person-centred health systems, decision-makers need to ensure their implementation as enforceable legal rights that enable people to exercise these rights. Not linking patients' rights legislation to actual enforcement mechanisms and procedures reduces related laws and frameworks to mere declarations or principles with little practical use and usefulness. This section explores how countries in Europe had defined and implemented patients' rights. It is structured according to the three clusters of the 13 core patients' rights we identified earlier in this chapter: self-determination and confidentiality; access and choice; and information and redress. We examine each cluster in turn.

Self-determination and confidentiality

All EU Member States have developed (or are developing) a legal approach to defining and implementing the traditional rights to self-determination and confidentiality, including the right to informed consent, to participate in clinical decision-making, to data confidentiality and to accessing one's medical record. These rights are often protected by multiple mechanisms.

Most countries have implemented strong mechanisms to protect the right to consent as it is fundamental to respecting a person's autonomy (Buelens, Herijgers & Illegems, 2016). There can be considerable variation in the way consent should be given (written, oral, implicit), although certain practices in place in some countries do not appear to be compatible with how informed consent is generally understood. For example, in Latvia, several hospitals require patients to sign a general consent form upon admission, which commits individuals to agree to any treatment recommended by the treating clinician. In practice this means that the consent given takes the form of a contractual obligation, that is, the patient can only be admitted to the hospital upon giving consent in advance. This further implies that the individual patient is being denied the right to be informed about alternative treatment options. This observation highlights the need for greater emphasis on self-determination in some European countries.

More generally, there is a growing perception that informed consent as a concept may be outdated in that it tends to overly rely on the notion of the patient as a passive recipient to whom certain information must be disclosed. Some commentators have argued for the development of a new ethical and legal standard that prioritizes patient autonomy in decision-making and which has been described as 'informed request' (Moulton et al., 2013). The right to actively take part in decisions about treatment options has so far been formally recognized in a limited number of countries, such as Finland, Germany, the Netherlands, Norway and Sweden.

In most countries the right to privacy and confidentiality is perhaps even more strongly protected than the right to informed consent, with various civil, criminal and constitutional protections in place, including complaint and redress mechanisms and penalties for violation of confidentiality and data protection. However, there have been instances where privacy and confidentiality have been violated despite new legal safeguards. Examples include lack of privacy during physical examination or inadequate protection of individual patients' health records. More systematic violations of confidentiality include the treatment of certain groups of people such as ethnic minorities, people with infectious disease or with substance abuse problems, and sex workers, with instances documented in a number of central and eastern European countries in particular that have been brought before the European Court of Human Rights (Talbot, 2013). Whether such cases point to weaknesses in legislation or lack of legal protection remains difficult to assess with certainty, however. There remains a small number of countries that do not specifically guarantee the right to privacy or confidentiality; instead, this right tends to be covered by data protection legislation.

The right to access one's own medical record is strongly provided for in most countries included in our review, although in some countries hospitals appear to restrict access in practice, through for example, charging administrative fees for people wishing to exercise this right. This right is crucially linked to the right to information while also serving as a means to monitor whether the right to privacy is being upheld.

Access and choice

The right to access medical care is intrinsically linked to the degree to which countries provide for universal coverage. It is for this reason that this right is generally addressed outside special patients' rights laws. Yet as we have seen in the Introduction to this book, there remain gaps in health care coverage in a number of European countries, with evidence of an increase in the gaps following the global financial crisis of 2007–8 as indicated by rising levels of unmet medical need in some countries (Reeves, McKee & Stuckler, 2015).

The right to receive safe and high-quality treatment in a timely manner is generally expressed as an obligation of the provider to adhere to a certain standard of care. The notions of 'standard of care' and 'adherence' are, however, not well defined in relevant legislation, ranging from 'meeting certain patients' expectation' to 'adhering to the current scientific medical knowledge'. Several countries have specified the right to receive treatment in a timely manner, with, for example, Denmark, Finland and Sweden defining maximum waiting times guarantees. Within the European Union, people are entitled to receive treatment in another EU Member State where that treatment cannot be guaranteed domestically within medically justifiable time limits (Palm & Glinos, 2010). This entitlement was reaffirmed in the aforementioned EU Directive on the application of patients' rights in cross-border health care.

The ability to choose a health care provider is increasingly acknowledged as a patients' right, although countries vary in the extent to which this right is realized. Provider choice can form an intrinsic value of the health system, or serve as a means to increase efficiency and improve quality and patient satisfaction (*see* Chapter 8). Under Directive 2011/24/EU, patient choice of provider is, within limits, extended to health care providers in another EU Member State irrespective of whether or not the provider in question is contracted by the publicly funded health system in that Member State. This can increase pressure on Member States to extend choice options and also allow reimbursement for non-contracted providers domestically. However, as shown in Chapter 8, provider choice can form an important source of inequity, especially for people living in rural and remote areas, and more importantly perhaps, for those who do not have the means to express choice and act upon it.

The right to a second opinion is less universally accepted, with only a small majority of countries having formally and unconditionally recognized this right. This implies that related costs will be covered under the publicly funded health system. In countries that do not permit free choice of provider, the right to a second opinion is often subject to strict rules and conditions, typically through strictly defined referral pathways requiring the explicit approval of the treating physician. Some countries only permit one referral per treatment or care process (Estonia, Norway, Slovenia, Spain) or a second opinion is limited to certain providers, usually public or contracted providers, or providers within the same provider organization (Slovenia), providers that are listed for a given pathology (some Italian regions), or as selected by the treating physician (Poland). In Estonia and Italy, a second opinion may also be obtained from a non-contracted provider or a provider outside the country, while elsewhere the right is restricted to certain (mostly life-threatening) conditions (Denmark, Italy, Spain, Sweden). In Denmark, the Health and Medicines Authority can establish a special second opinion panel for people with serious illness to assess the patient's eligibility for experimental treatment at a private hospital in Denmark or elsewhere, with the treating physician responsible for the final decision. In Italy, patients with a (suspected) rare disease can be evaluated by experts from the National Network for Rare Diseases, and this may include seeking scientific advice from outside Italy. Overall, clinicians tend to have a high level of discretion in deciding whether the patient will be able to exercise their right to a second opinion. In Poland, the right to a second opinion is framed as a right of appeal to a medical opinion or decision, which is to be filed to a Medical Commission operated by the Patient Rights Ombudsman's office. The Commission takes a decision on the basis of the medical records and any necessary examination. In 2013, 28 objections were filed but only two met the formal requirements and were forwarded to the Commission.

Information and redress

Informational rights are key to enable people to make informed decisions about their own care and to enforce other patients' rights. Their enforcement requires procedural rights that ensure the provision of *ex-ante* information to enable people to exercise their rights and *ex-post* information that involves redress procedures in case of violation of these rights. One major challenge in the delivery of health care more generally, and the clinician–service user relationship specifically, remains the imbalance of knowledge, frequently referred to as information asymmetry (*see also* Chapter 4). It is against this background that enhancing access to information about health and health care is seen as a priority in many health systems in order to help people make informed decisions. Within the EU context, the aforementioned European Directive on the application of patients' rights in cross-border health care emphasizes the need to improve information for cross-border patients, through, for example, establishing national contact points.

The right to information has three dimensions:

- *The right to information about one's health* is instrumental to the right to consent and the right to participate in (clinical) decision-making more broadly. Countries vary in terms of the content of information that should be provided and its dissemination. Typically, information should address the effectiveness, benefits and risks of any proposed treatment as well as alternative options, and it should be provided in a way that is understandable and suited for different people's needs, but this raises some practical and ethical issues (Entwistle et al., 1998). Importantly, the right to information also includes a right not to know, which needs to be respected where this is the individual's expressed preference (Laurie, 2014).
- *The right to information about health care providers* is instrumental for people to be able to exercise their right to provider choice. There are many challenges to realizing this in practice, such as the nature of the data and information that should be provided, approaches to data collection and validation, as well as their source and format (*see also* Chapter 7). Many countries have established an obligation for providers to publish information about various aspects, ranging from basic information about certification to practice to data about the quality of care provided, along with outcomes. A number of countries have invested in centralized web-portals to provide information about providers, but as discussed in Chapters 4 and 9, the evidence about the use and usefulness of this information by the public remains inconsistent.
- *The right to information about rights and entitlements* is instrumental to enforcing other patients' rights. Providing accurate and transparent information about citizens' rights and entitlements is part of good governance and is seen as a way to empower the public to access social services and demand the protection of their rights (Office of the United Nations High Commissioner for Human Rights, 2007). Governments have invested in improving access to information and reducing the administrative hurdles for people to claim and obtain the services to which they are entitled, including through central contact points, hotlines, web-portals, etc. The aforementioned EU Directive on cross-border health care specifies that the information provided should be easily accessible and made available by electronic means. It should include objective information about administrative procedures. While these provisions have been formulated in the context of cross-border care, people living in countries that have yet to establish public information systems may benefit, too.

Redress is the most critical aspect in the enforcement of patients' rights. It covers the whole spectrum of instruments to settle disputes that may arise in the context of the patient–provider relationship. Disputes not only result from harm inflicted on the patient, but also from their rights being violated, expectations unmet or miscommunication. We have noted earlier that as effective sanctions are lacking in many settings, redress is often regulated under more traditional legislation covering breaches of duty of care and negligence ('tort law').

Professional liability regulations provide a strong incentive for providers to act cautiously and they also provide for fair compensation for patients who have suffered harm. Yet reliance on professional liability also has several flaws. Patients seeking compensation carry the burden of proof, including the need to provide evidence of damage incurred as well as evidence demonstrating negligence (fault) on the part of the provider and of the causal link between the provider's action and incurred harm. Countries such as Sweden, Finland, Denmark, Norway, Iceland, France and Belgium have developed no-fault compensation schemes which grant financial compensation for medical injury without the need for the patient to establish evidence of negligence. While the modalities differ, no-fault out-of-court compensation systems are generally seen to be more fair and efficient, with some evidence pointing to reduced health care costs as a result of clinicians reducing the practice of defensive medicine (Vandersteegen et al., 2015). Relevant schemes may also benefit health systems more broadly by enhancing transparency around adverse events.

Redress based on medical malpractice is, however, not suited to address breaches of statutory rights which do not necessarily cause physical harm. Countries have thus developed alternative dispute resolution mechanisms that seek to prevent litigation through establishing complaint and mediation procedures. Several countries have introduced independent mediators, such as ombudsmen (Mackenney & Fallberg, 2004) or mediation councils, which act at provider level (e.g. Belgium, Finland), regional level (e.g. Norway, Slovenia), national level (e.g. Greece, Malta, Poland), or simultaneously at all levels (e.g. the UK). Outcomes range from out-of-court settlements, administrative or disciplinary sanctions, to explanations or apologies. The latter is typically done through providing a report to the complainant following an internal investigation by the health care provider or institution. If the outcome is not satisfactory, the patient can still decide to initiate a legal procedure. In order to address inequalities in the use of redress mechanisms, patients can be assisted or represented by patient advocates or patients' organizations, who sometimes act as their legal representative in court (Belgium, Estonia, France, Hungary, Italy).

Complaints are most commonly triggered by concerns about the quality of care, in particular safety, including poor communication, staff attitudes and undignified service. Complaints data, where collected systematically, can help steer quality improvement initiatives, although the evidence of impact of such systems remains weak (Pedersen et al., 2013). Complaints procedures can also contribute to monitoring the implementation of patients' rights. For example, Bulgaria, Greece, Hungary and Malta have introduced special patients' rights committees inside or outside the health ministry, which are tasked with monitoring the situation and advising on any changes. At the international level, monitoring mechanisms for individual and social human rights also contribute to the implementation of patients' rights. One example is the 1997 Biomedicine Convention described earlier, which can involve the European Court of Human Rights in giving advisory opinions on legal questions concerning the interpretation of the Convention, and the Court can also act directly if patients' rights that fall within the remit of the European Convention on human rights are being violated.

Conclusions and policy lessons

Patients' rights in Europe have become more widely acknowledged and accepted. The consolidation of patients' rights and their enforcement is expected to help raise awareness, to empower patients, and to guide policy-makers to support the achievement of broader health system objectives. However, evidence that patients' rights achieve any of these goals is generally lacking. In the Netherlands, an evaluation of the law on patient contracts (ZorgOnderzoek Nederland, 2000) found that the patient's perspective was taken into account and that a fear of legalizing the doctor–patient relationship proved to be unfounded (Leenen, 2001). An assessment of the implementation of the 2015 Patient Act in Sweden showed little evidence that it had improved the legal position of patients (Vardanalys, 2017) (*see also* Chapter 3). This was mainly because enforcement mechanisms were found to be inadequate and efforts at the various levels in the health care administration to implement the Patient Act had been limited. More generally, shortcomings in the implementation of a patients' rights framework could lead to reduced confidence in the health system, while also increasing inequalities where the mechanisms introduced only benefit that part of the population that is better able to take advantage of new opportunities afforded.

Increasingly the concept of patients' rights is interpreted in a broad sense; this includes the basic individual patients' rights rooted in human rights frameworks and the rights that are more closely linked to social and consumer protection frameworks. We find that fundamental patients' rights appear to have become well-established in most countries in Europe, while the implementation of consumer-oriented rights lags behind. The broader interpretation of patients' rights also includes greater attention to quality and safety in the health sector, and the responsiveness and efficiency of public services more broadly.

A broader notion of patients' rights that integrates these various dimensions is likely to help advance the notion of the patient as an individual who needs to be protected from unlawful intrusion into their personal sphere to an informed and active partner in the health care system. This increased recognition is reflected by recent moves in some countries such as Norway, which revised its Patients' Rights Act in 2011, to also include users of care services. Similarly, the 2014 reform of long-term care in the Netherlands explicitly includes stipulations on the participation and shared decision-making of service users.

However, while progress has been made, the implementation of patients' rights in European countries requires further development. A major challenge remains enforcement, with lack of awareness among different stakeholders seen as a major barrier towards achieving the intended aims of legislative frameworks. Effective complaints and mediation procedures as well as systematic monitoring of patients' rights compliance are important instruments to increase their impact on individuals and the system as a whole. International efforts can play an important role, such as the 2011 European Directive on cross-border care, which prompted several EU Member States to update their patients' rights legislation, at least the procedural rights around information and redress. Also, more effective European mechanisms for monitoring patients' rights development and compliance with the relevant international frameworks could help to support their further development, as well as the promotion of good practices in raising awareness and enforcing patients' rights nationally.

Appendix 13.1 *Patients' rights legislation in European countries*

Country	(Main) legal source	Category (*)	General comments and highlights
Austria	"Agreements on guaranteeing patients' rights" concluded between the Bund (Federal Republic) and the respective Länder (states)	IV	• The division of power between Federal and State level, lack of transparency and the more traditional approach to health care are hampering the development and enforcement of patients' rights. • Nine Federal States have so far concluded non-binding Patients' Rights Charter agreements: Burgenland, Carinthia, Lower Austria, Upper Austria, Salzburg, Styria, Tyrol, Vorarlberg and Vienna. • Next to rights drawn from constitutional, civil, criminal or administrative law, laws regulating different professions in the health care sector and court decisions play an important role, especially national supreme court decisions relating to rights and duties arising from the treatment contract (specifically relating to informed consent).

| Belgium | Law of 22 August 2002 | II | • The law of 22 August 2002 on the rights of the patient is mainly focused on traditional patients' rights as it derived from the discussion on the ratification of the Biomedicine Convention in the 1990s.
• In 2014 the right to receive limited information about the health care provider (insurance and registration status) was included, also under the impulse of the patients' rights directive.
• For its enforcement, patients are referred to standard liability procedures (civil, criminal, disciplinary).
• The patients' rights law also grants the right to a complaints and mediation procedure. All hospitals are required to appoint an ombudsman. The law also established a central liability for hospitals. |
| Bulgaria | Health Act (2004) | V | • Patients' rights are still rather in the stage of awareness raising. There is no special law on patients' rights.
• In 2009 the Public Council on the Rights of the Patient was established, an advisory and monitoring body within the Ministry of Health that is mandated to monitor and analyse all activities related to patients' rights and support the development of patients' rights legislation.
• Complaint procedures are established at various levels of the health system. |

Appendix 13.1 *(cont.)*

Country	(Main) legal source	Category (*)	General comments and highlights
Croatia	Patients' Rights Protection Act (2004)	III	• The Patients' Rights Protection Act provides for the establishment of a commission for the protection of patients' rights. • Apart from the criminal act that contains provisions about malpractice, enforcement is a weak point. • Within civil society the Croatian Association for the Promotion of Patients' Rights is pushing for the further improvement of patients' rights.
Cyprus	Safeguarding and Protection of Patients' Rights Law 1(I)/2005	III	• The law on the safeguarding and protection of the rights of patients (2005) includes 17 patients' rights and a mechanism for monitoring and resolving patients' complaints about patients' rights violations. • Enforcement of patients' rights still remains an important challenge, which is related to the subsisting paternalistic doctor–patient relationship that translates into relatively low awareness and sensitiveness levels among citizens.
Czech Republic	Act no. 372/2011 Coll. on Health Care Services	II	• The Health Care Services Act clearly defines the basic rights and obligations of each party and includes complaints procedures for patients and relatives as well as sanctions for providers. • The Act also sets adjusted monitoring and (quality) control requirements targeted at improvements in patient safety and the quality of care. • Additionally, a Specific Health Services Act (2011) specifies patients' rights related to specific situations such as sterilization, in vitro fertilization and organ donation.

| Denmark | Consolidating Health Act no.1202 (2014) | III | • In 2011 the National Agency for Patients' Rights and Complaints was established as an independent government institution.
• The Patient Insurance Scheme grants no-fault compensation in case of harm caused from medical treatment in the health system.
• In case patients cannot be treated in a regional hospital within two months they can benefit from an extended free choice of hospital. In 2013 a waiting time guarantee was also introduced for diagnostic assessment based on a referral by a General Practitioner. |
| Estonia | Law of Obligations Act 2001 (chapter 41 'Contract for provision of health care services') | I | • Estonia is still in the early phase of developing a comprehensive framework on patients' rights.
• The Estonian Patients Advocacy Association (EPAA) counsels and represents patients in mediation. Formal complaints can be lodged with the Health Care Quality Expert Commission, which acts under the Minister of Social Affairs as an independent and consultative body. |

Appendix 13.1 (*cont.*)

Country	(Main) legal source	Category (*)	General comments and highlights
Finland	Law No. 785 (1992) on the status and rights of patients	III	• Patients' rights are seen as essential in protecting the confidential relationship between patient and health care provider. • Each health care facility employs a patient ombudsman, whose duty is to inform patients of their rights and assist them, if necessary, in submitting a complaint, appeal or claim for indemnity. The most serious complaints are brought before the National Authority for Medico-Legal Affairs (NAMLA). • The 1987 Patient's Injury Act (amended in 1999) established a no-fault compensation scheme for unforeseeable injuries resulting from medical treatment or diagnosis. The scheme is managed by the Finnish Patient Insurance Centre. Unexpected adverse effects caused by pharmaceuticals (including from clinical trials) are covered under the Finnish Pharmaceutical Insurance Pool, a voluntary insurance taken by pharmaceutical companies operating in Finland.

| France | Act No. 2002–303 concerning the rights of patients and the quality of the health system (incorporated in the Code of Public Health) | III | • The Patients' Rights and Quality of Care Act established patient complaint and compensation procedures. Following the scandal of blood contaminated by HIV, a no-fault compensation scheme was introduced for all infections contracted through medical activities. For other therapeutic hazards, patients are compensated by their health insurance fund through the National Office for the Compensation of Medical Accidents.
 • Patients' associations have played an important role in the development of patients' rights. They also sit on hospital administrative committees and on research ethics committees. They can represent individual patients in court and before the Commission for indemnification. |
| Germany | Patients' Rights Act (2013) (*Patientenrechtegesetz*) | II | • To increase their transparency and consistency, patients' rights, which were formerly dispersed over various laws, were re-edited in the special Patients' Rights Act (2013).
 • A mandatory complaint management system was introduced for hospitals, but other institutions and health service providers have also started to use them on a voluntary basis as part of their quality management programmes.
 • A Charter of Rights for People in Need of Long-term Care and Assistance was developed in 2003 with the support of the Federal Ministry of Family Affairs, Senior Citizens, Women and Youth, and the Federal Ministry of Health. |

Appendix 13.1 *(cont.)*

Country	(Main) legal source	Category (*)	General comments and highlights
Greece	Law No. 2071/92 as amended by the Law of 17 July 1997 Law I. 3418/2005 on the Code of Medical Ethics	III	• The legal approach to patients' rights in Greece is still in the early stages of development. The status of enforcement still remains weak but recently case-law before the courts started to emerge. • Even if non-binding, the opinions and recommendations of the Hellenic National Bioethics Commission, established in 1998 as an independent advisory body of experts under the jurisdiction of the Prime Minister, are considered influential enough to fill any gaps in the legislation. • Also control mechanisms and institutions were created to support patients' rights implementation, e.g. the Ombudsman's office and the Office of Patient Rights in the Ministry of Health.
Hungary	Health Act CLIV (1997) Chapter II (Rights and obligations of patients) and Chapter VI (Rights and obligations of health care workers)	II	• The law also provides for non-litigious resolution of disputes between patients and health care providers through a Mediation Council. • The Commissioner for Fundamental Rights, the National Center for Patients' Rights, Children's Rights and Documentation (OBDK, established by government decree in 2012) and the network of patients' rights advocates all play a key role in the enforcement of patients' rights.

Iceland	Act on the Rights of Patients No. 74/1997.	III	• The Patients' Rights Act is to support the confidential relationship between patients and health care practitioners. It also accords patients the right to the best health service available for their condition, which also includes continuity of service and cooperation between all health care practitioners and institutions involved in their treatment. • In 2000 a Patient Insurance Scheme was established to compensate patients for any physical or mental damage in connection with health services.
Ireland	National Healthcare Charter 'You and Your Health Service' (2012)	IV	• The development of patients' rights in Ireland is mainly driven by national reform strategies, reports and controversies in the media, and constitutional jurisprudence of the courts. • The Human Rights Commission, established under the Human Rights Commission Act of 2000 and charged with promoting and protecting human rights as defined both in the Constitution and in international agreements to which Ireland is a party, is an important advocate for patient rights. • The National Healthcare Charter, established by the Health Service Executive and the Department of Health, sets out what users of health and social care services can expect from the Health Service, without calling them rights, as part of an exercise to improve its quality.

Appendix 13.1 (*cont.*)

Country	(Main) legal source	Category (*)	General comments and highlights
Italy	Law establishing the National Health Service (833/1978)	V	• Patients' rights are mostly derived from the constitutional right to health and the general principles of dignity, solidarity, autonomy and professionalism that underpinned the institution of the National Health Service.
			• Several initiatives at national and local level aim at raising patients' rights awareness. In 1980 Cittadinanzattiva, one of the largest Italian citizens' associations, created the Tribunal for Patient Rights (Tribunale per i diritti del malato), a network of citizens and professionals organized in local sections, to collect complaints from users of health care services and undertake action for patient participation in health care policy.
Latvia	Law on Patients' Rights (2010)	II	• The traditional paternalistic model of doctor–patient relationship still prevails in many respects and there is still a considerable gap between the legal situation and real practice. Despite a poor knowledge about patients' rights, they attract a lot of media coverage and public interest.
			• In practice, the main institution dealing with patients' rights is a non-governmental organization called the Patient's Ombudsman, which assists patients in mediation with providers. Formal patient complaints can be filed to the Health Inspectorate, under the Ministry of Health.
			• Since 2014 a Medical Treatment Risk Fund has been in place within the National Health Service to provide compensation in case of harm caused to a patient's life or health.

Lithuania	Law on the Rights of Patients and Compensation for the Damage to their Health No I-1562 (1996), included in Civil Code (2001)	I	• Patient complaints can be lodged at the provider level, or at the level of the Ministry of Health (the Commission on Evaluation of the Damage Caused to Health of Patients). The State Consumer Rights Protection Authority, which coordinates the activities of state institutions with regard to consumer protection, has a special division for paid medical services.
Luxembourg	Law of 24 July 2014 relating to the rights and obligations of the patient	II	• The special law was inspired by the patients' rights law in Belgium and France and was to some extent induced by the EU Directive on cross-border care.
Malta	National Patients' Charter of Rights and Responsibilities (2016)	IV	• The obligation to issue a Patient Charter was set out in the Health Act of 2013. • The Charter introduces a waiting time guarantee (maximum 18 months) that would give a patient the right to obtain treatment from a local private provider or in another European country in accordance with the Maltese Cross-Border Healthcare Regulations, under the Health Act. • In the interests of patients' rights, the Government established three commissioner functions: the Commissioner for Health, the Commissioner for Mental Health and the Commissioner for the Elderly. These officials act as ombudsmen in dealing with grievances and concerns from the public in their respective areas.

Appendix 13.1 (*cont.*)

Country	(Main) legal source	Category (*)	General comments and highlights
Netherlands	Medical Treatment Contract Act (1994)	I	• There is an elaborate system of complaints, mediation and compensation. In 2016 a new Patients and Clients Rights Act was adopted containing new rules aimed at ensuring good and effective complaints and disputes management in health care as well as promoting quality of care. • With the 2006 health care reform, the Dutch health care system assigned a more significant role to patients with greater opportunity for them to influence the quality of services and a more pronounced right to receive information needed to make an informed choice of health care provider.
Norway	Patients' Rights Act No. 63 (1999)	III	• The Patients' Rights Act has been amended several times. The heading of the Patients' Rights Act was revised in 2011, adding "users of care services". In 2013 the Patients' Rights Act was amended to simplify the priority-setting process for specialized health care. The severity of the condition will only be used to determine the maximum waiting time. • Every county must have a Health and Social Services Ombudsman (POBO), who assists users of care services with information, advice and guidance. • The Norwegian System for Patient Injury Compensation (NPE) instituted by the Patient Injury Act (2001) handles compensation claims for patients who have sustained an injury while accessing statutory as well as private health care services. Its binding decisions can be appealed to the Patients' Injury Compensation Board.

| Poland | Act of 6 November 2008 on Patients' Rights and Patients' Rights Ombudsman | II | • The Law on Patients' Rights and the Patients' Rights Ombudsman gathered all dispersed patients' rights in one well-defined legal act and established the post of Patient Rights Ombudsman. All patients' rights regulations are to be interpreted in compliance with the Polish Constitution of 1997.
• The Office of the Patient Rights Ombudsman, a central government authority appointed by the prime minister, acts independently of the Minister of Health and the President of the National Health Fund, aiming to ensure that patients' rights are protected and providing support in exercising those rights. Nevertheless, the state of enforcement of patients' rights is still considered to be weak in reality. |
| Portugal | Law no. 15/2014 on the rights and duties of the Health Care System beneficiaries | III | • Despite growing attention and monitoring by the regulatory health authorities, the level of implementation at the level of health care institutions still seems weak. Also the judicial system seems to be hesitant in sanctioning patients' rights violations and enforcing medical liability. |

Appendix 13.1 (*cont.*)

Country	(Main) legal source	Category (*)	General comments and highlights
Romania	Law 46/2003 related to patients' rights	III	• Given the poor patients' rights knowledge among the population and the fragmentation in complaint and redress procedures, enforcement remains weak. However, media reports about shortcomings in the health system, including poor conditions and cases of neglect in long-term and mental care facilities, have stirred the public debate. It also encouraged citizens to set up or join patients' organizations that provide counselling, support and practical guidance (even to seek treatment abroad).
Slovakia	Act No 576/2004 Coll. on health care, health care-related services and on the amendment and supplementing of certain laws	I	• Complaints about inadequate care can be lodged with the Health Care Surveillance Authority, an independent body which has become a credible advocate of patients' rights. • A non-governmental organization called the Association of Protection of Patients' Rights also deals with patients' rights.
Slovenia	Patients' Rights Act No. 15/2008	III	• General awareness among patients, doctors and other medical professionals is still quite low. Also the enforcement of patients' rights is weak but improving gradually. • In 2002 the ombudsman for patient rights was appointed for a period of six years. This person, however, is only responsible for the population of the eastern part of the country. • The nongovernmental Slovene Consumer Association is involved in the development of legislation relating to patients' rights, patient satisfaction and quality of health care services.

| Spain | II | Basic Law 41/2002 on the Autonomy of the Patient and Rights and Obligations with regard to Clinical Information and Documentation | • Within the framework of Basic Law 41/2002, all Autonomous Communities have developed their own Patients' Rights and Duties Charters, in some cases as part of the regional health act.
• Regions have established specific structures and procedures to monitor and enforce patients' rights and deal with complaints through Patient Support Services (Servicios de Atención al Paciente) or User Complaint Units (Unidades de Atención al Usuario).
• Most regional health systems have also introduced a patients' ombudsman. Their reports have a certain influence in safeguarding patients' rights due to their impact in the media. |
| Sweden | III | Patient Act (2015) | • The idea of the Patient Act was to gather all statutes regarding patients into one single law in order to improve transparency to care providers, patients and their family members.
• The Patient Act needs to be interpreted along with other relevant acts and frameworks, e.g. the Health and Medical Services Act, the Patient Safety Act and the Patient Data Act.
• Since 1997 a no-fault patient injury insurance scheme compensates any person suffering an injury in connection with medical or dental care in Sweden under the terms of the Patient Injuries Act. |

Appendix 13.1 *(cont.)*

Country	(Main) legal source	Category (*)	General comments and highlights
United Kingdom	NHS Constitution for England (based on Health Act 2009) Scotland: Patient Rights Act (2011)	IV	• The NHS Constitution for England, which is regularly updated, outlines the principles and values of the NHS, as well as the rights and responsibilities of patients and NHS staff in England. • The Scottish Charter of Patient Rights and Responsibilities was published in 2012, after legislation required it. Wales introduced the idea of a charter for patients' rights as early as 2007, but to date one has not been published. There is no charter in Northern Ireland. • Patients who want to file a complaint can get assistance from the Patient Advice and Liaison Service (PALS), which is located in all hospitals in England. They can also contact their local Healthwatch branch, a statutory body established under the Health and Social Care Act 2012 and hosted by the Care Quality Commission. Complaints that cannot be solved at the provider level can be addressed to the Parliamentary and Health Service Ombudsman.

Note: (*) I = 'sui generis' private contract legal rights model; II = generic private contract legal rights model; III = vertical quasi-legal rights model; IV = moral rights model; V = split rights model

References

Active Citizenship Network. European Charter of Patients' Rights. Available at: http://ec.europa.eu/health/ph_overview/co_operation/mobility/docs/health_services_co108_en.pdf (accessed 2 November 2017).

Barendrecht JM et al. (2007). *Principles of European law. Service Contracts.* Oxford: Oxford University Press.

Buelens W, Herijgers C, Illegems S (2016). The view of the European Court of Human Rights on Competent Patients' Right of Informed Consent. Research in the Light of Articles 3 and 8 of the European Convention on Human Rights, *European Journal of Health Law*, 23:481–509.

Care Quality Commission (2015). Guidance for providers on meeting the regulations. London: CQC.

Council of Europe (1997). Convention for the Protection of Human Rights and Dignity of the Human Being with regard to the Application of Biology and Medicine. Oviedo, 4 April 1997.

den Exter A (2002). *Health care law-making in central and eastern Europe. Review of a legal-theoretical model.* Mortsel: Intersentia.

Emanuel E, Emanuel L (1992). Four models of the physician–patient relationship. *JAMA*, 267:2221–6.

Entwistle V et al. (1998). Evidence-informed patient choice: practical issues of involving patients in decisions about health care technologies. *International Journal of Technology Assessment in Health Care*, 14:212–25.

European Commission (2018). Patients' Rights in the European Union Mapping Exercise. Final Report. Brussels: Directorate-General for Health and Food Safety (SANTE).

Ezer T, Cohen J (2013). Human rights in patient care: a theoretical and practical framework. *Health Human Rights*, 15:1–19.

Fallberg L (2000). Patients' rights in Nordic countries. *European Journal of Health Law*, 7:123–43.

Hart D (2004). Patients' rights and patients' participation. Individual and collective involvement: partnership and participation in health law. *European Journal of Health Law*, 11:17–28.

Laurie G (2014). Recognizing the right not to know: conceptual, professional, and legal implications. *Journal of Law, Medicine & Ethics*, 42:53–63.

Lawler M et al. (2014). A Bill of Rights for patients with cancer in Europe. *Lancet Oncology*, 15:258–60.

Leenen H, Gevers J, Pinet G (1993). *The rights of patients in Europe: a comparative study.* Kluwer Law and Taxation.

Leenen H (1994). The rights of patients in Europe. *European Journal of Health Law*, 1:5–13.

Leenen J (2001). Het patiëntenperspectief aan het begin van de 21e eeuw. *Tijdschrift voor Gezondheidsrecht*, 25:1–5.

Mackenney S, Fallberg L (eds.) (2004). Protecting patients' rights? A comparative study of the ombudsman in healthcare. Oxon: Radcliffe Medical Press.

Moulton B et al. (2013). From informed consent to informed request: do we need a new gold standard? *Journal of the Royal Society of Medicine*, 106:391–4.

Nys H, Goffin T (2011). Mapping national practices and strategies relating to patients' rights. In: Wismar M et al. (eds.) *Cross-border health care in the European Union. Mapping and analysing practices and policies.* Copenhagen: WHO Regional Office for Europe on behalf of the European Observatory on Health Systems and Policies, 159–216.

OECD (2017). *Caring for quality in health: lessons learnt from 15 reviews of health care quality.* Paris: OECD.

Office of the High Commissioner for Human Rights (2000). CESCR General Comment No. 14: the Right to the Highest Attainable Standard of Health (Art. 12). Available at: http://www.refworld.org/pdfid/4538838d0.pdf (accessed 2 November 2017).

Office of the United Nations High Commissioner for Human Rights, the World Health Organization (2008). *The Right to Health*. Geneva: Office of the United Nations High Commissioner for Human Rights.

Office of the United Nations High Commissioner for Human Rights (2007). *Good governance practices for the protection of human rights*. New York/ Geneva: Office of the United Nations High Commissioner for Human Rights.

Palm W, Glinos I (2010). Enabling patient mobility in the EU: between free movement and coordination. In: Mossialos E et al. (eds.) *Health systems governance in Europe: the role of European Union law and policy.* Cambridge: Cambridge University Press, 509–60.

Pedersen JS et al. (2013). *The puzzle of changing relationships. Does the changing relationship between healthcare service users and providers improve the quality of care?* London: Health Foundation.

Reeves A, McKee M, Stuckler D (2015). The attack on universal health coverage in Europe: recession, austerity and unmet need. *European Journal of Public Health*, 25:364–5.

Roscam Abbing H (2004). Rights of patients in the European context? *European Journal of Health Law*, 11:7–15.

Roscam Abbing H (2014). Twenty year WHO principles of patients' rights in Europe, a common framework: looking back to the future. *European Journal of Health Law*, 21:323–37.

Talbot S (2013). Advancing human rights in patient care through strategic litigation: challenging medical confidentiality issues in countries in transition. *Health and Human Rights*, 15:69–79.

Vandersteegen T et al. (2015). The impact of no-fault compensation on health care expenditures: an empirical study of OECD countries. *Health Policy*, 119:367–74.

Vardanalys (2017). *Act without impact. Assessment of the Swedish Patient Act 2014–2017. Summary*. Stockholm: Vardanalys.

Will JF (2011). A brief historical and theoretical perspective on patient autonomy and medical decision making: Part I: The beneficence model. *Chest*, 139:669–73.

ZorgOnderzoek Nederland (2000). Evaluatie Wet op de geneeskundige behandelingsovereenkomst. Available at: Available at: https://www.zonmw .nl/uploads/tx_vipublicaties/3_evaluatie_wgbo.pdf (accessed 2 November 2017).

Index

Note: The suffix n after a page number denotes information found in a footnote.

For EU product safety concerns, contact us at Calle de José Abascal, 56–1°,
28003 Madrid, Spain or eugpsr@cambridge.org.

9 781108 790062